.ope Renewed

Oils cannot be wholly pressed into a rational, scientific box. Categorizing and labeling are foreign to any living thing. This is just as true of plants as it is of people. Every living thing has its own subtle beauty and inherent strengths.

While I categorize, label, and dissect essential oils in this book, please remember the following:

First: My husband and I (he does this better than I do) look at the plants—every one, and perhaps the rocks and minerals, too—as personal messages from a loving Heavenly Father. Because He understood that we would not always ask for, or even recognize, His help in our lives, He endowed the various plants with His own healing capacities and invited us to partake of them to balance and heal our own lives. Plants affect us, not just on a physical (vitamin and molecular) level, but on a spiritual plane as well. It is impossible to use an essential oil to heal the physical body without partaking of its ability to bring light and wisdom, healing and peace into your life. The peace and wisdom will be multiplied many times over if you use the oils with thanksgiving to the Creator and an acknowledgement of the role of the Atonement in the healing of both physical and emotional (spiritual) pain.

Secondly: Plants are living things. To feel the living spirit and intelligence of each plant is the true foundation of herbal medicine. Just as each plant can exemplify the attributes of our loving Father, so can the plants personify some lessons about the operation of the body and the soul. The possibilities for learning are endless. To think 'herbally' is to think differently; we must think as nature does—holistically. Nature emphasizes the whole, rather than the precise piece, and nature has an inherent logic and wisdom.

Last, and to me, most important: I have found that essential oils are many times more effective if used with gratitude, and especially gratitude to a loving Creator who established this world in such a way that the things we need for balance and health in every aspect of our lives are everywhere around us. This need for gratitude has been brought home to me in a myriad of ways over the years. I don't believe that God requires our gratitude for His glory. The commandment to be grateful is an example of God explaining to us what is best for our own souls. If you don't do it already, try doing all that you do in this alternative medical world with a large measure of gratitude.

Essential oils are sensitive by their very nature. Our sensitivities are the vehicle through which we can touch others emotionally for good. It follows, then, that if essential oils are to heal our hearts, calm our nerves, revive our hope, and ground our fears, they must be sensitive.

THEY ARE!

There are tears in your eyes and a lump in your throat about now if you have used essential oils with faith and gratitude. I do not know how, but I know that essential oils have sensitive natures.

Love your oils, pray for and with your oils, and use them with gratitude. If you do this, they will bless you abundantly.

Butterfly Miracles with Essential Oils

LaRee Westover

butterflyexpressions.org
butterflymiracles@hotmail.com

ISBN-0-9818396-3-0
Revised August 2010

Legalese

There is absolutely no substitute for caution and common sense!

This oil booklet is written for general information and education only. It is not my intent to diagnose or prescribe for any ailment whatsoever. Your use of the information contained in this book is entirely at your own discretion and is, also, entirely your own responsibility. My goal is, simply, to bring to your attention things that, when I became aware of them, seemed to make significant changes in the quality of my life. It is not meant to be training in psychology, psychotherapy or medicine of any kind. You are advised to apply the techniques and information along with the assistance of competent professionals.

You have managed this far in your life without that oil you are considering and you can manage another day or two while you start slowly to determine the correct oils and the correct dosages for your own needs.

There are details concerning the safe use of essential oils that cannot be contained in any book. Before using an essential oil the reader is advised to seek the assistance of a competent professional.

The statements and products mentioned in this booklet have not been evaluated by the FDA. They reflect traditional and anecdotal usage and data from recent scientific studies.

***The essential oil blends referred to in this document are proprietary blends made and distributed by Butterfly Express, llc.**

I hope you come to enjoy and love essential oils as much as I do!

Rev 8/10

TABLE OF CONTENTS

Introduction

'My father took down some bottles from over the fireplace and mixed several liquids in a bowl. He then made a compress by folding a small piece of flannel, soaked it in the liquid and placed it on the man's side. Within half an hour the pains had gone and his face was no longer screwed up out of all recognition as it had been. Gripping the table in my excitement I couldn't take my eyes off him: it was a miracle!!

' "Papa, did you do that?!"

' "Mon cheri, he who causes the plants to grow is the one who did it." '

Of Men and Plants *Maurice Messegue*

This same excitement in the face of a 'miracle' is exactly the way I felt when I first became acquainted with essential oils, and a little gratitude is always a good thing. I had been using herbs and homeopathics for many years and was already doing foot-zone therapy for friends and family, but there were some health concerns in my family with which we had made great progress but seemed to be 'stuck' at that level. The inclusion of essential oils into the programs made such a phenomenal difference that I was immediately hooked on essential oils for life. I should warn you right now that essential oils are addictive. Once you learn to love them, you just can't have enough of them!!

This book is a very personal sort of journal for me. Although I have quoted authoritative articles, books and journals freely, I have also continually expressed my own opinions, preferences and experiences. The use of essential oils, much like homeopathic remedies, is very person specific. No one can–or should–tell you exactly how to use an essential oil. Your likes and dislikes, your core personality, your personal body chemistry, and the circumstances of your life at this particular time will influence what works for you, the particular aroma of each individual oil, and what oils you will fall in love with and find useful. These factors will also influence what oils you may, occasionally, react to negatively.

Essential oils are made from plants; they are very highly concentrated plant material, in fact. Because they are plant material, you may have or develop what may appear to be an allergy to a particular oil. An oil that you used with no adverse effect one day may cause a negative reaction on another day, even under what appears to be similar circumstances. This is true even of oils that are not on anybody's list of "oils not to use or to use with caution." The use of essential oils must be based on common sense and the basic principles of natural therapeutics. The more you know, the more success you will have. The facts are that the use of essential oils, with even a little bit of common sense, is not in the least 'dangerous', unlike the practice of putting toxic chemicals into the body in an attempt to make it 'well.'

History

Essential oils have been in use in both religion and medicine for thousands of years. We know this because reference is made to them in many manuscripts of ancient date. In addition, there are, as near as I can tell, nearly 200 references to essential oils in the Bible. Essential oils were used extensively in Renaissance Europe and in ancient India. In fact, India is probably the only place in the world where this tradition and art was never lost. With several thousand years of continuous practice, Ayurvedic medicine (including the use of aromatic oils) is the oldest continuous form of medical practice. Much of what is known about the medicinal properties of essential oils comes from these sources.

The arrival of modern science in the 19th century brought about the decline of all forms of herbal medicine. This suppression, if you study history even a little, appears to have been deliberately brought about by people who stood to gain financially. Scientists, quite probably with the best of intentions at first, began the practice of isolating the main active ingredient of plants and then reproducing them in laboratories. In this way, penicillin (derived from mold growing on bread), aspirin (naturally present in birch, wintergreen and meadowsweet), antibiotics, and so on came into wide-spread usage.

There is obvious value in many scientific discoveries, but it must also be acknowledged by any open-minded person that these isolated compounds, such as those found in drugs and synthetic therapeutic oils, have many serious side effects and can be easily abused. Every plant and, therefore, every essential oil contains hundreds of chemical compounds, most of them in very small amounts. We know that certain trace elements are fundamental for life, and the human body often requires one in order to assimilate another. Rational thought, and now scientific study, shows clearly that there is an undeniable corollary to this in medicine. The power of living products (herbals and essential oils) lies in the combination of their elements, and the trace components are every bit as important as their main constituents. In fact, it seems to be that the minor constituents have a synergistic (controlling and strengthening) effect on the main constituents, enabling the herbal or oil to heal more efficiently and without the nasty side effects experienced when using the synthetic reconstructions (drugs or oils) that do not contain the trace elements.

With pure essential oils and herbal medicines in their complete state
you can heal and nourish without the traditional side effects of drugs!

Aromatherapy, in our time, can be said to have began in France in the early 1900's. England and European countries learned of it quickly and it is a basic part of even mainstream medicine in most countries of Europe and Asia, as is the use of homeopathic medicines. Aromatherapy did not exist in any significant way in the United States until the early 1980's and can be classed into two separate and distinct movements: pure and genuine essential oils for therapeutic use, and a mass-market approach to perfumery, etc. Because of the prevalence of mass-marketing techniques, much of what you hear and see in the media and in promotional material is outright blarney, and what you buy is often synthetic substitutions. Education and personal experience are your best tools in this market; an oil source that you have come to trust is also invaluable.

Schools of Thought

As noted on the previous page, essential oils have been used throughout the years and throughout the world, but not always by utilizing the same methods of application and/or use. There are large gulfs of difference between what is considered safe and the best method of application between countries and schools of thought.

For the most part, aromatherapists trained in **Germany** consider inhalation as the best and most effective way to use essential oils. Essential oil molecular structure is such (small molecules with low atomic weights) that they pass directly into the blood stream when breathed into the lungs. At the same time they are also moving directly into the brain through the olfactory nerves which are connected to the brain's central portion.

In **Britain** and other English speaking countries, the skin is the primary avenue of absorption and utilization of essential oils. The emphasis is on massage with carrier oils containing only 2-5% of essential oil. The early proponents of aromatherapy in England were not therapists nor health-care practitioners, and often the oils used and studied were perfume or food-grade rather than therapeutic-grade essential oils. In addition, the British tend to rely heavily on scientific research. This sounds good in theory, but in practice the research has been almost exclusively done using low quality food-grade oils, synthetic reproductions, adulterated oils and isolated compounds rather than the whole oil. ***Their data, and the advise and cautions generated by it, is invalid in relation to unadulterated therapeutic grade essential oils.***

The British place a great deal of emphasis on the potential problems with essential oils. Their lists of cautions are extensive for nearly every oil and their lists of oils that should never be used is also quite lengthy. Formally trained aromatherapists in the United States tend to lean heavily in the British direction, probably because studying English texts is easier for us than studying French or German ones. I consider myself guilty of this bias to a great extent in my early days using essential oils.

It should be noted here that most essential oils contain compounds that are toxic individually. Myrrh oil contains many such compounds, yet it is one of the gentlest, safest, mildest oils in nature. The Bible says that Esther was massaged with oil of myrrh every day for 6 months to prepare for marriage to the king. Some British aromatherapists believe that this cannot be correct since studies of the individual components of myrrh *obviously* show some of these components to be hazardous, especially when applied day after day. (Interesting how scientists are so prone to believe their own prejudices rather than revealed word.)

An interesting fact, noted in The Chemistry of Essential Oils Made Simple by David Stewart, Ph.D., D.N.M., is that myrrh essential oil is used to protect skin from the rays of the sun. This is amazing because myrrh contains more furanoid compounds than any other essential oil. Furanoid compounds are implicated in studies as amplifying ultraviolet light and are said to make an oil phototoxic (meaning that it can potentially cause sunburn and skin damage when exposure to sunlight occurs after application). This is a perfect illustration of the difference between a complete oil and its individual components.

The **French** recommend the use of essential oils in just about any way you can imagine. They particularly emphasize the taking of essential oils orally. Many people, using only pure therapeutic grade essential oils, are doing this with good result and no reported problems. As is emphasized in this book, I do not recommend the oral consumption of essential oils. The fact remains that ***every*** incident in which harm from essential oils has been documented has been with internal consumption, either intentionally or accidentally. Oils absorb so rapidly when inhaled or placed on the skin and I have had such great success with those methods that I have rarely felt the need to recommend internal use.

My recommendation is to use oils consistently, sensibly, with joy and thanksgiving, and by any method whatsoever that you choose. My thinking certainly follows French thought more closely than English.

Basic Principles and Information about Essential Oils

Essential oils contain the nutritive values and healing properties of plants in a very concentrated form. They often heal the body, mind, and spirit, while regenerating damaged tissue and bringing oxygen to deprived cells. The use of essential oils also seems to improve overall immune function.

Frequency Every organ of the human body has a frequency range at which it operates when healthy; the human body has an overall bio-electrical frequency. During illness or with impending death, the body's frequency drops significantly. Essential oils have frequency ranges that are several times greater than the frequency of herbs and food. The application of essential oils can quickly raise the body's overall frequency or stabilize the frequency of a struggling organ (LeVabre, Higley, Stewart).

Studies have been conducted showing that, without question, negative things such as coffee, negative thoughts, stress, poor nutrition, etc. lower the body's overall frequency (imagine that!). Essential oils often restore the body to normal ranges within seconds and improve over-all feelings of well-being.

Each essential oil (single) has a frequency range that is attractive or healing to particular organs, meridians, etc. of our bodies. In general, and this varies quite a bit, oils with lower frequencies are considered to make physical changes in the body; oils with mid-range frequencies to effect emotional changes; high frequency oils, nearly always 'blossom' oils, bring about spiritual changes.

A well-done blend can contain oils in all three frequency ranges and creates a profound and deeply healing environment. Blends are less likely to cause a negative reaction because each individual oil is only a percentage of the whole, and sometimes only a very small percentage.

Learning to mix your own blends can be a tricky undertaking. Professionals often go to several years of school and then practice, practice, practice before they get it right. Playing around with blends can be more fun than cooking creatively, but it can be an expensive experience.

Oils have to go into a blend in a particular order and in very specific quantities. If a book of recipes does not mention this, the author probably does not understand it (or does not know how to explain it). Either way, unless you get the order correct, your blends will not turn out very well.

The order in which oils go into a blend depends on things called 'notes' and other things called 'properties.' The term 'notes' refers to a combination of aromatic pungency and the longevity of the therapeutic qualities and is relative to the other oils in the blend. Many oils can be considered either middle notes or high notes depending on quantity and what other oils are in the blend.

Understanding the properties of each single oil, whether it is considered a base, an equalizer, an enhancer, etc., is also necessary for you to understand how the oils you have chosen will react to each other and which should be put in first and in what quantities.

Synergy The term used to express the idea that single oils blended together achieve a product that is more than just the sum of its parts. A blended essential oil is better able to reach the various layers of spiritual, physical, and emotional healing and do all this with less chance of negative results.

Bacteria and Viruses, etc. Essential oils are antibacterial, anti-fungal, antiviral, anti-infectious, anti-tumoral, anti-parasitic, and antiseptic. This is not a matter of some oils being one and other oils being another; all essential oils have these properties to one degree or another. These properties could be the result of the unique oxygen/nutrient carrying capacity of essential oils as described above. Essential oils have been shown in laboratory studies and clinical trials to destroy or seriously inhibit tested bacteria and viruses and to do so without causing harm (unlike drugs) to cells, organs, tissues, or body systems.

Aromatic Essential oils are aromatic (volatile). This means that their small molecules are able to be diffused readily into the air and absorbed into our bodies through our olfactory and respiratory systems. It is an interesting fact that although we may not be able to detect all of an oil's fragrances because our nose has no receptor sites for particular molecules, all of the molecules can enter our systems through the nose. From the nose they can go directly into the central brain or they may go into the lung and from there directly into the blood stream.

Because of their small molecular structures, when diffused they purify the air in the following ways: removing metallic particles and toxins from the air, increasing ozone and negative ions which inhibit bacterial growth, destroying odors from mold, cigarettes, animals, etc., and filling the air with a fresh, beautiful, healing and uplifting scent.

Applying Externally and Benefitting Internally Because of the molecular structure of essential oils, they can act on internal organs when applied externally to the body. This ability is explained by Hilton's Law of Physics, which states that the nerve which supplies a joint also supplies the muscles which move the joint and the skin over the joint. This law also applies to organs and the tissues surrounding them. Massage therapy and other modalities operate using this principle. Essential oils work through the skin on nearby organs, on the nervous system, and then throughout the entire body. Essential oils quickly penetrate the tissues of the skin reaching the organs and joints.

Penetrate Cell Walls One great benefit of essential oils is that they are capable of moving through cell walls even when the cell walls are hardened because of damage or scarring. Essential oils reach areas of the body far from where the oil was applied, and they do so in just a few minutes. The oils are then metabolized by the body in the same way that other nutrients are metabolized.

Cell Regeneration Most essential oils are cytophylactic; this means that they stimulate the generation of new cell growth following burns, surgeries, or wounds of any nature. Of particular note in this category are lavender, patchcouli, neroli, ravensara, coriander, and helichrysum.

Skin Care The skin is a barrier between our bodies and the outside world, but it is not the impenetrable barrier that it was once thought to be. The skin absorbs and filters both nutrients and pollutants and expels various waste materials through the sebaceous glands. The skin is supposed to do all this amazing work while staying moist, healthy and glowing. Essential oils can be of great help to the skin in accomplishing this amazing work. Your skin care regimen need not be elaborate or time consuming to make a significant difference to both the beauty and functionality of your skin.

Circulation Essential oils are rubefacient, which means that they activate capillary circulation. Increased circulation to the capillaries prevents tired, achy legs and the slow healing experienced by diabetic people, as well as muscle tenseness and strain.

Expectorant Most essential oils are expectorants to some degree. They improve the function of the lymphatic system by causing mucous to become more fluid, and thus, more easily expelled from the lungs and mucous membranes.

Cleansing Effect All essential oils have a cleansing effect on the human system, whether it be on the skin, in the blood, in the lymphatic system, or on a person's accumulated cellulite. One of the things that appears to happen when essential oils are used regularly is that toxins, free-radicals, cellular debris, heavy metals, pharmaceutical drugs, petrochemicals, renegade cells, fungi, bacteria and even viruses attach themselves to the cellular structure of the essential oil and are then excreted from the body in natural and harmless ways. This cleansing effect on cellular receptor sites increases our ability to absorb and utilize vitamins and minerals.

Anti-oxidants Essential oils are powerful anti-oxidants. By their very nature they aid the body in eliminating free radicals and the damage they cause. This is explained further in the section on essential oils and security scanner in Chapter 3 on page 9.

Oxygen and Nutrient Transport Oxygen is the carrier of nutrition throughout the human body. Essential oils contain molecules which help transport nutrients to starving or undernourished cells. Disease begins when a cell lacks the oxygen for proper nutrient assimilation. By providing needed oxygen, essential oils strengthen every cell in the body, including those necessary to the immune system.

Balance or Homeostasis Many essential oils are adaptogenic, meaning they will instigate a reaction in the body to bring about a state of balance. For example, hyssop normalizes either high or low blood pressure; peppermint is found on lists both as a stimulant and as a sedative, and this is accurate; lemon acts on the nervous system either as a sedative or a tonic, as needed. This is true of the various plants in herbal form, as well. Essential oils are simply stronger and the effects more immediately recognizable.

Blood/Brain Barrier Some essential oils, those containing sesquiterpenes, cross the blood/brain barrier. According to Connie and Alan Higley in Reference Guide for Essential Oils, The American Medical Association (AMA) determined that if they could find an agent that would pass the blood/brain barrier, they would be able to cure alzheimer's disease, Lou Gehrig's disease, multiple sclerosis, and Parkinson's disease. In June of 1994, it was documented by the medical Universities of Berlin, Germany, and Vienna, Austria that sesquiterpenes have the ability to go beyond the blood/brain barrier. This should have been met with the world-wide awe that the scientific team who discovered it expected (Higley). Perhaps the world is fortunate that doctors are NOT attempting to make drugs cross this barrier with the use of essential oils.

The blood/brain barrier is the membrane between the circulating blood and the brain that prevents certain damaging substances from reaching the brain tissue and cerebrospinal fluid. Oils such as frankincense and sandalwood, high in sesquiterpenes, cross this barrier and bring increased amounts of oxygen and their healing properties to the limbic system of the brain.

Essential oils containing sesquiterpenes in significant amount are as follows: cedarwood, patchouli, sandalwood, ginger, blue cypress, myrrh, vetiver, vitex, chamomile German, black pepper, spikenard, ylang yland, and yarrow. Frankincense, which is world-renowned for this, actually contains far less than the oils listed above. It does, however, contain other components that make it very effective overall.

Acupressure and Energy Work Essential oils are considered the life force or the energy of the plant. They are used in many parts of the world in energy and acupressure work. This type of work is finally catching on in the United States. Specific essential oils can be associated with the meridians and chakras. (There is further information on the meridians and chakras in Chapter 8.)

Variety of Action People are a complex combination of mind, body and spirit. Essential oils seem to have the ability to affect all three areas at the same time and in a balanced and beneficial way. The various levels of action of essential oils are not exclusive from one another. You cannot say, "I will use this oil today because it has astringent properties for my oily skin," and not encounter, for example, the antiviral properties of the chosen oil. <u>When working on any physical ailment, there will also be beneficial effects seen on the emotional and energy levels, etc.</u>

Spiritual and Emotional Dimensions The spiritual and emotional dimensions of essential oils are well known and have been used by people throughout recorded history.

Some oils are calming; others bring sharpness and clarity to thinking processes and stimulate memory; still others bring a sense of contentment, well-being and faith in the future. The phenomenon of improved mood and mental/spiritual clarity has been experienced and described by many.

Releasing Emotional Trauma Present in the limbic system of the brain is a gland called the amygdala. This gland is directly connected to the olfactory bulb and is stimulated by the sense of smell and by our thoughts. Studies conducted recently on the meditation techniques of Tibetan monks indicate that the amygdala is the brain's 'solution center.' Present it with a problem and it immediately begins to come up with possible solution scenarios. It is now known in scientific circles that every cell of our bodies contain memories, even memories that have passed along family lines, much like the tendency to a certain eye color or curly hair. The aroma of essential oils reaches into this level of the body and aids us in releasing patterns that are not serving us well.

Response to Words, Thoughts, and Prayer In studies conducted by Bruce Tainio, participants were asked to direct negative thoughts toward several essential oils. The frequency of the oils was measured before and after the thought directing. The overall frequencies of the oils went down by an average of 12 MHz following negative thought. The frequencies of the same oils went up by an average of 10 MHz when positive thought energy was directed at them. Interestingly, the average increase in resonant frequency went up by 15 MHz when the oils were prayed for consistently.

Anecdotal evidence has been produced showing that oils amplify our intent. The intent of the user will move molecules of oil to where they are most needed more quickly. Oils respond with an increase (or decrease) in frequency and effectiveness according to the attitudes and intentions of the producer, handler, distributor, experimenter, shipper, and end user (you). Love your oils, pray over and for them, and for yourselves, use them with a firm intention set in your mind of what you need them to do and you will notice an increase in the effectiveness of the oils and, I believe, in your health and well-being.

The powerful properties displayed by essential oils make perfect sense to the student of molecular biology and have been proven in clinical trials and practical usage. Essential oils, being derived from whole plants which are part of God's marvelous creation, contain some amazingly well-designed molecules that work in consistently predictable ways. There is nothing 'magical' about the way that essential oils work.

Pure Essential Oils

For effective therapeutic use it is absolutely crucial that only good quality, natural essential oils be used. It is worse than pointless to buy any other product, and sometimes it is downright dangerous to use them. No matter how pleasant the aroma might be, reconstituted or diluted products lack the constituents necessary to achieve good therapeutic results. Synthetic copies are not only ineffective, but they cannot be metabolized and utilized by the body, nor can they be excreted by the normal pathways of skin, kidneys, colon etc.

Because the largest buyer of aromatic oils is the perfume and cosmetic industries and these industries are not the least bit interested in the medicinal value of the oils, the driving criterion for the production and marketing of essential oils has been aroma and uniformity and not the maintenance of medicinal value. Growers and processors tailor their product to the buyer, naturally, and sometimes corners are cut to save money and expense.

Under the current laws, many products come under the heading 'essential oils' and can be marketed as such even if they have been diluted with vegetable protein oils and even if they are deadly synthetic reproductions with a little pure oil added. In addition, because some pure oils are very expensive to produce, some companies mix two or more oils together to mimic the aroma of an expensive oil. Some of these blends have wonderful (and sometimes similar) fragrances and frequencies. If blended by someone very experienced in medicinal oils, the constituents can occasionally be matched quite closely, but this accomplishment is very rare. Butterfly Express, llc, has a blend of melissa which is very good. They also sell a rectified melissa with very good medicinal properties. Pure melissa oil is out of reach, price-wise, for most people.

Unscrupulous or unknowledgeable dealers will sometimes dilute a pure essential oil in a carrier base and try to pass it off as pure and natural. These fakes are quite easily spotted because the base oil is oily, while essential oils, for the most part, are not. Most pure essential oils, when dropped on blotting paper, will absorb rapidly into the paper; a stain may remain but there will be no oily patch. A pure oil will not clog the motor of a fountain, although balsams and resins, because of their viscous nature, need to be cleaned from your fountains after each use. If a carrier oil has been added, the oil will most definitely cause problems with the motor of even your most expensive fountains.

The production of pure essential oils can be very costly. This makes the cost of some good quality essential oils quite high. Some of the 'blossom' oils require two to three tons of plant material to extract 1 pound of quality oil. Time of day, weather conditions, and many other factors affect the chemical composition of the oils and must be carefully monitored in order for a satisfactory medicinal- quality oil to be produced. For example, climate, altitude, and distillation methods drastically affect the amount of thymol in the final product when distilling *Thymus vulgaris.* The amount of thymol in the finished product drastically affects how thyme essential oil can be used because thymol is very strong and quite caustic.

When buying essential oils, you should begin with shops or suppliers that are concerned with nutrition and health, rather than ones concerned with perfumery and cosmetics. Eventually your nose and your energy will become very discriminating: 'good' oils will feel and smell good to you and 'bad' oils will not! It is not that 'good' oils will always smell pretty; it is that they will smell 'right', even if you do not care for the aroma of that particular type of oil.

Understanding Tests and Standards for Therapeutic Oils

Analytical Tests and Techniques

It is important that we remember that it is not possible, even with the most powerful of today's microscopes, to see the living molecules of essential oils.

Chemical formulas denote how many atoms of this and how many atoms of that are in each component of an oil, and can be determined by the techniques used by modern chemists. But chemical formulas are only the introductory pieces of a complete analysis of any essential oil. The next things that you need to know are the percentages of each compound that are in that particular oil and, then, the actual structure of those compounds. The percentages and structures are ***very*** important!

The industry standard for analysis of the *percentage of each component* is the gas chromatograph (CG). There are several variations of this tool: the high performance liquid chromatograph (HPLC), the gel liquid chromatograph (GLC), and the thin layer chromatograph (TLC). These instruments separate the components of an oil into individual compounds so that the percentages of each can be measured.

There are ***three things*** that need to be understood about this technology that is so often relied on and quoted as proof that an oil is pure and up to a proper standard.

The ***first*** thing to know is that ***only the main components of an oil can be measured by any of these chromatographs.*** Most of the components of the oil go undetected and uncounted with each test. Most often the compounds that are measured and counted do not comprise even 50% of the entire oil and, in many oils, it is one or more of the trace components, *which are not shown by the test*, that really matter. In grapefruit oil, for instance, the component that accounts for its distinctive aroma is found in amounts of less than 1 part per billion. Trace components *which the tests do not record* are vital to both the aroma and the therapeutic properties of every essential oil.

Synthetic and chemically altered compounds are **not** going to show up in a chromatograph unless the percent of the 'fake' that has been added is quite high, and then only if the technician is both very good at his job and very lucky. Only if the analysis is well done and the amount of the both the natural compound and the fake is high enough to register will the adulteration be detected by chromatograph technology.

The ***second*** thing that impacts the usefulness of these tests is that there is a lot of skill, artistry, and just plain judgment that goes into interpreting a chromatogram. There is a lot of room for error and misinterpretation. Experience and skill on the part of the lab technician, greatly impacts the reliability of the results. Some labs and some technicians, of course, do a better job than others.

Third, it is so easy to 'fake' a paper. I once ordered read-outs on lavender oil from a 'reputable' dealer three years in a row and was sent exactly the same sheet. Perhaps I was being sold very old oil by the third year, the papers did not apply to the oil I was purchasing, or the papers were just plain 'faked' to convince me that what I was purchasing was a very good oil. I say this with confidence because it is impossibe to keep growing conditions so nearly identical from year to year as to produce identical results legitimately. Most likely, the same results sheet was used each year, with only the date changed, to save the money that the testing would have cost. Since they knew the growing and production procedures they had used, they were probably confident that it was a good oil. Nevertheless, I have learned to treat all spec sheets with a healthy dose of skepticism. A spec sheet does not guarantee a good oil.

The mass spectrograph (MS) is the most often used tool to analyze the *structure of the molecules* in an essential oil. The mass spectrograph bombards the molecules of the oil with high energy electrons which causes the molecules to separate into atoms. The atoms are then analyzed to determine the angles of the original connections and the original shapes of the molecules before the use of the spectrograph. The illustration used by David Stewart in his book, *The Chemistry of Essential Oil Made Simple* is stepping on a bunch of Lego creations and then trying to put them all back together again without even knowing how many items there were let alone the basic structure of each piece. Is this possible? Maybe, or maybe not. But here again, the skill of the technician, and his patience, has a lot to do with the accuracy of the results obtained. To quote Dr. Stewart, it takes 'an incredible amount of technological effort, mathematical deduction, intuition, serendipity, patience, money and sweat' to identify what is the proper structure for the molecules of an essential oil. An equal amount of effort, mathematical deduction, intuition, etc. will have to be put into identifying and analyzing an oil to determine if the structures in a particular oil are, in fact, natural and not synthetic, man-made, non-living and non-healing fakes.

Standards and Standardization

I shall try to make this complicated topic simple and, maybe, fairly brief.

There is no government agency in North America who publishes any kind of standard for non-synthetic essences. The United States Pharmacopoeia Convention (USPC) was founded in 1830 to set basic standards for the medicinal preparations of that day. At that time, a large portion of the remedies prescribed by doctors were herbal in nature and included a few essential oils. At that time essential oils and herbal products could be marketed as 'USP grade.' This grading system and label has not been in use for a long time, but there is pressure being applied to re-establish grading standards. The USPC today is mainly concerned with echoing every opinion of the FDA relating to vitamins and nutritional supplements.

The USPC today is also responsible for the standardization of medical formulas. There is another organization which sets the codes for additives, coloring agents, binders, syrups, carrier oils, and other non-active ingredients. These two organizations have recently merged in theory, and now cover both the active and inactive ingredients in prescription and nonprescription drugs. They also set the standards for dosage amounts and the forms the dosages should be in. Since 1995, their work has been expanded to include dietary supplements, medical devices, and other health care products, including tests, procedures, and labeling requirements. The National Formulary branch of this joint organization is lobbying to place botanical medicines under their jurisdiction. In fact, the NF is currently devising standards for growing, distilling, and packaging essential oils. There are those who think that this could be a good thing. Before making up your mind, let us look at the standards set by some European countries and their inherent limitations.

AFNOR (Association Francaise de Normalization) is a French agency that sets standards for, among other things, essential oils. The ISO (International Standardization Organization) in Geneva, Switzerland and the EC (Eurpoean Community) has adopted the AFNOR standards.

AFNOR authorities are quick to point out that their standards are meant only to be a ***base-line*** profile of ***some*** of the compounds, and the amounts of those compounds, that should be contained in an essential oil if it is to be labeled as a therapeutic grade oil of a particular species. Let us use peppermint (*Mentha piperita)* oil as an example. To be labeled as *Mentha piperita* according to AFNOR (or ISO or EC) standards, peppermint oil must contain 35-45% menthol, 10-20% menthone, 4-9% methyl acetate, 3-7% 1.8 cineole. Sounds straightforward enough, right? But there is a serious problem:

There are only four compounds listed and monitored, out of the hundreds of compounds present in the complete, natural essential oil of Mentha piperita. This fault is the same for all AFNOR standards on all essential oils; AFNOR standards usually look at no more than 6 compounds for any particular species. This leaves plenty of room for an unethical company to substitute man-made 'fakes' for both these basic compounds and the ones not monitored at all. Because synthetics are so much cheaper to produce they are sometimes even added to a suitable filler oil in the listed proportion and then sold as a natural oil with no living, growing plant ever involved in the process at all. They still meet the AFNOR standards and, if well-crafted, can be difficult to detect until your 'nose' has become quite sensitive. These 'fakes' are worthless as healers; only God can make a tree or a plant capable of healing the human body. Only life begets life!

In addition, in the United States and many other countries at this time, a product need only have a small percentage of natural (non-synthetic) material in it to be labeled as 'natural.' As explained above, being labeled as "natural and meeting the AFNOR standard" does not in any way indicate whether the compounds in the labeled oil are natural or synthetic, and does not tell you anything about its therapeutic value. The AFNOR standards will guarantee you the fragrance and taste of peppermint (or whatever oil you are referring to), but it does not guarantee that the oil has any healing properties at all. To achieve the healing properties that you need, you must allow time and space for God and the plant to complete the creation process, and then you must harvest, distill, process, and package the oil appropriately. The oil will then contain hundreds of constituents, most of them in trace amounts that are measured in fractions of percents. As stated several times in this booklet, it is often the trace amounts that are responsible for both the aroma and the therapeutic properties of an essential oil.

There is nothing wrong with producing perfume or cosmetic grade oils. The problem comes from labeling them as pure *therapeutic grade* essential oils when they are not. This mislabeling is fraud. Adulterated or chemically altered oils do not have the same healing properties as pure essential oil.

Recommended Study

For an in-depth discussion and information on why you should use only pure therapeutic grade essential oils (and why not to use laboratory produced 'fakes'), I would recommend The Chemistry of Essential Oils Made Simple by David Stewart, PH.d. D.N.M.

This big book is in three parts: The first part is, as the title indicates, an explanation of chemistry relating to essential oils put as simply as possible. The second part is an excellent reference of single essential oils, their constituents, and many other facts and bits of information. The third part, titled *Beyond Chemistry*, is a series of four fascinating articles on such topics as the nature of matter and the limitations of the scientific methods of study in understanding the universe.

Following are two short quotes from the introductory section of Dr. Stewart's book. He expounds further on this topic in the third section of the book in the lecture that is titled ***The Limits of Science:***

> *What developed was a philosophy of separation between church and science. . . . Religion was for the sanctuary and science was for the laboratory. The two were not to mix. As a result, today we have materialistic science and secular medicine, both of which claim no relationship to God in their practice. At the same time, we have religion that does not know how to incorporate science into its theology and has lost its healing ministry.*
>
> *But the 'separation' of science from religion is a false dichotomy. To deny God as the source of healing makes medicine impotent, ineffective, and incapable of true healing. To deny the spiritual as an integral part of the material makes science incapable of discerning the true nature of the universe.* ***Both science and medicine have confined themselves inside a materialistic container where the ultimate answers they seek are all on the outside.***

In other words, it is completely impossible to understand the universe without acknowledging the one who created it all. Albert Einstein, when asked why he became a scientist, is said to have replied that it was because he "wanted to understand what God was thinking." That is what science should be, a seeking to understand the present, the past, the future, and the world around us. To study, or give credence to, only the physical would be failing to acknowledge that there are such things as magnetic force, gravity, etc. and totally ignoring that the material world is subject to these unseen and unexplained forces. I say 'unexplained' because the explanations tell you *how* magnetism works, but they do not explain *why* in any adequate fashion. In science, there is the creation of artificial boundaries. Chemistry deals with this little bit, physics with this other little part, and quantum physics with some of the less material aspects and forces that the others do not get into at all. What is needed is science as Albert Einstein and other great scientists, then and now, view it. Dr. Stewart says the following:

> *Healing with essential oils is intuitive and spiritual, a gift acquired by one's receptivity to the Divine. Intellectual study with a secular attitude, unappreciative of the source of all things, will block intuition. Such study is spiritually harmful. Such study will reduce and limit your finer sensitivities and right brain capabilities. This is the kind of study that dominates our schools and universities today. There is a better way.*

Dr. Stewart points out that the "science of prayer" is always going to be the best method for studying and applying essential oils in our own lives. Being taught by God, in whole sentences, is the closest we are likely to come in this world to the broader picture.

He also shows, by the science of molecular structure, that it requires an intelligent life essence, a living plant operating by God's laws of nature, to make a 'healing' essential oil (or an herbal, for that matter). Laboratories and scientists have been unable to imitate what God has designed and set in motion. What man produces through scientific methods in a laboratory will contain molecules of unnatural dextrorotary (right) isomers*, along with other isomers that contain the same atoms but in slightly different structural configurations and formations. It can be accurately stated that these molecules have the same formulas, but the human body has no receptor sites for these man-made, backwards rotating, oddly structured molecules. These molecules cannot be utilized without producing side effects. They are impossible to metabolize and very difficult to eliminate from our bodies. Most often they gradually accumulate, acting as toxins that contribute to or cause disease.

**An isomer is a compound with the same chemical formula but different structural formats. Some isomers occur naturally but many, and certainly the ones discussed above, are the result of man tampering with a naturally occurring molecule in a laboratory.*

Shelf Life

In order to understand the shelf life of a particular oil you must first determine which category of *scented* oils the oil belongs to. So let us take a moment here to discuss these basic classes of oils.
1) Essential Oils: In the vernacular of the industry, true essential oils are those products that are the result of distillation. The methods used in the distillation process have a huge impact on the final quality of the essential oil. Distillation methods should be given close attention.
2) Citrus Oils: Oils derived from the fruits or the rinds of citrus fruits are cold pressed or expeller pressed, not distilled. They are commonly referred to as 'essential oils' all over the world, but in a technical sense they are not since they are not processed by distillation.
3) Absolutes: Oils extracted by chemical solvents, rather than distilled or expressed, are referred to as absolutes. The phrase 'chemical solvents' can make you think that someone has 'messed up.' This is not necessarily true and certainly not true of most solvents used to extract essential oils. To produce an oil with all of the properties that you value when working with jasmine, neroli, onycha oils, and some types of rose, solvents are necessary. The properties of the oils do not 'pull' any other way and the solvents used are ones that can then be removed most easily and completely. Additionally, the best medicinal properties of these plants would not survive the heat of the distillation process.
4) Carrier Blend Oils: Carrier oils are explained in some detail on pages 7 and 9 of this chapter. The oils referred to here are the ones which, by British standards and wording are called an 'essential oil,' but are really at least 95% carrier oil with the remaining 5% being pure therapeutic grade essential oil. This dramatically changes the properties of the oil and certainly impacts the shelf life of these 'massage' oils. The essential oil deteriorates until the healing properties are just not there and the carrier oil itself goes rancid after a short time.

The various categories of scented oils above are impacted differently by such things as heat, cold, light, and air. They also work differently in diffusers and when placed in water and have their own characteristics when absorbed into the body.

Heat

It is a basic law of chemistry that chemical changes, if a change is going to occur at all, happen faster at higher temperatures.
Distilled essential oils: When talking about the first category above—true essential oils—you do not need to be concerned at all if such oils are temporarily exposed to high temperatures, even up to the 140° F which is found in vehicles on a hot day. True essential oils are the product of distillation at higher temperatures than 140°. They are substances that were created by high temperatures. Each oil has a point at which the lightest components separate from the rest of the oil. However, when the bottle is returned to lower temperatures, these components condense, becoming liquid again, and then mix back into the rest of the oil with their chemical composition unaltered.

From a practical standpoint this means that if your pure distilled oils get too warm, leave the lids on until they have cooled back down. This separation of the lightest components is what makes steam inhalation of essential oils effective.

Storing the distilled category of oils at room temperatures is sufficient to preserve their quality. Storing these oils at cooler temperatures offers no advantages and does not increase shelf life.

Expressed citrus oils: Citrus oils can be damaged by temperatures in excess of 100° F. This sensitivity has a lot to do with the molecular size of some of the components. The larger the molecule the more likely it is to break down as temperatures rise. The plants used to make expressed oils produce molecules which are larger than those found in plants that are used for making distilled oils. The larger molecules have little or no fragrance in their complete, un-deteriorated state, but as they break down they produce a variety of smells, usually unpleasant. Both the fragrance and the therapeutic properties of citrus oils would be altered by the heat of the distillation process, so an expeller method is employed. This distinction also applies to all blends of essential oils with citrus ingredients. Having deeper note oils like sandalwood and myrrh included in the blend stabilizes the larger molecules of the citrus oils. Oils with deeper notes slow, and even prevent, this breaking down process. Expressed citrus oils include bergamot, grapefruit, lemon, lime, mandarin, orange, and tangerine. Citrus oils need to be stored at temperatures below 100° F. If they ever get too hot, let them cool before opening the bottle.

Absolutes: Absolutes are slightly more sensitive to heat than expressed citrus oils. It is best to keep them at cooler temperatures; at least no higher than normal room temperature. Absolutes have also not passed through the higher temperatures of distillation because they also contain some larger molecules that can be damaged and broken down by heat. For maximum quality you should read the labels of your blended oils and be aware of the categories of the oils contained in them. Or you can just make it a habit to keep all of your oils at no warmer than moderate room temperatures.

Carrier Oil Blends: These are carrier oils such as almond, coconut, or grapeseed, etc. with some of the other three categories of oils added to them. There is a lot of controversy here because there is a wide range of percentages being used around the world by otherwise reputable companies. There are those who claim that adding a little bit of carrier oil causes only an insignificant amount of damage and the trade-off for convenience and ease of application is worth it. I do not agree!! Logically, the reason citrus oils and absolutes break down is because of the larger molecules (proteins, amino acids, etc.). Adding proteins, etc. with even their larger molecules can only increase the rate of breakdown. While the addition of essential oils slows the break down of the molecules in the carrier oil (they do not smell rancid as quickly), the therapeutic properties of the essential oil are still altered as the larger molecules break down. There are studies that back this position up very soundly, but every day, practical experience with these diluted oils has been enough to convince me. It is best to keep your carrier oils separate and mix them together as you use them. The only possible reasons that I can see for the practice of mixing pure oils with carrier before the time of sale are: 1) that the oil would be a little easier to apply in a hurry over a large area and, 2) since carrier oils are cheaper than essential oils, more profit could be made by their sale. I believe that the profit factor is the bottom line here, since mixing as you use them is not that difficult or inconvenient.

Flames and Candles: The heat of a candle, flame, or heat ring is in excess of 300° F. This will be damaging to your essential oils of any type. Using heat to vaporize oils is said to cause the most volatile compounds to disperse into the air first with the heavier molecules dispersing later. Is this the problem? No. The volatile components of any oil always disperse into the air first anyway; heat just makes this more pronounced. To minimize this effect, try placing your oils in distilled water and then over the source of heat. Scentsy™ candles warmers work well if used in this way. Just leave out the wax, use distilled or spring water, and add your oils to the water. The problem is that heat destroys some of the therapuetic properties of the oil.

Cold

Even extremely cold temperatures do not damage the therapeutic properties of oils. They may become congealed, waxy, or even semi-solid. If your oils get cold, do not apply any heat to warm them up. Just keep the lids on and let them warm up gradually to room temperature. They will be just fine.

Light

Essential oils of any category (distilled, expressed, or absolute) should be stored in dark-colored bottles, in specially lined metal containers or in hard plastic of very specific specifications. Exposure to light causes the small molecules of an essential oil to polymerize. Polymerization means that the light sets in motion the processes by which the small molecules of the essential oil bind together to make larger molecules. Since it is the small molecular sizes that enable essential oils to penetrate tissues and enter cells as well as diffuse into the air, the creation of large molecules makes the oil less therapeutic in irratic ways. Put very simply, light will eventually destroy an essential oil by chemically altering it into a substance that is neither aromatic or therapeutic. A few minutes, or even a few hours, of exposure to light will not substantially alter the makeup of your oils; exposure to light over days, weeks, and months will destroy any essential oil.

Air

The most damaging thing that happens to an essential oil when it is exposed to air is the loss of the most volatile components, the high notes. Essential oil bottles for daily use are small in size and typically come with a dropper cap that minimizes the circulation of air into the bottle when the screw down top caps are off. Nevertheless, with most essential oils, you can smell the aroma of the oil the minute you remove the outer lid. Make it a habit to put the screw top lids back on each time you use an essential oil. Do not worry over much if they are off for a few minutes, while you are applying the oil, but do not leave a bottle open if you can avoid it. If you have removed the hard plastic, push-in applicator section of the cap, do not leave it open any longer than is absolutely necessary.

The second thing that happens to an oil through exposure to air for an extended period of time is that the oil begins to oxidize. Oxidation is the taking on of extra oxygen atoms by the molecules of the original substance. When this happens to metal you get rust. When this has happened to an essential oil, there will have been changes in the molecular structure and the compounds present in the oil.

Store essential oils intended for long-term storage in larger bottles with ordinary phenolyic non-dropper caps. The bottles should not be opened every day. Use the larger bottles to refill the smaller bottles that you will use every day. Each time a bottle of essential oil is opened, the oil inside is exposed to light, air, and contaminants. For the best therapeutic quality and to keep the high notes intact, the lid needs to remain on the bottle as much as possible.

Water

Most of the components of essential oils do not mix well with water. They will either float or sink, but they will not mix in. This is only a problem if a drop of a strong oil comes in contact with some sensitive part of your anatomy. I use essential oils in the bath frequently. I love it and have had no serious incidents. I do believe that the frequency of the essential oil in the water creates a homeopathic effect, magnifying the best properties of the oil. Water is an amazing way to utilize the therapeutic properties of essential oils.

In summary, only people who are using adulterated, synthetic, or oils to which carrier oils have been added need worry about shelf life. Some references in the British school of thought recommend throwing away all your oils every six months and purchasing a fresh bunch. Such a recommendation may be appropriate for oils that are 95% carrier oil, but certainly does not apply to pure aromatic oils that were properly distilled. It does not even apply to expressed oils or absolutes. The fact is, that some oils actually improve with age if properly handled and stored.

Stored properly, the shelf life of pure essential oils is longer than is generally believed. Some oils found in the tombs of Egypt are still wonderfully viable. Remember, however, that oils are sensitive to the ingredients in cosmetics, soap, shampoos, etc. and can be damaged by light, air, and heat if not properly handled. They should also be stored away from electrical appliances.

Essential Oils and security Scanners

Will x-ray scans in an airport damage your essential oils? The answer is probably yes, but the damage will be minor and whatever damage occurs is easily repaired, and by the oils themselves.

Being subjected to x-rays and other high frequency electromagnetic energy is not a big problem for essential oils. What can happen in an oil is that a few molecules that took a direct hit may fracture into pieces. Fragmented molecules are called free radicals and, as we have been told, free radicals are not good things to have floating around in your body. Because they are unbalanced electrically they will grab up electrons and atoms from your tissues to complete their structures and bring them back to a balanced state. This process accelerates the aging process, damages organs and tissues, and sometimes causes cellular mutations that are the fore-runners of cancers. Your tissues and organs need their electrons and atoms! They don't need to become unbalanced themselves because fractured molecules are racing around scavenging from others to make themselves better balanced.

Percentage wise, in an oil, there will not be many damaged molecules from passing through an x-ray scanner. This is because essential oil molecules are small and have spaces between them, to begin with. And the atoms and electrons are in constant motion. It is like they are all traveling around the neighborhood, visiting, at high speeds. It is this 'traveling' that gives an oil its frequency. Only a few of these traveling molecules will take a direct hit.

Antioxidants are substances that remove free radicals from our bodies and neutralize their effects. Essential oils are among the best antioxidants. Some of them are nearly off-the-charts in their free radical removing capabilities. What this means to the damaged molecules of an x-rayed oil is that the broken-apart pieces, with the help of the undamaged molecules, will immediately begin to repair and rebuild themselves.

If you pass your oils through airport security, just give them a little time and they will repair themselves. I have always felt this (and the muscle test has consistently confirmed it). What an illustration that "God is in his heaven and all is right with the world." I find this an appropriate time for a prayer of petition and of gratitude. A little bit of love, gratitude, and prayer always improves essential oils.

Essential oils have the capability of repairing themselves and cleaning up free radicals within themselves, just like they clean up free radicals throughout your body and help to repair you!

Carrier Oils

Carrier or base oils are often applied in conjunction with an essential oil. The common industry term for carrier oils is 'fixed oils.' These oils are made from vegetables, nuts or seeds and often have therapeutic properties of their own. The carrier oils used in therapeutic settings should be cold pressed and organically grown rather than produced by chemical methods. This is an important distinction, as some of the carrier oil will be absorbed into the body along with the essential oil. Some of the more common carrier or base oils are as follows: almond, grapeseed, sunflower, olive, jojoba, safflower, apricot, avocado, borage, carrot, coconut (both fractionated and whole), corn, evening primrose, sunflower, wheat germ, and arnica.

Carrier oils are used for several different reasons. One major reason is because pure essential oils are often too concentrated to be applied undiluted to skin. Adding essential oils to a carrier also allows the oil to be spread over a larger application area and to be absorbed more evenly. Many essential oils are quite expensive and, because they are so highly concentrated, one or two drops may be all that you need. The use of a smaller quantity is often more beneficial than a larger quantity and is certainly less likely to cause any type of reaction.

My husband explains one of the needs for carrier oil when using essential oils in this way. Imagine putting an alcohol-based primer on hot asphalt prior to painting it. That would be almost impossible since the alcohol would evaporate almost before it touched the road. Essential oils behave in a similar manner. They are made of several different constituents, some of which evaporate at lower temperatures and faster rates than the others. Place these essential oils on the skin (90 - 95 degrees) and the higher, more volatile notes are gone before they can be absorbed. A carrier oil stabilizes the essential oil, holding onto all the constituents until they can be absorbed. The chemical composition of the oil remains intact.

Each carrier, or protein oil as they are sometimes referred to, has its own characteristics and ways of reacting to the various essential oils. For example, olive oil, jojoba oil and avocado oil, while excellent for use in skin and beauty care because of their emollient and nourishing properties, are less easily absorbed and not usually used by themselves.

Sweet almond oil is easily the most popular for many reasons. It is inexpensive and absorbs quickly, usually in 5 to 10 minutes. Almond oil has a light, non-offensive aroma.

Fractionated coconut oil is another popular choice. Like almond oil, coconut is inexpensive, absorbs quickly, has almost no aroma at all and has the added advantage of a long shelf life at room temperature without rancidity.

Grapeseed oil is another excellent choice, as is safflower oil. Safflower, however, tends to rancidity if not refrigerated. Sweet almond, grapeseed and safflower can be used by themselves or in combination with small percentages of other oils.

Plant-based salves, like the Miracle Salve or the BHM salve marketed by Butterfly Express, llc, are also excellent mediums for applying essential oil. The essential oils should, as always, be added to small portions of the salves and always added as close to the time of use as possible.

Certain carriers should never be used by themselves. Because of their characteristics they are better as part of a blend of carrier oils with their proportions kept to 10 to 20%. Some of these oils are borage, carrot, evening primrose, black cumin and even jojoba. Very dry skin or skin that has been severely traumatized can greatly benefit by the use of these oils as part of a carrier.
Arnica oil is an oil tincture made by soaking fresh arnica blossoms in almond oil. It is used for bruising, swelling and/or inflammation with amazing results. Arnica oil can cause swelling in exposed muscle tissue, so it is never used on open wounds or deep abrasions.

Black Cumin *(Nigella sativa)* This oil is sometimes referred to as an essential oil but, because of the methods by which it is produced and the size of its molecules, it is more properly classified as a carrier oil. Black Cumin is variously called fennel flower, nutmeg flower, Roman coriander, black caraway, and just plain blackseed. The plant is, in fact, not a cumin at all. Its many uses have earned it a name in Arabic which means 'seed of blessing.' In Islam, it is regarded as one of the greatest of the healing medicines available and is listed as a natural drug in the "Medicine of the Prophet (Muhummad)." The Prophet Muhammad is said to have counseled someone, while traveling, to crush the seeds, add a little oil, and place the mixture in the nostrils with the comment that 'This black cumin is healing for all diseases except death.' (Crushing the seeds this way would be an effective and simple way to release the essential oils and gain their medicinal values temporarily.)

Black cumin seed oil has been used as a digestive aid (flatulence, colic, indigestion, and constipation), as a medicine for colds, asthma, bronchitis, deep coughs, headaches, toothaches, and infections. Black cumin is also used traditionally for circulatory ailments, to strengthen the urinary system and aid in the removal of toxins and excess fluids. This oil is also used as an immune stimulant, and to clear lymphatic congestion. It is listed in many texts as a nervine for the relief of nervous exhaustion, tiredness, debility, insomnia, lethargy, and migraine headaches. Black cumin is used for rheumatism and related inflammatory diseases and to increase milk production in nursing mothers. Black cumin makes an excellent carrier oil for skin conditions such as eczema and boils. It is recommended in protocols for hepatitis.

Scientific research into the individual components of this oil indicate that it protects from histamine-induced bronchial spasms, explaining its use in asthma, bronchitis, and coughing; the presence of beta-sitosterol, and anti-tumor sterol, gives credence to its traditional use in treating abscesses and tumors of the abdomen, eyes, and liver; studies show that black cumin is effective in treating opioid dependence; researchers at the Kimmel Cancer Center in Philadelphia have used that one ingredient, thymoquinone, to block pancreatic cancer cell growth and killed the cells by enhancing the process of programmed cell death (apoptosis). These studies are in the very early stages, but are showing great promise, perhaps as a preventative for those at risk for cancer.

Black Cumin, like the carrier oils referred to above, is too 'heavy' to be used alone. It is best mixed about 1 part black cumin to 4 parts of almond or grapeseed oil, etc.

Distilled water is a great carrier for essential oils. Even bath water will give astonishing results. Water is especially effective in carrying essential oils under the nail bed when fighting a toe-nail fungus. The bath is one of the best ways to carry anti-inflammatory or pain relieving oils to the deep tissues of the body.

Yet Another Reminder

Never mix your pure essential oils into a carrier oil and then store them that way! The therapeutic properties of the oil break down rapidly and you are left with a massage oil of low quality that does not even smell as good as the original essence. Instead, place a small amount of the carrier in the palm of your hand, then add 2 to 4 drops of the essential oil and apply. Following this method allows your essential oils to stay vibrant for long periods of time. It also makes your bottle of essential oil last much longer.

Safety Guidelines

Every book you will ever find on essential oils has a section of cautions and safety guidelines, a fact that could be considered very helpful if any of them agreed on anything and if they were based on facts gleaned from valid studies! In Chapter 1 on page 2, we discussed the major schools of thought concerning essential oils. Most of the books published and sold in America lean to the British way of thinking. Perhaps this is because of the language barrier between texts written in French and the English-speaking people who are reading them.

If you follow the studies quoted in the majority of aromatherapy books written from the British point of view, you will find that the studies were done on animals, or were done with single components of an oil (essential oils which were broken down and, therefore, altered in a laboratory before the testing began), or were done using non-therapeutic, perfumery grade oils for the test. The concerns raised as a result of these tests are of very questionable validity when discussing the subject of pure therapeutic grade essential oils. In fact, I doubt it applies at all.

Please refer back to the discussion on page 2 of Chapter 1, and always consider the bias of the book you are reading. There are books full of cautions that really do not apply to your every day use of therapeutic grade essential oils. On the other hand, essential oils are very concentrated plant material and are biologically active. They penetrate into the tissues and cells of the body. Because they are active agents, essential oils can, of course, be misused and even over-used. The relative safety of essential oils is different depending on the method of use.

It would be difficult, probably impossible, to inhale a lethal dosage of any essential oil, or to absorb such a dosage through the skin. You may irritate your nostrils or lungs, break out in a nasty rash, or trigger a cleanse response by the body, but you will not do yourself serious harm if the oils you are using are pure and non-synthetic. The drugs you have taken play a factor in the nastiness of a cleanse reaction.

The oral ingestion of essential oils is another matter altogether. ***I do not recommend the taking of essential oils internally.*** The proponents of internal ingestion will tell you that when serious over-doses (meaning death) have occurred it was either deliberate on the part of the person or was an accident with a child. The death of a child is always a tragedy and being accidental does not mitigate that. In addition, the 'accidents' I have read of with children would be better termed 'criminal stupidity.' When a substance is making a child seriously ill it is time to stop using it and find an appropriate antidote and a way to cope with the over-dose! Nevertheless, because essential oils are very concentrated, enough of an overdose to cause illness and harm to a child with internal use would be very easy to accomplish. Even with an adult, a great deal of caution and thought should be taken.

The rest of the story is that in studies conducted at universities in both Germany and Austria, essential oils were placed on the feet and then detected on the tongue in 20 minutes. Essential oils absorb so readily into the body and pass through the cells to the needed areas so efficiently that it would rarely be of any additional benefit to take them orally. There are even studies indicating that the rate of travel and the site targeted are responsive to the thoughts and intents of the user.

I have been using essential oils for many years with grand results, and I have never felt the need to use them internally. I brush my teeth with them. I gargle with them and, occasionally, I even use them in a water pick. If I need them somewhere internally I trust the oil itself to find the best path there from use in an external application of some kind.

The purity of the oil does not change the fact that they are extremely concentrated plant material and can be easily overdosed when taken internally. Being a therapeutic grade essential oil does not make that oil automatically safe to be taken internally. Therapeutic grade does eliminate a host of ills unrelated to concentration and strength. Synthetic, man-made versions are *extremely dangerous* taken internally and just plain *dangerous* used otherwise!

With that said, I would like to add that the essential oils sold by Butterfly Express, llc, are therapeutic grade essential oils. The choice, and the responsibility, for their use internally is all yours. Just remember, they, and certainly I, do not advocate internal use of essential oils.

I can find no record of recent deaths, or even serious injuries, linked to the proper use of essential oils. This is true in spite of the fact that more and more people are using them every day. The American Medical Association, in reports of their own, admit that hundreds (some claim thousands) die every year from ***properly*** applied pharmaceutical drugs. Essential oils are among the safest and most effective of all therapeutic modalities. They are safe enough for amateurs and novices to use with only the remotest possibility of causing harm to themselves and others. As always, the more you know the more effective and safe you will be.

Here are a few guidelines and suggestions for the safe use of essential oils

Children The very first rule is, of course, to keep your oils out of the reach of children. Think of and store them just as you would any other therapeutic product containing active ingredients. This means that you do not leave bottles of oil sitting on the side of the tub or anywhere else.

When applying oils to infants and small children, always dilute with a carrier oil. 1 to 3 drops of essential oil in 1/2 teaspoon (or even more) of a carrier oil will do the job nicely without the risk of skin irritation or overdose. If a child does get hold of a bottle of oil and either dumps it in the tub or all over themselves, the solution is carrier oil applied liberally and frequently. The carrier oil will dilute the oil, slow down the rate of absorption into the body, and relieve much of the discomfort of the skin irritation.

Vegetable protein oil (carrier oils) such as olive, almond, grapeseed, safflower, etc. are excellent to use whenever too much oil has been used or an oil has reached the wrong place (the eyes, the mucous membranes of the nose, or other sensitive areas). Do not use water. Water amplifies the effects of the oils and carries it even more quickly into the body.

Phototoxicity Many oils which contain furanoids are phototoxic. This means that if the skin where the oil was applied is then exposed to a source of ultraviolet light, it will absorb more UV radiation at a faster rate. This is true even when the oil was diluted with a carrier oil to be applied. Please note that the ***oil must have been applied to skin which is then going to be exposed. Putting a phototoxic oil on your chest or feet and then exposing your arms and face to sunlight does not create a problem.***

Apparently, furanoids can resonate with UV light in two opposing ways: either to magnify the UV waves, or the furanoids can result in the destruction of the UV radiation. In myrrh oil, for example, there are compounds that quench the solar amplifying properties. Ancient Egyptians applied myrrh oil on their skin daily. Myrrh is an example of how the compounds of living things change their behavior according to the company they are in. ***Testing individual components for toxicity does not tell you much of anything useful!***

Oils which are considered to be phototoxic include angelica, bergamot, orange, bitter, grapefruit, lemon, lime, petitgrain, and rue. Some sources include fennel, aniseseed, and cumin on this list. Notice that not all of the citrus oils are included. Oils of mandarin, orange sweet, tangelo, and tangerine are **NOT** considered phototoxic.

Pregnancy Essential oils are very beneficial for many of the conditions of pregnancy, but caution, of course, should be used. Pay close attention to the lists of oils which are contra-indicated for pregnancy, but do factor in the bias (British, French or German) of the book you are consulting. Always begin with only half the dosage that you would ordinarily use. Remember that blends, because of the smaller percentage of the stronger oils, are usually safer than single oils, especially during pregnancy.

Oils that are known to have estrogenic/hormonal properties should be avoided during pregnancy, or at least used with great caution. These oils include clary sage, sage, calamus, aniseseed, myrtle, wild tansy, and fennel. Blue tansy, tarragon, and cypress should also be used with caution and consideration.

Other oils listed in books of the British persuasion include basil, cinnamon, juniper, marjoram, rosemary, thyme (red and linalol), oregano, clove, nutmeg, bay, pimento berry, cistus, hops, valerian, spikenard, black pepper, cedarwood, hyssop, myrrh, peppermint, mace, cumin, parsley seed, wintergreen, and birch. I am sure that all of these oils have a high risk of creating a problem if they are synthetic, rather than therapeutic grade essential oils. Synthetic oils are a risk to everybody!

A pregnant woman is responsible, for a time, for a life other than her own. She should always be cautious and sensible, especially with substances as concentrated as essential oils.

During my daughter's pregnancies she worked with me continually in our essential oil business. We muscle tested every step of the way and found very few times and very few oils that she could not handle in reasonable quantities. Nevertheless, I handled all the oils that are listed as having hormonal effects. Here is an interesting note about an experience that we had. During her first pregnancy, ylang ylang (which is not listed on cautions lists) opened anywhere in her vicinity would drop her blood pressure immediately to scary levels. During her second pregnancy she used ylang ylang daily to help repair a muscle in her abdomen that was struggling. She did not have any trouble whatsoever with her blood pressure when using it. Experience, caution and paying attention to the cautions lists (which are based on someone else's experience) are the best ways to remain safe in the use of essential oils.

Oils that should never be used, whether you are pregnant or not (listed here so pregnant women do not miss them), include bitter almond, boldo leaf, yellow camphor, horseradish, jaborandi leaf, mugwort, mustard, pennyroyal, thuja, tansy, rue, sassafras, savin, southernwood, wormseed, wormwood.

People with epilepsy or other serious nervous or seizure disorders and people with a history of drug abuse or who are taking potent prescription medications Always proceed with caution. A cleanse from these substances (described in item #1 on page 4 of this chapter) can be a nasty, possibly even deadly, experience. Always use small amounts of the essential oil and space the time of usage out well, at least for the first few days. The detoxification method suggested on page 4 can also be helpful in avoiding problems or dealing with the less drastic ones should they arise.

A Few Last Words

Essential oils are very powerful substances that should be treated with respect. They are highly concentrated plant extracts and should not be used rashly and without knowledge or thought. Each drop is equivalent to at least one ounce of plant material. In most cases, essential oils are more effective in infinitesimal amounts, anyway. Increasing the dosage or amount applied will not usually increase effectiveness.

Begin with a small amount. You can always add more to the bath, to the skin, to the diffuser. You, or the person you are working with, have survived this long without using that particular oil. Another day or two, to gradually bring up the dosage to your personal tolerance level, will be time well spent.

When an oil causes discomfort it is usually for one of two reasons:

1) The use of the oil has triggered a cleanse in the body. Toxins, heavy metals, chemicals, poisons, parasites or mucous are being pulled from cells, particularly the liver, and then filtered through the body's eliminative organs. This can cause a stress reaction in the kidneys and bowels or manifest as a rash if the body uses the skin to eliminate the poisons. Support the eliminative organs (kidney, colon, skin) in any way that you know how and consider slowing down the use of the oils until your system catches up. When the body is detoxifying at too fast a rate, the toxins that cannot be eliminated simply return to storage in new places—often the brain stem—and have to be dealt with all over again later.

A suggested detoxification method:
Run a tub of warm water (quite hot, but not hot enough to be debilitating). Add 3 Tablespoons of *redmond clay or 1 cup sea salt (or Epsom Salts–sea salt is preferable) and soak for at least 20 minutes. Allow time to rest afterwards as you may feel weak and tired for a time.

Soaking just the feet in hot water to which 2 Tablespoons of redmond clay has been added is almost as effective and not as debilitating as soaking the entire body. Be sure to keep the water quite hot.

2) The second reason that a person might have a negative reaction to a particular oil is a simple allergy or an intolerance to the plant from which the oil was made. Oils are made from plant material and they are very concentrated; hence, a person may not realize that they have a problem with a particular plant until they use the oil. Allergic reactions are quite rare in working with essential oils and usually mild when they do occur. An allergic reaction can often be minimized, or dealt with altogether, by using basic energy procedures, massage therapy, or you might try the following:

A. Put [Le]Unity on the palms of both hands.
B. Place one hand over the thymus (heart chakra) and the other hand over the navel.
C. Take 3 deep breaths and switch hands, then take 3 more deep breaths.

There is no substitute for common sense and caution. Only you are responsible for your own health and welfare, and you must use these wonderfully beneficial substances responsibly.

*Redmond clay is the type of diatomaceous earth clay that I usually purchase. It is, of course, acceptable to substitute your favorite one instead.

Methods of Use

One of the nicest things about essential oils is the grand variety of things you can use them for and the stunningly wide range of ways in which you can use them. I have tried to break these many methods down into categories and give you simple instructions for each method.

Direct/Topical Application

Because of the molecular structure of essential oils (the molecules are extremely small and the chemical structure is quite simple), they absorb readily into the body through the skin. This effect can actually be increased by the use of a good carrier oil. A good carrier oil allows you to use less of the more expensive essential oil with the same, or even increased, therapeutic effects.

A few guidelines and suggestions for topical application:

- **Directly on the area of concern** Apply the oils directly to the skin using 1 to 6 drops of essential oil, almost always with a carrier oil. More oil is not necessarily better since a large amount of oil can trigger a detoxification of the surrounding tissue and blood. Such a quick detoxification can be somewhat uncomfortable. To achieve the desired results, 1 to 3 drops of oil is usually adequate.

  Layering is the process of applying one oil, rubbing it in, and then applying another oil immediately. There is no need to wait more than a few seconds between oils as absorption occurs rapidly. A good example of this is the use of the blends ^{Le}Warm Down (for muscle relaxation and inflammation) and ^{Le}Paine or ^{Le}Deeper (for pain relief and healing). Layering them makes them more effective for muscle injuries than either one used alone. Another good example is ^{Le}Woman Wise (for hormone balance) and ^{Le}Deeper (deep tissue muscle spasms) for menstrual cramping and pain.

- **Feet** Placing oils on the feet is a very fast way to get them absorbed into the body because the feet have abnormally large pores. The feet also seem to be an area least likely to be sensitive. Other areas of quick absorption are behind the ears and on the wrists. (The wrists are nice because they are constantly waving in front of the nose as we go about our day.) 1 - 4 drops per foot/ear/wrist are adequate.

- **Acupressure points** have been used for centuries as a means of accessing and correcting imbalances in the energy systems of the body. Essential oils applied to these points can be very effective, and certainly less invasive and scary than needles, as well as less cumbersome than holding the points or placing magnets, etc. on them.

  There are many good books showing these points and how and when to use them. Two of my favorites are <u>Reference Guide for Essential Oils</u> by Connie and Alan Higley and <u>Releasing Emotional Patterns with Essential Oils</u> by Carolyn L. Mein.

- **Wash** You can use an essential oil, diluted in distilled water, to wash infected areas such as wounds, grazes, cuts and for other body and facial treatments.

- **Lotions** Essential oils can be added to prepackaged lotions and creams or to ones of your own making. Be sure that the lotion you use is perfume free. Buy the simplest, purest product you can find. I find essential oils in a little distilled water or light carrier oil are more effective than any lotion.

- **As perfumes or colognes** Some single essential oils and many of the blended ones at Butterfly Express, llc. have a nice enough aroma to wear as perfumes or colognes.

- **Auricular Therapy** This is a method of applying the oils to the rims of the ears and, occasionally, to the earlobes. This is well-documented in the books by Higley and Mein referred to previously.

- **Compresses** Fill a bowl with hot water. Add the desired essential oil. Stir the water vigorously and wait a few moments for any oil to rise to the top. A few essential oils mix very well with water, so you might not be able to see anything if you have used one of those oils. Lay a towel across the top of the water. After the towel is completely saturated, wring out the water. This will leave much of the oil, and all of its frequency, in the moist hot towel. Place the towel over the area needing the compress. Cover with a dry towel and apply a source of heat. Leave on location for one to two hours.

- **Shampoo or Scalp Treatment** Oils such as sage can treat or prevent hair loss. Chamomile Roman prevents (or covers to a certain extent) gray hair in lighter hair colors; rosemary does the same for brunettes. There are many other oils for hair and scalp treatment. Just mix the oil into the shampoo or conditioner–preferably a fairly natural one. I do this one application at a time by putting the conditioner into my hand and then adding the essential oil.

- **Massage** The human body holds every thought, feeling, trauma, pain, distress, tension and emotional crisis within its muscular structure. Massage can release much of this negativity, and a massage with a well-chosen essential oil can be of particularly great benefit. Massage can also help improve circulation and essential oils can aid in this process also.

  The chart below shows which parts of the body are most likely to hold certain types of stress. I hope you find it useful and informative.

Body Area	Emotions
back of the neck	difficulty expressing feelings
throat	difficulty expressing emotions
upper chest	sadness and/or regret
outer shoulder	afraid of letting go
back of shoulder	fear and/or sadness
upper arm - biceps	fear
forearm	anxiety and/or insecurity
hip - outer thigh	too much responsibility
upper thigh (front of the body)	feeling overburdened
outer thigh	persistent sadness
lower chest - center (solar plexus chakra)	fear of love - abuse issues
head/neck/solar plexus/tailbone	stress and tension
inner ankles	depression
calf muscles	feeling overwhelmed

Olfactory Administration

Odor molecules travel to the top of the nasal cavity and fit like little puzzle pieces into specific receptor cells on the nearly ten million olfactory nerve cells. These millions of nerve cells serve to transfer electric impulses to the olfactory bulb which, in turn, sends those impulses along to the amygdala and then to the limbic system of the brain. The amygdala is directly responsible for storing and releasing emotional trauma and responds only to odor. Recent studies indicate that it is the area of the brain that produces solutions when we are presented with a problem that needs solving. Because the limbic system is directly connected to those parts of the brain that control the autonomic nervous system, essential oils can have profound physiological and psychological effects. The autonomic nervous system controls the heart rate, blood pressure, breathing, memory, stress levels, and hormones. It is believed by many people that we have no conscious control over these areas but events in recent scientific and practical arenas are showing us the error of this type of thinking.

Our sense of smell is very sensitive and highly developed. We can detect as little as 1 part of fragrant material in 1 billion. Our noses can differentiate several hundred different odors at the same time. Fragrances such as those of essential oils can bring about the deepest emotions and sensations in us. The smell of something familiar from your past, such as the aroma of baking bread, can take you by surprise and bring you either memories of times when you were happy and safe, or take you back to scenes of severe distress.

The sense of smell is closely related to memory; olfactory memories are very accurate and almost indelible. Since the olfactory system is, literally, the doorway to the subconscious, it would be logical to use aroma in psychotherapy. This is being done, but the research is in early stages and made difficult by the fact that every person's olfactory associations are different. There are some oils, however, that seem to have similar effects on most people. You will, no doubt, quickly develop your own list of favorites.

- **Diffuser:** There are a wide range of diffusers on the market. They can be divided into two basic groups: heated and non-heated. Heat and essential oils was discussed in some depth in the chapter on shelf life (Chapter 3). For a simple method, place a few drops of oil into a bowl and pour warm water over it. Oil molecules in the air remain and are effective for healing purposes long after the aroma has vanished.

  There are non-heated diffusers on the market that have specially designed filters to disseminate the molecules. These work well, but are extremely expensive and often no better than cheaper methods and equipment.

  One of my favorite types of diffusers are simple fountains, bought inexpensively at Wal-Mart, etc. The literature will tell you that you need fountains with specially designed motors so that the essential oil will not ruin it. Essential oils are not really oily, except when they have been adulterated with a carrier oil. Most pure essential oils do not clog motors, although the resins and balsams require that you clean your fountain or diffuser well after each use. I have had some of my diffusers for years and they are still going strong, day in and day out! Learn to read labels carefully because many, if not most, essential oils (not those sold at Butterfly Express, llc, however) have a little almond oil, etc. added to them.

A Scentsy® candle warmer, with water substituted for the wax, is my new favorite way to diffuse essential oils. Put water in the dish part and add a few drops of essential oil. Oil placed directly into the dish (without water) gets too hot. This damages the therapeutic properties of the essential oil and makes a sticky mess of he dish.

- **Sniffing:** This is the simplest method imaginable. Simply open the bottle and take a whiff. Or you can put a little on a cotton ball and place it in a vent or in front of a fan. I have put the cotton ball into a zip-lock bag and carried it with me. Placing some oil in a tissue or handkerchief also works well. I love to place a drop or two of oil on my pillow at night.

- **Inhalation**: Place a few drops of an essential oil in a bowl and add hot water. Place a light cotton dish towel, or something similar, over your head and hang your head over the bowl. Inhale deeply. This is a great method for oils such as eucalyptus and blends like ^{Le}Breezey, ^{Le}Mariah and ^{Le}Aspire.

- **Inhalers:** Small plastic tubes with a cotton core onto which an essential oil may be placed are convenient ways to have the aroma of an essential oil with you at all times. A drop or two of oil added as needed will refresh the inhaler very quickly. This is a very good way to sniff an essential oil in a public place without the aroma of the oil dispersing all over the room and being obvious to everyone around you.

- **Room Sprays**: Put warm water into a plant mister, add the essential oil and shake vigorously. Avoid spraying over furniture and fabrics or anything that could be damaged by water. This is very effective at removing odors and for disinfecting purposes.

Water Magic

Essential oils and water do not mix readily in most cases. As was explained in the section on diffusers, pure essential oils are not really oily at all, and most of them (the balsams and some of the resins are an exception) mix well enough with water to accomplish your purposes. In any case, the frequency of the oil seems to be imbued into the water whether or not it is mixed in well or is just floating there in droplets or even sinking to the bottom of the tub.

In the last few years there have been several studies done verifying the homeopathic nature of acqueous solutions. Some of these studies, involving the filtering of bacteria from distilled water, clearly demonstrated that an 'imprint' of the bacteria remained in the water after all of the bacteria had been removed. While science may be at a loss to explain this phenomenon, homeopathy relies on it millions of times every day. Put a couple of drops of an essential oil in your bathtub, enjoy a 10 minute soak, and you will have experienced this phenomenon, too.

Water is an excellent conductor of electricity, which is an important point to keep in mind when you consider that the human brain is 90% water and brain activity is electrical in nature. It is known that substances put into bath water often enter the body by osmosis. This is good news for the use of essential oils and alarming when you consider the chemicals present in our water!

- **Baths** Run the bath as usual, then add the drops of essential oil and swish the water around. One interesting bath method is to place the oil in milk powder and then place the milk powder in the bath. Milk is popular and well-liked because it makes the skin feel so soft and smooth. Diluted oils used in the bath are gentle to sensitive skin and give aromatherapy effects at the same time. 2 - 5 drops is enough. More than that of some oils will cause skin irritation!

- **Foot bath** Fill a large bowl with warm water and add the essential oil, being sure to swish it around some. This method can be used to pull toxins from the body or, by using soothing/ calming oils can facilitate relaxation and sleep. Other oils could be used to stimulate the immune system or to increase circulation. This is one of my favorite methods. Again, 2-5 drops is enough.

- **Hot tub or jacuzzi** Use as you would in a tub. Here again, the literature says that an oily residue may be left on the pipes and jets. This may be true with heavy balsamic or resin oils, but because of their basic nature, these oils are not typically used in the bath anyway. <u>If the oil is pure and undiluted with a carrier or extender oil</u>, there should be no problem with any oil residue which water will not readily wash away when the tub or jacuzzi is drained.

- **Shower:** Place a few drops in the bottom of the tub or shower. The hot water will diffuse it upward in a very pleasant manner and the therapeutic effects will absorb through the large pores of the feet and be very effective. It helps if you close the drain and let 2 or 3 inches of water build up in the bottom of the tub.

Miscellaneous Methods:

- **Gargle** Although I do not recommend essential oils for internal use, some oils make excellent gargles and mouth washes. Mix the essential oil of your choice (LeDeliverance, LeSpice-C or Spearmint are good choices) into water. Some people like mixing the oil into a teaspoon of honey, then diluting with warm water until the honey is thoroughly dissolved. I liked this, but it was way too much work and I didn't like the idea of something that sweet being left on my teeth and gums and feeding any unwanted bacteria in my throat. I prefer not to swallow the oil, or the oil and honey mixture, and I never use more than 1 - 3 drops of any oil.

- **Toothbrush** During times of illness or when other members of the family are ill, I often put a drop of LeDeliverance oil on my toothbrush as a way of fighting bacteria. A friend of mine who often foot-zones very ill people has been doing this for some time and has greatly reduced the number and duration of the 'bugs' she catches. Never use more than a drop or two.

- **Dishwasher, Dishwater, Washer, Dryer** Unadulterated essential oils can be added to the dishwater or put into the dishwasher (1-2 drops is sufficient) to clean, disinfect and fight bacteria when family members are ill. I use them in the laundry to fight the smell of oil, grease and gasoline. They can also be placed on dryer sheets. My favorite oils for this are LeSunburst and LePurify. You should avoid the resin oils, listed in Chapter 10.

- **Internally** Occasionally, I will add a drop or 2 of essential oil to 5 gallons of distilled water, or even run a drop or two through my distiller to freshen, clean and sanitize it. The machine must then be cleaned and copious amounts of water ran through it if you wish to eliminate the flavor of the essential oil. Lemon, lime, grapefruit and orange are particular favorites of mine and cause the least complaining about the residual taste.

- **Cooking with essential oils** There are all sorts of recipes out there for cooking with essential oils. The oils referenced here have been purchased oils in culinary shops to be used in cooking, rather than in a health oriented shop for their therapeutic properties. These are essential oils which have been mixed with carrier oils such as almond for ease of use. There is nothing unethical about this practice; they are not being represented as anything other than what they are. Just don't confuse them with pure, unadulterated, therapeutic essential oils and expect them to be healing. They are meant to be cooking ingredients.

  I have tried cooking with pure essential oils. The recommended number of drops is **way too much and too strong!** One drop of mandarin, lemon or lime in a batch of frosting or cookie dough is offensively strong. 3 drops of peppermint in a whole batch of 'green herbal drink' gives your mouth a real cooling sensation! I have tried mixing a drop with a tablespoon of cooking oil and then using it in much the same way as you would use the extracts you can buy. I have been quite pleased with the results.

  Less than a single drop of oil is often needed when cooking with essential oils. This can be easily accomplished by placing a drop of oil on a toothpick and then immersing the toothpick in your batch. Immerse the toothpick again if the flavor is not quite strong enough for your taste.

  Pure, undiluted, high-quality essential oils, in my personal opinion, are not meant to be taken internally. While not usually dangerous there is usually no need to do so!

Essential Oil Charts*

Action of Essential Oils on Skin:

Property	Essential Oil	Special Applications
Antiseptic	LeMela Plus, LeNo-More, LeSunburst, tea tree, eucalyptus, lavender, geranium	Cleansing, protecting and treating acne-prone skin
Cytophylactic (cellular stimulatation and protection)	LeMillenia, myrrh, frankincense, rose, sandalwood, geranium, rosemary, lavender, neroli, helichrysum	Treatment and healing of minor skin lesions and blemishes, mature skin
Rubefacient (capillary circulation)	LeMillenia, LeWarm Down, LeWoman Wise, LeVisibility, juniper, grapefuit, rosemary	Toxin elimination, lymphatic drainage, treatment of sluggish conditions
Astringent	LeInsight, LeWeightless, geranium, lemongrass, lemon	Skin toner, treatment of oily skin
Regulator	LeInside Out, LeEndo Relief, LeLife Force, LeTurmoil, sage	Sebaceous secretions, oily skin
Protectant	LeBaby Me, LeWarm Down, palmarosa, sandalwood, myrrh	Protect skin, help it retain moisture
Soother	LeBaby Me, LeMillenia, chamomile, neroli, rosewood, rose, ylang-ylang	Sensitive skin, broken capillaries

Essential Oils for Skin Care:

Skin type/problem	Essential Oils
Normal skin	clary sage, geranium, lavender, ylang-ylang, rosewood
Dry skin	clary sage, cedarwood, sandalwood, rose, palmarosa
Oily skin	lavender, lemon, geranium, frankincense, rosemary, ylang-ylang
Inflamed	chamomile German, chamomile Roman, clary sage, helichrysum, jasmine, lavender, myrrh, patchouli
Sensitive	chamomile Roman, chamomile German, rosewood, neroli
Acne	cajeput, tea tree, juniper, lavender, lemon, palmarosa, rosewood, yarrow
Eczema	cedarwood, chamomile German, lavender, sage, patchouli, rose, benzoin
Rejuvenation	LeMillenia, frankincense, sandalwood, cedarwood, geranium, lavender, myrrh, rosemary, helichrysum
Seborrhea	bergamot, lavender, cypress, patchouli
Broken capillaries	LeVisibility, rose, ylang-ylang
Wrinkles	lemon, palmarosa, myrrh, frankincense, patchouli, rose, rosewood, clary sage

*These charts have been compiled from many reliable and well-respected sources detailing the traditional use of these oils. It is meant for informational purposes only and is certainly not meant to diagnose or prescribe in any way.

The blend LeBaby Me is excellent for all skin types and most problems

Therapeutic Properties of Essential Oils

Property	Essential Oils
Adrenal Stimulants	LeInside-Out, LeLife Force, LeVitality, basil, geranium, rosemary
Analgesic	LeBreezey, LeDeeper, LeMy-graine, LePaine, LeTenda Care, birch, clove, eucalyptus, geranium, lavender, peppermint, marjoram, rosemary
Anti-inflammatory	LeCypernium, LeWith-In, LeTenda Care, LeVitality, LeWarm Down, chamomile German, chamomile Roman, lavender, basil, peppermint, birch, coriander, cypress, helichrysum, ravensara, spruce
Antiseptic/Antiviral	all essences are antiseptic to one degree or another; some of the most effective are: LeDeliverance, LeInsight, LeMela Plus, LePurify, LeSunburst, bergamot, eucalyptus, juniper, cajuput, citronella, oregano, peppermint, sage, cedarwood, hyssop, lemongrass, marjoram, myrrh, thyme, tea tree, cinnamon, clove, garlic, lavender, ravensara, sandalwood
Antispasmodic	LeAspire, LeBalance, LeMillenia, LeTenda Care, LeWarm Down, basil, berga-mot, chamomile Roman, cypress, eucalyptus, hyssop, lavender, marjoram, melissa, peppermint, rosemary, sandalwood
Carminative	LeBalance, LeInside-Out, basil, black pepper, chamomile Roman, chamomile German, clary sage, fennel, frankincense, hyssop, juniper, lavender, marjoram, melissa, myrrh, peppermint, rosemary, sandalwood
Cephalic	LeDeeper, LeMy-graine, basil, peppermint, rosemary
Cytophylactic/ Vulnary	LeMillenia, lavender, neroli, helichrysum, yarrow, bergamot, chamomile Roman, chamomile German, eucalyptus, frankincense, geranium, hyssop, lavender, myrrh, rosemary
Digestive	LeBalance, LeInside-Out, basil, bergamot, chamomile German, chamomile Roman, clary sage, frankincense, hyssop, marjoram, melissa, neroli, rosemary
Diuretic	LeBalance, LeMillenia, chamomile Roman, chamomile German, cedarwood, cypress, eucalyptus, frankincense, geranium, hyssop, juniper, lavender, rosemary, sandalwood
Energizing/ Stimulant	LeEnergy, LeVitality, LeRevitalize, LeWake-Up, peppermint, ginger, nutmeg, peppermint, rosemary, lemon, eucalyptus, pine
Expectorant	LeAspire, LeMillenia, basil, bergamot, cedarwood, eucalyptus, fennel, hyssop, marjoram, myrrh, peppermint, sandalwood
Hypo/Hyper-tensor	LeGood-Nite, LeVitality, clary sage, hyssop, lavender, marjoram, melissa, ylang-ylang
Nervine	LeDeeper, LeLife Force, LeMillenia, LePaine, LeTenda Care, basil, chamomile German, chamomile Roman, clary sage, hyssop, juniper, lavender, marjo-ram, melissa, peppermint, rosemary
Sedative (taken in moderate dosages)	LeBelieve, LeDreams, LeEverlasting, LeGood-Nite, LeMeditation, LeMy-graine, LeSolitude, LeTranquility, benzoin, bergamot, chamomiles, cedarwood, clary sage, cypress, frankincense, geranium, hyssop, jasmine, juniper, lavender, marjoram, melissa, myrrh, neroli, patchouli, rose, sandalwood, ylang-ylang
Sudorific	basil, chamomile German, chamomile Roman, hyssop, juniper, lavender, melissa, peppermint, rosemary

Base Oils/Fixed Oils		
Sweet almond oil	Good for all skin types. Helps relieve itching, soreness, dryness, and inflammation	can be used as a base oil 100 percent
Apricot kernel oil	all skins types, especially prematurely aging, sensitive, inflamed, and dry skin	can be used as a base oil 100 percent
Avocado pear oil	all skin types, especially dry and dehydrated; eczema	use as an additive to a base, no more than 10 percent
Borage oil	all skin types; multiple sclerosis, menopausal problems, heart disease, psoriasis and eczema, prematurely aged skin. Good for regenerating and stimulating the skin.	use as an additive to a base, no more than 10 percent
Coconut oil	all skin types but really nice for dry or damaged skin; low rancidity factor; less oily residue than other carriers; very little odor	excellent used 100 percent; not suitable as an addition to a carrier oil blend
Carrot oil	premature aging, itching, dryness, psoriasis and eczema. Rejuvenating, reduces scarring	***Do not use undiluted*** use as an additive to a base nor more than 10 percent
Corn oil	soothing on all skin types	can be used 100 percent
Evening primrose oil	multiple sclerosis, menopausal problems, heart disease. Excellent in the treatment of psoriasis and eczema. Helps to prevent premature aging for the skin	use as an additive to a base no more than 10 percent
Grapeseed oil	all skin types	can be used 100 percent
Hazelnut oil	has a slight astringent action; good for all skin types	can be used 100 percent
Jojoba oil	inflamed skin, psoriasis, eczema, acne, hair care, all skin types; highly penetrative	use as an additive to a base no more than 10 percent
Olive oil	rheumatic conditions, hair care, cosmetics; soothing	a heavy oil use as an additive to a base no more than 10 percent
Peanut oil	all skin types	can be used 100 percent
Safflower oil	all skin types	can be used 100 percent
Sesame oil	psoriasis, eczema, rheumatism, arthritis all skin types	use as an additive to a base no more than 10 percent
Soya bean oil	all skin types	can be used 100 percent
Sunflower oil	all skin types	can be used 100 percent
Wheatgerm oil	eczema, psoriasis, prematurely aged skin; all skin types	use as an additive to a base no more than 10 percent

Definitions of Basic Essential Oil Terms

absolute — An oil that is extracted by a complex process using solvents such as alcohol or hexane. The solvent is then removed. This extraction method is used when there is very little essential oil in the plant part being used or when a more concentrated or complex fragrance is desired.

attar (otto) — This term is used to describe the steam distillation of rose petals. It is also an Indian term for the oil obtained from the co-distillation of rose and sandalwood.

balsam — A balsam is a water insoluable, viscous or semi-solid substance which is exuded from some types of trees and bushes. A balsam is similar to a gum resin.

cold pressed — Cold pressed refers to a process of extraction used for citrus and fixed oils. The process of pressing uses minimal heat to prevent harm to the therapeutic properties of the plant material. Heat is usually under 120 degrees Fahrenheit.

concrete — Concretes are extracted in a manner similar to an absolute. The final product, however, is a semi-solid wax rather than a liquid essential oil.

CO2 extraction — This refers to extraction methods using carbon dioxide (CO2). One method uses low pressure cold extraction with a dense liquid CO2. The other method involves heating the CO2 to just above 87 degrees Fahrenheit, making it a dense fog. CO2 is the most desired of solvents because it leaves no toxic residues behind. Low pressure is the best CO2 extraction method for obtaining high quality results.

deodorized — An oil is considered deodorized when unwanted fragrance or flavor materials have been removed from a botanical product.

distillate water — Distillate water is another term for floral water or hydrosol and is the by-product of steam distillation.

distillation — Distillation is a heating process which separates and purifies a liquid mixture. Different components have different vapor pressures. The process involves vaporization of the more volatile components and then condensation of the vapor back to a liquid.

expeller pressed — A machine pressing process for plant materials which operates at around 140 to 210 degrees Fahrenheit.

essential oil — Essential oils are volatile oils, typically fragrant, which are extracted from botanicals using steam distillation. Normally liquid, but some may be solid at cooler temperatures. For commercial purposes expressed oils and absolutes are usually identified as essential oils, while technically they are not.

extraction — Extraction is a process of removing botanical components from a raw material through the uses of distillation and/or solvents. The solvent containing the extracted materials is filtered and the solvent removed. The extract contains non-volatile as well as volatile components. Oleoresins, resinoids, concretes, and absolutes are all produced by varying forms of extraction methods.

exudate — Exudates are non-cellular, natural raw material that is secreted by plants. This can occur spontaneously or after damage or cutting of the plant. Balsam oils are an example of an exudated substance.

FCC FCC stands for Food Chemicals Codex and is the industry standard listing of food grade ingredients.This label indicates that the substance is considered safe for use in food and cosmetics.

fixatives a material which slows down the rate of evaporation of the more volatile components in perfume composition and natural product formulation.

fixed oils These are non-volatile oils derived from plant materials, commonly referred to as vegetable oils These oils are often referred to as carrier oils.

fractional distillation In the fractional steam distillation process, the essential oil is collected in batches over the distillation period at set times. The oil yield taken initially is referred to as 1st, thereafter 2nd and 3rd. A blend of all the batches is referred to as 'complete.' Ylang ylang is harvested in this manner.

gum resin absolute An oil soluble, purified exudate consisting mostly of resinous constituents, gums and small amounts of volatile components. Examples are myrrh, galbanum, and opoponax.

hydrosol see distillate water

isolate The separation of a particular aroma chemical from an essential oil via: distillation (mechanically), hydolysis (chemically), or by other partitioning methods. Example: eugenol from clove leaf oil.

oleoresin An extraction, usually of natural spice or flavoring materials, using selected solvents to remove the vital components. An oleoresin will contain the essential oils plus other important non-volatile components responsible for the flavor, color and other aspects of the starting raw material.

rectified This term indicates that a material was re-processed or distilled a second time. Sometimes a rectified (or redistilled) oil will be added to oil from a first distillation. This is not done to commit fraud, but to enable an oil such as melissa to be produced less expensively so that people will be able to afford to use it. These oils often have amazing healing properties, although the first distillation would be better.

refined Refined describes the removal of impurities from the natural, crude botanical product.

solvent extraction Some natural raw materials are too delicate to process using steam heat. These are processed using various solvents and the solvent is then filtered out of the product. The extract will contain both non-volatile as well as volatile components. Oleoresins, resinoids, concretes and absolutes are all produced by solvent extraction.

terpeneless The complete or partial removal of monoterpenes or hydrocarbons by distillation. This is done to:

a) improve solubility in diluted alcohol or food grade solvents,
b) increase stability of the oil and prevent the appearance of rancid notes.

water miscible/dispersible This means that the substance can be uniformly mixed with water.

water soluble A substance that will dissolve in water.

winterized A cold-filtering process which removes substances which cause cloudiness at cooler temperatures.

wonf A wonf is an essential oil or flavor to which 'other natural flavors' have been added to enhance specific notes, properties, or aroma.

Glossary of Therapeutic Terms

Analgesic: Reduces pain sensations in tissues and nerves

Antibiotic/antibacterial: Prevents bacterial growth

Anti-oxident: Capable of inhibiting free radical damage in the cells of the body

Anti-catarral: Reduces inflammation and phlegm in mucous membranes that have resulted from infections or allergic reactions

Anti-coagulant: Prevents the clotting of blood

Anti-diarrheal: Prevents or reduces the symptoms or causes of diarrhea

Anti-emetic: Aids in the relief of vomiting

Anti-fungal: Prevents fungal growth

Anti-histaminic: Histamine is part of the body's natural response to foreign pathogens. When our immune systems are out of balance, an over-reaction can occur. A substance that is anti-histaminic neutralizes the action of histamine or inhibits its over-production in the body

Anti-infectious: Prevents the growth and spread of infections

Anti-inflammatory: Reduces *excess* redness and swelling in damaged tissues

Anti-microbial: Prevents or inhibits the growth of miro-organisms such as bacteria, fungi, or protozoans.

Anti-neuralgic: Prevents inflammation of nerves and nerve endings

Anti-parasitic: Acts against insect parasites

Anti-putrescent: Prevents or inhibits the putrefaction and destruction of tissues

Anti-rheumatic: Acts against the pain or the cause of painful joint disorders

Anti-seborrheic: Acts to prevent *excessive* secretion of the sebaceous glands. The sebaceous glands are microsopic glands in the skin which secrete what we refer to as oil to lubricate the skin and hair.

Antisclerotic: Prevents hardening of cells and tissues

Antiseptic: Destroys microbes on surfaces and prevents their further development

Antispasmodic: Prevents or relieves muscle spasms, convulsions, contractions, and coughs

Anti-sudorific: Prevents or inhibits sweating

Anti-tumoral: Inhibits the growth of tumors

Anti-tussive: A substance which relieves coughs

Anti-venomous: Acts in the body against venom

Antiviral: Prevents viral growth

Aphrodisiac: Acts to increase sexual desire or pleasure

Astringent: A substance that constricts and tightens body tissues. Some examples of the benefits of taut tissues in the body would be shrinkage of mucous membranes of the lungs to expel mucous during infectious illnesses; the prevention of calcium deposits (stones) in the kidneys or gallbladder; the healing of skin problems such as stretch marks, scars, and acne.

Balsamic: Soothes the irritation of sore throats, coughs, etc.

Bronchial dilator: Opens the bronchial tubes in the lungs for relief and ease of breathing in respiratory infections

Calmative: Sedative, calming agent

Cardiovascular tonic: Tones and strengthens the heart and veins

Carminative: Relieves flatulence, easing abdominal pain and bloating

Cephalic: Pertaining to the head, specifically headache

Cerebral stimulant: Stimulating to the brain and central nervous system

Cholagogue: Promotes the evacuation of bile from the gall bladder and gall ducts

Cicatrisant/cicatrisive: Aids in the healing of wounds

Circulatory stimulant: Increases the circulation of blood throughout the body

Corticosteroid: Steroid hormones produced in the adrenal cortex. They are involved in stress response, immune response and the regulation of inflammation, carbohydrate and protein metabolism, blood electrolyte levels, and aspects of our behavior

Cortisone-like: A substance with properties similar to cortisone. Cortisone suppresses undue immune response, thus reducing inflammation, pain, and swelling at the site of an injury.

Cytophylactic: Promotes cell regeneration at the site of an injury, which speeds healing and reduces scarring

Depurative: Eliminates toxins and purifies the system

Diaphoretic: Induces a sweat. Used when the immune response of fever and sweat by the body has been insufficient to kill infectious microbes.

Disinfectant: Destroys harmful micro-organisms

Diuretic: Promotes the removal of excess water from the tissues of the body. This usually increases urine output by the kidneys.

Emmenagogue: Induces or regulates menstruation

Emollient: A substance that soothes and softens the skin

Endocrine stimulant: The endocrine system consists of glands which secrete various types of hormones to regulate body functions. It also includes the information system which communicates hormone needs between different organs and system. An endocrine stimulant acts to increase the action of some or all of the endocrine system.

Estrogenic: While estrogen is a necessary female hormone, too much estrogen is associated with several unwanted things including breast and cervical cancers.

Expectorant: Promotes removal of mucus from the body

Febrifuge: An agent that controls fever, keeping it at optimum levels for killing microbes but not too high.

Fungicidal: A substance that acts against fungi.

Galactagogue: Induces the flow of milk in nursing mothers

Hemostatic: Inhibits or stops bleeding and hemorrhage

Hepatic: Acts on the liver to balance and to cleanse

Hormonal: An agent that brings the hormone levels of the body back into balance.

Hyper/Hypo-tensor: Stabilizes the blood pressure, whether the blood pressure is too high or too low.

Immuno-stimulant: Stimulates the action of the immune system

Insecticide: Agents and substances that control insects.

Laxative: Substances that induce bowel movements or loosen the stool.

Lymphatic decongestant: A substance that cleanses and drains the lymph

Menstrual regulator: Substances that balance the hormones and regulate the timing of the menstrual cycle.

Mucolytic: Agents that liquefy mucous and help the body carry it off

Muscle relaxant: Relaxes the muscles and calms cramping sensations

Neuralgic: Neuralgics help heal the nerves and quiet spasmodic pain that runs along the nerves

Neuro-muscular: A neuro-muscular agent aids the healing of a muscle and the nerves that feed it.

Nervine: Acts on the nerves; relieves nervous disorders

Pectoral: Beneficial for diseases or conditions of the chest and respiratory system

Prostate decongestant: Decongests and strengthens the function of the prostate.

Regenerative: Aids in the re-creation of lost or damaged tissue

Restorative: Stimulant for nerves and adrenal cortex

Revitalizer: Providing energy and health to the body and mind

Rubefacient: Dilates and opens the capillaries, improving circulation to the extremities and to the skin

Sedative: Reduces mental excitement or physical activity

Soporific: Induces, or tends to induce, sleep and relaxation

Stimulant: Increases the function of an organ or body system; increases alertness or wakefulness

Styptic: An astringent that promotes the contracting of tissues and blood vessels for the control of bleeding

Stomachic: Good for the stomach; gastric tonic, digestive aid

Sudorifice: Produces a sweat or a 'healthy' germ-killing fever

Tonic: Invigorates, refreshes, and restores bodily functions

Tranquilizing: Relieving anxiety or tension; promoting calm

Vasonstrictor: Causes the blood vessels to contract; slows blood flow through capillaries

Vermifuge: Expels intestinal worms; anti-parasitic

Vulnerary: Promotes the healing of wounds and sores by external application

Warming: Increases overall circulation and the movement of energy throughout the body

Suggestions and Practical Uses

Abscesses, dental	LePurify, LeMela Plus LeDeliverance, spearmint	apply to gum area; may want to dilute
Abundance	LeBountiful, LeAcknowledge LeUnity, cardamom, myrrh, patchouli	diffuse; wear as perfume; use in the bath; apply to wrists or temples
Abuse - physical sexual	LeAngel, LeHeart Song, LeInsight, rose	diffuse; wear as perfume; use in the bath; apply over heart area; on wrists; consider carrying an essential oil inhaler
Accidents	LeTurmoil, LePatches, LePaine, LeDeeper	dilute and apply to the site of the injury
Acne/Skin	LeSego Lily, LeBaby Me, rosewood, grapefruit, cajeput, laurel, lemongrass, niaouli, litsea cubeba, rose geranium	dilute in distilled or clear spring water and sponge on skin with clean cotton balls (do not use carrier oils as they will feed any bacteria that may be contributing factors)
Addictions	LeRevitalize, grapefruit, patchouli, petitgrain	diffuse; carry an essential oil inhaler
Adrenal Glands	LeEnergy, LeHeart Song, LeEndo Relief, LeTrust, LeVitality, spruce, basil, geranium, rosemary, sage	dilute well and apply locally or to the feet; dilutes particularly well with LeEnergy
ADHD	LeMillenia, LeTranquility	dilute and apply LeMillenia along the spine and/or feet; diffuse LeTranquility, especially during the early hours of the night; carry an essential oil diffuser of either one, or both
Aftershave	LeMillenia, LeEverlasting, sandalwood	massage coconut oil (the more solid variety) onto the face and then add a little bit of essential oil
Allergies	LeAcknowledge, LeBreezey, LeUnity, LeExhilaration (applied down the sternum), LeAspire, LeLife Force, LeSego Lily, lavender, elemi (for rashes), melissa, eucalyptus, patchouli, chamomile Roman, niouli, patchouli	inhale; diffuse; wear
Alignment *physical structures and electrical energies*	LeMillenia, yarrow	dilute and apply locally, but especially along the spine; use in a bath; on feet (little boys like this because no one can smell it at school); yarrow for spiritual alignment
Alzheimer's	LeMeditation, LeAcknowledge, LeMagi, LeIQ, LeTrust, LeUnity, frankincense, sandalwood, galbanum	dilute and apply on the back of the neck and on the temples; use in the bath; diffuse throughout the day

Analgesic	LePaine, LeDeeper, birch, eucalyptus, black pepper, peppermint	dilute and apply locally; a few drops in a tub is particularly effective; *dilute black pepper particularly well and use only 2 drops in the tub*
Anemia	LeLife Force, LeRevitalize, carrot seed, lavender, lemon	dilute and apply to the chest and the bottoms of the feet
Anorexia	LeHoliday Spirit, LeEZ-Traveler LeSunburst, LePurify, LeMela Plus, LeMillenia, LeWeightless, coriander, grapefruit	apply to stomach and to the bottom of the feet; might be advisable to also diffuse or wear any of the oils used for depression, etc.
Anger	LeExpressions, LeInsight, LeLetting Go, LeRevitalize, LeTranquility, LeTrust, LeTurmoil, LeUnity, LeWisdom, bergamot	most of these work well as a perfume; dilute and apply, particularly over the heart area; use 2 or 3 drops to relax in a bath; diffuse into the air
Antiviral	LeDeliverance, LeDiscernment, LeMariah, LeSpiceC, cinnamon, clove, oregano, garlic (sparingly, less than 1 drop at a time!!)	as a gargle, on your toothbrush, dilute and apply to throat or the bottoms of the feet; *Remember to use these as a preventative, not just when you are sick*
Anti-inflammatory Anitspasmodic	LeWarm Down, LeDeeper, LeTenda Care, LePaine, LePatches, LeVitality, birch, black pepper, coriander, cypress, helichrysum, patchouli, peppermint, petitgrain, spearmint, spikenard, spruce, wintergreen, anthopogon, opoponax	dilute and apply to affected muscles or joints
Antiseptic	LeMela Plus, LePurify, LeDiscernment, LeSunburst, LeDeliverance	all essential oils are antiseptic to some degree. This is just a list of my favorites.
Anxiety	LeAngel, LeAssurance, LeDreams, LeFaith, LeInner Peace, LeLetting Go, LeWhispering Hope, LeVision, bergamot, frankincense, jasmine, lavender, lime, melissa, rose, sandalwood, patchouli, chamomile Roman, spruce, tangerine, ylang ylang, rose geranium	a few drops on a cotton ball (in a small plastic bag) carried with you at all times is very good or carry an inhaler such as the ones from Butterfly Express, llc; diffuse, wear on the wrists or as a perfume; in a bath
Aphrodisiac/libido	LeMoonlight, LeLetting Go, LeBeloved, LeExpressions, jasmine, neroli, rose, sandalwood, ylang ylang	diffuse or wear as a perfume

Arthritis	LeVitality, LeWarm Down, LeUnity LePaine, (w/LeMillenia), LeDeeper, LeMela Plus, LeTranquility, LePatches, birch, celery seed, cajeput, opoponax, peppermint, pine needle, rosemary, sage	apply (usually diluted) on location; diffuse; particularly effective when used in a bath
Asthma	LeBreezey, LeAspire, LeStefanie, LeMariah, LeEverlasting, peppermint, cedarwood, eucalyptus, thyme, hyssop, lavender (for babies), myrtle, peppermint	apply over lungs (front & back) & throat; diffuse. Put on cotton ball or cloth, inhale. (Many other singles are listed as helpful) place on pad of foot (not inhaled during attack)
Athlete's feet	LeSunburst, LeSpiceC, LeMela Plus, LeNo-More, LeDeliverance, cypress, tea tree, thyme, manuka, myrrh, patchouli	apply to feet (may want to dilute with distilled water)
Auto Immune disorders	LeLife Force, LeRevitalize, LeGrateful Heart, cistus, patchouli	dilute and apply to the chest area and to the bottoms of the feet; diffuse
Babies (in general)	LeBaby Me, dill (gentle digestive), chamomile Roman (for sleep) lavender (calming, too much is stimulating)	for babies, always dilute essential oils well
Back Pain & Trouble	LeMillenia, LeDeeper, LePaine, LeTenda Care, LeWarm Down, LePatches, helichrysum	dilute and massage along the spine
Belching, Bloating	LeInside-Out LeEZ-Traveler LeRevitalize	dilute and massage over stomach and abdomen
Bladder Bed-wetting Infection (Cystitis)	LeEndo Relief, LeDreams, LeMeditation, LeBeloved, cypress, cedarwood, celery seed	apply over kidneys; best as a hot compress rub on abdomen at bedtime
Bleeding (stops)	LeVitality, LeKadence, yarrow, cistus, helichrysum, rose, myrrh, cayenne pepper	apply, undiluted, to the area
Blisters	lavender or lavender/chamomile	apply 1 drop, blot gently with a clean cloth
Blood Pressure	LeAngel, LeBenediction, LeVitality, LeEZ-Traveler, LeFaith, LeKadence, marjoram, lavender, rosemary, peppermint (usually low pressure), ylang ylang, hyssop, lime, litsea cubeba, marjoram	apply over the heart; diffuse; cotton ball in vents; in a relaxing bath
Bone Spurs	LeAspire, LePaine, LeDeeper birch/wintergreen	if possible, use arnica oil as a carrier and apply these oils topically. Arnica deals with the bruising, which is often the source of most of the pain. It takes a little time, but this has been known to dissolve spurs

Bronchitis	LeBountiful, LeLife Force, LeDeeper, LeBreezey, LeStefanie. LeAspire, LeDeliverance, LeSpiceC, LeMariah, thyme, eucalyptus, peppermint, melissa, myrtle, niaouli, oregano, rosemary	dilute the oils mentioned in a carrier and apply to the chest; diffuse; place on the pillow
Bruises	LePaine, LeMela Plus LeTenda Care, LeMillenia, LeDeliverance, LeSpiceC, LePatches, marjoram	best if applied in a base such as arnica oil
Burns	LeVallee, lavender, helichrysum. carrot seed, lavender, niaouli, rose geranium	nothing beats lavender applied to a burn, except the healing salve sold by Butterfly Express, llc. with extra helichrysum and lavender added; LeVallee is for rebuilding of skin and muscle tissue after the wounds have closed
Bursitis	LeWarm Down, LeDeeper LePaine, LeMillenia LeTenda Care, LePatches	dilute and apply to the shoulder area
Calcium absorption	LeEternity, LeEZ-Traveler, LeKadence, LeWarm Down, calamus	inhale; diffuse; dilute for full body massage; use in bath; wear on body as perfume or cologne
Callouses	LeMela Plus, LeVallee, oregano, carrot seed, chamomile Roman	dilute with carrier oil and apply frequently to the callused area
Candida	LeCandila, LeInside-Out, LeEndo Relief, LeMela Plus, anthopogon, bergamot, manuka, patchouli	dilute with massage oil; apply on stomach area, feet or over abdomen; can also be diluted (well) and used as a douche
Canker/Cold Sores	LeDeliverance, LeSpiceC, LeRefresh-Mint, LeDiscernment, LeSimplicity, hyssop, laurel, chamomile—all types, myrrh, tea tree, opoponax, oregano, manuka	rinse mouth with water in which a drop of oil has been added
Capillaries	LeCypernium, LeVitality, LeMillenia, LeWarm Down, LeSoliltude, LeVisibility, lavender, chamomile German, lemongrass	dilute with carrier oil and apply topically to the area; use as a compress or in a bath
Cardiovascular Health	LeVitality, LeEternity, LeKadence	dilute and apply to chest; inhale; diffuse
Cartilage	sandalwood (regenerates), fir siberica (relieves pain)	dilute and apply to the area
Cavities (teeth)	LeDeliverance, LeMillenia, LeSpiceC, spearmint	use to brush teeth or add a drop to toothpaste on your toothbrush

Cellulite	LeWeightless, LeSego Lily, spearmint, grapefruit, juniper, lemongrass, lemon, orange bitter, rosemary	dilute and apply topically; 2 or 3 drops added to the tub
Chakras	see Chapter 11 page 18	
Charley Horse	LePatches, LeWarm Down, LeTenda Care	dilute and apply to the area
Cholesterol	LeRevitalize, helichrysum, ginger	dilute and apply to the bottoms of the feet
Chronic Fatigue	LeEternity, LeEverlasting, LeInner Peace, LeRevitalize, LeIQ, LeDeliverance (to kill Epstein Barre virus)	These oils should be diluted and applied to the chest and the feet. LeEternity and LeEverlasting are for the absorption of nutrients: LeRevitalize and LeIQ will help with energy; LeInner Peace for emotional strength and balance. All of the oils will be of benefit if diffused
Circulation	LeVitality, LeEnergy, LePaine, LeSunburst, LeTranquility, LeDeeper, LeHeart Song, LePatches LeVisibility, LeVitality, bay, copaiba balsam, geranium, lemongrass, pine needle	diffuse; use in a bath; massage; compress over specific area
Cleaner, household	LeSunburst orange, sweet	diluted makes a great disinfectant; can be applied undiluted to most surfaces (check on a small area first); works amazingly well on grease
Colds	LeJourney, LeBreezey, LeAspire, LeDeliverance, LeEndo Relief, LeSpiceC, LeMariah, LeStefanie, LeSimplicity, basil, melissa, oregano	diffuse; place on a tissue and sniff; use in a tub; place on forehead, temples, back of neck, and chest. One recommendation: LeAspire on the back, LeBreezey on the chest, with LeDeliverance on the feet, all diluted well, of course
Colic	LeInside Out, chamomile German, chamomile Roman, bergamot, cardamom, carrot seed, fennel, coriander, dill, ginger, marjoram, melissa, orange sweet, peppermint, black pepper, spearmint	dilute and apply to abdominal area
Colon	LeInside-Out, LeLetting Go, peppermint	dilute LeInside Out or peppermint and apply to abdomen or use then as a compress; LeLetting Go can also be diffused or sniffed
Complexion	jasmine, orange sweet for general use; tangerine for dull complexion; bergamot, orange sweet for oily skin	dilute with a very light carrier oil or with distilled water and apply to the face, neck, and abdominal area
Concentration	LeWake-Up, LeCrystal Clear, LeIQ, LeFocus, LeKadence, rosemary, frankincense, cardamom, niaouli	inhale: diffuse; apply to wrists or forehead

Concussion	LeTurmoil, cypress	apply to the back of the neck and to the feet on the underside of the big toe (the narrow, bony part, not the fleshy pad)
Confusion	LeEverlasting, LeIQ, LeCrystal Clear, LeInner Peace, LeInsight, LeUnity, LeWisdom, LeMillenia, cypress, frankincense, peppermint, rose, marjoram, rosewood, ylang ylang	Often the aroma, diffused or inhaled, is all that is needed; can also be applied to the bottoms of the feet
Constipation	LeInside Out, carrot seed, turmeric, mandarin, patchouli	dilute and massage over the abdomen
Cradle Cap	LeDelicate	dilute and massage into the baby's scalp with a very soft brush, leaving it on for a few minutes, then gently shampoo—repeat as often as necessary
Crohn's Disease	LeInside Out, LeLife Force, basil	dilute and apply to the abdominal area
Cuts, Bleeding	LeMela Plus, yarrow, neroli, helichrysum	dilute LeMela Plus in water; it is very strong; apply yarrow undiluted then bind the wound, brings edges of cut together; helichrysum promotes tissue regeneration
Cuts, infected	LeDeliverance, LeMela Plus, lavender, niaouli	apply diluted, usually with water
Cystitis bladder infection	basil, cajeput, cedarwood, eucalyptus, fennel, pine, frankincense, hyssop, juniper, chamomile German, sage, sandalwood, rosewood, thyme	dilute and use for an abdominal massage or add a drop or two of the oil of your choice to a bath
Cysts	LeBeloved, LeWoman Wise, LeBalance	dilute and apply frequently to the abdominal area and to the insides of the ankles
Dandruff	LeDandy, laurel, lavender, sage	add a few drops to your normal shampoo
Debility	LeTurmoil, LeRevitalize, LeVitality, LeKadence, cardamom, cumin (nerves), nutmeg, sage, lavender, patchouli	dilute and apply to the chest or to the bottoms of the feet
Dental Infection	LeDeliverance, LeSpiceC, LeRefreshmint, LeTenda Care, spearmint, myrrh, sage	apply to jaw and gums, diluted; place 2 drops in water and swish around the mouth
Deodorant	LeBenediction, LeWarm Down, leDreams, LeEndo Relief, LeUnity, LeHeart Song, LeTranquility, LeLetting Go	dilute with carrier oil and apply to the underarms

Depression	LeBeloved, LeBelieve, LeHeart Song, LeMy-graine, LeTranquility, LeAcknowledge, LeBaby Me, LeUnity, LeMeditation, LeTurmoil, LeLetting Go, LeSego Lilly, LeGrateful Heart, basil, bergamot, ylang ylang, rose, geranium, lavender, chamomile Roman, lemon, jasmine, neroli, allspice, benzoin, howood, orange bitter, rose geranium	diffuse, w[illegible] to heart chakra; us[illegible] inhaler wh[illegible]
Detoxification	LeAngel, LeEndo Relief, LeRevitalize, LeLetting Go	diffu[illegible] the f[illegible] to a [illegible] soak o[illegible] aid the detox)
Diabetes	LeDeliverance, LeEndo Relief coriander, dill, eucalyptus	coriander is said to lower glucose/insul[illegible] levels; dill supports the pancreas and controls glucose levels in the blood; LeDeliverance and LeEndo Relief support immune and endocrine system function and eliminates bacteria; the oils may be diffused, applied to the back, chest, feet, or over the pancreas; consider carrying an essential oil inhaler with you
Diaper Rash	LeBaby Me lavender w/yarrow	dilute with carrier oil and massage on the rash with each diaper change (calendula oil or Miracle Salve make excellent carrier oils for any type of rash)
Diarrhea	LeInside Out, cardamom, ginger, carrot seed, mandarin, orange bitter	dilute and apply to the abdomen. There are homeopathic remedies that are effective; contact Butterfly Express, llc
Digestion	LeInside-Out, LeBalance, LeRevitalize, LeEZ-Traveler, peppermint, basil, carrot seed, celery seed, caraway, litsea cubeba	dilute and apply to stomach and colon area; apply along spine or on the bottoms of the feet
Dish Washing	LeSunburst	add a few drops to dishwasher or dish water
Disinfect/ Deodorize	LePurify, LeSunburst copaiba balsam, cedarwood	in vacuum cleaner; diffuse; add to water and mist; use diluted or as a cleaning solution
Diuretic	LeBalance, LeMillenia	dilute with carrier oil and apply to the abdomen
Dizziness	LeEZ-Traveler, LeKadence, melissa, melissa blend	massage diluted oil behind the ear on the hard, bony area (temporal bone)
Eating Disorders	LePurify, LeWeightless, grapefruit, juniper	the aroma seems to be the key, so diffuse or wear on wrists to be accessible to the olfactory bulb

Earache	LeMela Plus, LeLife Force, LeMillenia, LeEndo Relief, basil *garlic*	dilute 1 drop in carrier oil and put in ear and then massage behind the ear. LeMela Plus, LeEndo Relief or LeLife Force for infection and LeMillenia for inflammation or any disturbance of structure in the ear canal or inner ear. BBL, a tincture sold at Butterfly Express, LLC, will help with pain and inflammation—a must have! *Garlic* ***must*** *be diluted very well!!! 1 drop of garlic oil is enough for at least 5 ml of carrier oil. You can dip a toothpick in 1 drop of oil and then stir the toothpick into a few drops of carrier. This mixture can then be put in the ear.* ***Garlic essential oil is <u>much</u> different than the garlic capsules you can purchase in health food stores. It is strong enough to cause serious burns undiluted.***
Eczema	LeBaby Me, LeSego Lily, LeSolitude, carrot seed, juniper, lavender, myrrh, patchouli	dilute with distilled or spring water and apply to the affected areas
Emotional Imbalances	LeFaith, LeAngel, LeBeloved, LeTrust, LeHeart Song, LeUnity, LeInsight, LeTurmoil, LeAcknowledge, LeMeditation, LeTranquility, LeTomorrow, LeMagi, LeBelieve, LeGrateful Heart, LeSanctuary, LeWisdom, lavender, lemon, rose, cedarwood, orange sweet, mandarin, sandalwood	diffuse; dilute and apply over heart, on the crown of the head, on the wrists, behind the ears; wear as a perfume; use in the tub; carry an essential oil inhaler
Endocrine Balance	LeEndo Relief, LeBalance, LeWoman Wise	diffuse; use as aromatherapy; apply to lymph areas of the body (essential oils can act as hormones or stimulate the body to produce the needed hormones)
Energy, protection	LeBenediction, LeHeart Song, LeAngel,	protection: apply to shoulders and wrists
Energy, improvement of	LeEnergy, LeRevitalize, LeBountiful, LeWake-Up	dilute and apply to bottoms of feet
Environmental Toxins	LeLife Force	dilute and apply to the feet or along the spine
Expectorant	LeDeliverance, LeSpiceC, ravensara, benzoin	dilute and apply to throat and chest areas
Eyes	LeMillenia, cypress, frankincense, lemongrass, carrot seed	dilute and apply along the back of the neck and sides of the temples; may also be helpful inhaled

Fainting (see shock)	LeIQ, LeCrystal Clear, LeKadence LeTurmoil, black pepper, peppermint, rosemary, lavender	hold one of the listed oils under the nose; dilute and apply to the bottoms of the feet
Fatigue	LeRevitalize, LeWisdom, LeVitality, LeWake-Up LeWarm Down, LeKadence peppermint, rose	LeVitality: diffuse or smell frequently. Vitality and rose: high frequency oils which help with 'energy' fatigue. Warm Down: 1 or 2 drops in bath; dilute for massage, especially for tired muscles. Peppermint: aroma is very stimulating; dilute for massage
Fever	LeLife Force, LeTherma-Care lavender (babies), eucalyptus, yarrow yellow	Life Force: dilute and apply to spine. Lavender and LeTherma-Care: dilute, apply to back of neck and the feet
Fibromyalgia	LeDeeper, LeLife Force, LePaine, LePatches, birch, wintergreen	Should be diluted and applied to the body; add 1 or 2 drops in a tub and soak
Flatulence	LeInside Out, angelica, aniseseed, bergamot, cardamom, coriander, cumin, fennel, ginger, carrot seed, lavender, nutmeg, benzoin, peppermint, chamomile Roman, rosemary, tarragon, hyssop, orange bitter	dilute and apply to the abdomen
Flu	LeDeliverance, LeEndo Relief, LeMariah, LeStefanie, LeBreezey, LeAspire, LeRevitalize, LeLife Force, LeInside Out, LeJourney LeEZ-Traveler, LeTherma-Care, melissa	Apply to thymus area, chest, back, feet and wherever the flu has settled creating aches and pains. You should also apply LeInside-Out, diluted, to the abdomen.
Food poisoning	LeInside Out (homeopathic Arsenicum album)	dilute and apply to the abdominal area; It would be very helpful to use the homeopathic, Arsenicum Album, in addition to the essential oil.
Gallbladder Gallstones	LeTrust, LeRevitalize, LeLetting Go, LeVision, grapefruit, rose geranium, lemon, lime	apply the listed oils as a compress over the gallbladder area; apply on the feet
Gas	LeInside Out, angelica, aniseseed, bergamot, cardamom, coriander, cumin, fennel, ginger, lavender, nutmeg, benzoin, carrot seed, hyssop, peppermint, chamomile Roman, rosemary, tarragon	dilute and apply to the abdomen

Gingivitis/Gums	LeTrust, LeUnity, LeMela Plus, LeDeliverance, LeSpiceC, LeRefresh-Mint, LeTenda Care, spearmint	apply on throat and gums; dilute in water and swish around the mouth
Gout	LeMeditation, LeDeeper, LePaine, LeRevitalize, LeVitality, lemon, anthopogon, birch, celery seed, hyssop	dilute and apply to the back; use a drop or two in water to soak the feet; add a drop or two to the tub.
Gratitude	LeGrateful Heart	diffuse, wear as perfume; enjoy in the tub; dilute as a massage oil
Grief	LeSego Lily, LeHeart Song, LeFaith, LeWhispering Hope, orange sweet	diffuse, especially at bedtime, wear as a perfume; enjoy in the tub; diluted as a massage oil; apply to wrists
Hair, color	chamomile Roman, for blonde hair Rosemary for brunettes	2 or 3 drops added to clear water, shampoo or conditioner and massaged into hair 1 or 2 times a week
Hair, health Hair, loss	LeDelicate, LeEternity, LeDandy, lavender, rosemary	2 or 3 drops added to clear water, shampoo or conditioner and massaged into the scalp 1 or 2 times a week. Can be added to an almond oil/jojoba oil carrier, massaged into the scalp and then a warm towel placed around the head, just like a salon hot oil treatment, only much better
Headaches	LeAngel, LeVitality, LePatches, LeWarm Down, LeCrystal Clear LeBaby Me, LeWoman Wise, LeDeeper, LeBalance, LeMy-graine, LeMillenia, LeBeloved, LeEZ-Traveler, LeBenediction, calamus, marjoram, rosemary, peppermint, rosewood, bay	there are as many different kinds of headaches as there are people (most people even have more than one kind of headache). Massage an oil from the list onto the arteries in the neck until you find what works for you; using diffused is also effective; consider carrying an essential oil inhaler
Heart muscle	LeKadence, LeVitality, LeMariah	dilute and apply to the chest
Heart, palpitations	LeVitality, LeBelieve, LeBeloved, LeBenediction, LeKadence, marjoram, neroli, orange sweet, petitgrain	apply, diluted, to chest; aroma; place on temples
Heartburn	LeInside Out. LeRevitalize, LeBaby Me, peppermint	LeInside Out and peppermint: apply diluted over stomach and colon; Baby Me should be diluted and applied on chest over the thymus
Hematoma	LeDeeper, LeMillenia, cypress, helichrysum, lemongrass	dilute and apply to the affected areas
Hemorrhoids	LeCypernium, LeVitality, LeVisibility, geranium	dilute well in carrier oil or KY Jelly, apply (with a Q-tip, if necessary) to affected areas
Hernia	LeWith-In, LeMillenia	dilute and apply to the area
Herpes virus	LeSimplicity, melissa	dilute and apply along the jawline, along the spine and on the feet

Hives/ Allergic Rashes	LeBaby Me, LeSego Lily, LeMela Plus, peppermint, chamomile German, yarrow	dilute in carrier oil, massage over area 4 drops in 1/4 cup of baking soda in the bath
Hormone Balance	LeBalance, LeAcknowledge, LeVitality, LeCrystal Clear, LeWoman Wise, LeEndo Relief, LeDeeper, jasmine, patchouli melissa (sterility in women), petitgrain	apply to thymus area; inside of ankles (around the bone); lower back; thyroid area; along the spine; the clavicle area; diffuse
Hot Flashes	LeEndo Relief, LeBalance, yarrow green	apply these oils, diluted, around the bone on the inside of the ankles
Hyperactivity	LeSunburst, LeTranquility, LeTurmoil, LeMillenia	apply to the feet; diffuse; wear anywhere on the body
Hypoglycemia	LeBaby Me, LeGrateful Heart, LeEndo Relief, LeWake Up, LeDeliverance, coriander, dill, eucalyptus	apply over pancreas area on body or feet; diffuse
Immune Stimu-lant	LeDeliverance, LeBountiful, LeJourney, LeBreezey, LeSpiceC LeRevitalize, LeLife Force, hinoki, ledum, orange sweet, oregano	massage any one of the listed oils on feet and body; diffuse; use in the bath
Insect Bites/ Stings	LeMela Plus, LePurify, tea tree, basil, lavender, manuka, niaouli	apply 1 drop, undiluted, to the area
Insect Repellent	LeAway, LePurify, citronella, peppermint, opoponax	dilute in water or Miracle II Neutralizer and apply, either by misting or rubbing on. Avoid contact with the eyes
Insomnia	LeBelieve, LeGood-Nite, LeTranquility, LeSunburst, LeVision, LeSolitude, LeDreams, basil, myrtle	LeTranquility is for the 'chattering mind' type of insomnia and is excellent diffused or worn; apply any of these oils to big toes, bottom of feet, around navel and on the back of the neck; diffusing or placing on the pillow is easier and often just as effective
Irritable Bowel Syndrome	LeInside Out, LeRevitalize, aniseseed, peppermint	dilute and apply to the abdominal area
Jaundice	LeRevitalize, rose geranium, geranium	dilute and apply, or use in a compress, over the liver
Jet Lag	LeIQ, LeCrystal Clear, LeEnergy, LeWisdom, LeMillenia, grapefruit	Apply to temple, thymus area of the chest and to the feet. Always eat lightly when travelling and drink plenty of water.
Kidneys	LeAcknowledge, LeVitality (congestion) LeEndo Relief, LeRevitalize, LeLetting Go, LeMeditation birch (stones), grapefruit, bergamot, ledum, ravensara	apply as a compress over the kidneys; be sure to drink plenty of distilled water

Laundry	LeSunburst, anything citrus or the evergreens, any smell you especially like	add a few drops to the water in the washer or place a few drops on the dryer sheet that you ordinarily use. Essential oils destroy bacteria and provide a fresh clean smell
Laxative	hyssop, jasmine, tangerine	Apply to the abdomen; inhale
Lice	LeDeliverance, LeMela Plus, tea tree	dilute with non-chlorinated water, making the mixture as strong as can be tolerated, and apply frequently to scalp and hair; use to wash combs, bedding, etc.
Ligaments, torn	LeWarm Down, LePaine, LeTenda Care, LePatches, birch, wintergreen, peppermint, fir siberica, lemongrass	dilute and apply to the affected areas; consider layering one oil on top of another
Liver Cleanse & Support	LeRevitalize, LeLetting Go LeEZ-Traveler, LeAngel, helichrysum, carrot seed, angelica, celery seed, grapefruit, lemon, lime, rosemary	dilute and apply to liver area and along the spine; add to redmond clay and water, soak the feet
Lupus (an auto-immune disorder)	LeInside Out, LeLife Force, LeMillenia, LeWisdom, LeDeliverance	Lupus is an auto-immune disorder—please see that section
Lymphatic Congestion	LeDeeper, LeDeliverance, LeEndo Relief, LeVitality, LeSunburst, LeRevitalize, LeDeliverance, birch, lemon, orange sweet, ravensara	diffuse; dilute for massage or apply to lymph drainage areas of the body; excellent in the bath
Massage	LeBaby Me, LeHeart Song, LeExpressions, LeSego Lily, LeWeightless, LeTenda Care, LeWhispering Hope, LeWarm Down, eucalyptus, peppermint	dilute with your favorite carrier oil; massage is good for tired muscles and circulation but since essential oils absorb readily and rapidly into the skin on contact, there is really no need to work them in
Memorization	LeCrystal Clear, LeIQ, LeWake-Up, LeFocus	inhale; apply to wrists and forehead
Menopausal Symptoms	LeBalance, LeEndo Relief	dilute and apply to chest, abdomen, and feet
Menstrual Symptoms	LeWoman Wise, LeBeloved, LeFaith, LeBaby Me, marjoram	apply over abdomen & back; in a bath; particularly effective used with a BBL (B&B) tincture, an old Dr. Christopher formula
Mental Confusion	LeInsight, LeSunburst, LeRevitalize, LeFocus, LeIQ, LeWake-Up, LeWeightless, basil	inhale; diffuse; apply to wrists, forehead and back of the neck
Mental Alertness	LeEnergy, LeFocus, LeRevitalize, LeWake-Up, LeIQ, LeWeightless basil, cardamom, howood, peppermint	inhale; diffuse; apply to wrists, forehead and back of the neck

Metabolism	LeEndo Relief, LeWeightless, LeEZ-Traveler, oregano, pine needle	dilute and apply to throat and thymus area; diffuse; inhale; add to bath
Migraine	LeMy-graine, LeBeloved, LeBelieve, LeEZ Traveler LeWarm Down, LePaine, LeTranquility, LeMillenia, LeDeeper, LeLetting Go LeDeliverance, LeAngel, LeBalance, birch, grapefruit, peppermint, rosemary	apply to the back of neck (a few drops in a bowl of water, then soak a washcloth, wring out and place at back of neck); apply to underside of big toe just below the fleshy part; diffuse; to smell, carry a cotton ball, soaked with LeMy-graine, in purse or pocket; try LeDeliverance for headaches
Mold/Mildew	LeDeliverance, LeSunburst, LePurify, LeNo-More, manuka	place a few drops in a squirt bottle, spray into the air or directly onto walls, window-sills, any place mold grows in your house
Mononucleosis	LeEndo Relief, LeRevitalize, LeMillenia, LeDeliverance, clary sage	use in tub; dilute and apply to bottoms of feet; soak feet; carry an essential oil inhaler
Morning Sickness	LeInside-Out, LeEZ-Traveler orange sweet, grapefruit	place a drop or two of oil behind ears; inhale
Motion Sickness	LeEZ Traveler LeInside Out, LeMy-graine peppermint	apply to feet, temples, and wrists; Place on palms of hands, hold to nose and breathe deeply
Mouthwash	LeRefreshmint, LeDeliverance, LeSpiceC, LeTrust, wintergreen, spearmint	dilute and rinse the mouth for a few seconds
Muscle Relaxant	LePaine, LeTenda Care, LeBreezey LeWarm Down, LePatches, cajeput, peppermint, opoponax	dilute with carrier oil and massage the affected areas
Muscle Spasms	LePaine, LeTenda Care, LeBreezey LeWarm Down, LePatches, marjoram, myrrh, niaouli, peppermint	dilute with carrier oil and massage the affected areas
Multiple Sclerosis	LeCrystal Clear, LeInner Peace, LeMagi, LeMeditation, LeWarm Down, frankincense, peppermint, sandalwood	dilute and apply to the bottoms of the feet, the spine, and/or the chest; add 1 or 2 drops to the bath; diffuse; inhale
Nausea and Vomiting	v LeEZ-Traveler, LeMy-graine, LeInside Out, orange sweet, basil, cardamom, lavender, peppermint	apply over stomach and colon; apply behind ears; place on cotton ball (in purse, etc) and sniff frequently
Nerve Pain	LeDeeper, LePaine, birch	dilute and apply to the affected areas

Nervous system	LeTranquility, LeIQ, LeBelieve, LeInside-Out, LeExpressions, LeDreams, LeTrust, LeInner Peace, LeUnity, LeFaith, LeHeart Song, LeAssurance, LeLetting Go, LeSanctuary, LeTurmoil, cedarwood, frankincense, sage, geranium, fir balsam, jasmine, lavender, marjoram, palmarosa, petitgrain chamomile Roman, sandalwood, spruce, valerian, vetiver, howood, orange sweet	dilute and apply to the chest, the back of the neck, or on the feet; diffuse
Neuropathy	LeDeeper, LePaine, birch	dilute and apply to the affected areas
Nightmares	LeDreams, LeBelieve, LeGood-Nite	diffuse; place a drop or two on the pillow
Nursing	caraway, fennel	dilute and apply to the breasts and the feet
OCD Obsessive Compulsive Disorder	LeAcknowledge, LeEverlasting, LeFaith, LeTrust, LeSanctuary, LeMillenia, LeTurmoil, LeCrystal Clear	diffuse; inhale; place a drop on the pillow at night; carry at all times in an inhaler; dilute and apply to the chest and the bottoms of the feet
Odors, purifying	LePurify, LeSunburst, LeInsight, pine, lime	diffuse; dilute in water and spritz into the air using a plant mister
Osteoporosis	LeWarm Down, LeBelieve, LeDeeper, LePaine, LeKadence LeEternity,LeTranquility	dilute for massage; use in a bath; supplement Tri Boron or other quality calcium; use wild yam cream or other natural progesterone
Overwhelmed	LeAcknowledge, LeBeloved, LeWhispering Hope, LeConnection, LeMillenia	diffuse; wear as perfume; use in a bath; use on acupressure points on the ears
Pancreas	LeEndo Relief	Dilute and apply to the chest, abdomen, and feet
Panic Attacks	LeTranquility, LeHeart Song, LeBeloved, neroli	inhale; diffuse; wear as perfume; place over thymus or heart chakra
Parasites	LeInside Out, LeRevitalize, bergamot, turmeric, bergamot	dilute and apply over abdominal area
Pineal & Pituitary	LeInner Peace, LeEZ-Traveler, LeEndo Relief	dilute and apply to back of neck
Pleurisy	LeVitality, LeTrust, LeBreezey, LeHeart Song, LeAspire, LeMariah, cypress, thyme	apply diluted over the lungs—front & back; diffuse or sniff deeply
PMS	LeBalance, LeWoman Wise, LeDeeper	Dilute and apply to the abdomen and the small of the back
Pneumonia	LeBreezey, LeAspire, LeMariah, cajeput, hyssop, oregano	inhale; place on back and chest
Prostate	LeBalance, LeEndo Relief, LeWoman Wise, basil, myrtle, peppermint	dilute and massage inside of ankle around the bone

Protection, Energy & Psychic	LeBenediction, LeUnity, LeSanctuary, LeHeart Song, LeMillenia, clove, cypress, fennel, fir, frankincense	Wear on the body, particularly over the heart Chakra, but also on wrists, etc. if massaging or body working; diffuse; inhale
Purify Air	LePurify, LeDeliverance	diffuse; add to water and mist into the air
Purify Water	LeSunburst, lime, grapefruit	add 1 drop per gallon
Rashes	LeBaby Me. carrot seed, lavender, myrrh, patchouli, rosewood, howood	depending on the type of rash, dilute with either distilled water or a carrier oil
Relationships	LeBeloved, LeExpressions, LeMoonlight, jasmine	diffuse; wear as perfume; use in the bath; apply to wrists or temples
Respiratory Ailments	LeBreezey, LeAspire, LeBountiful, LeSanctuary, LeHoliday Spirit, marjoram, orange sweet, oregano, ravensara	inhale; diffuse; dilute and apply to lung area on both the back and the chest
Restless Leg Syndrome	LeSolitude, LeVisibility	support the thyroid and adrenal glands using LeEndo Relief and herbal supplements to increase the body's ability to absorb calcium; increase your intake of good quality calcium
Ringworm	LeNo-More, LeDeliverance, LeSpiceC, LePurify, geranium, manuka, tea tree, myrrh, thyme, patchouli	Ringworm is a fungal infection; dilute the oils with distilled or purified water and apply with a cotton ball or soft sponge—a vegetable protein based carrier oil may give the fungus something to feed on, making the situation worse
Sanitize	LeSunburst, LeDeliverance	dilute with water and use everywhere
Scarring	LeBaby Me, LeVallee, geranium helichrysum, lavender, rose, hyssop, jasmine, palmarosa, patchouli, rosewood	dilute and apply often and generously
Sciatica	LePaine, LeVitality, LeBaby Me, LeMy-graine, LeDeeper, LeMillenia, LeTenda Care, celery seed	dilute one of the listed oils and massage onto the lower back, across the hips and down the side and back of the leg; can be used in the bath or as a compress
Self-Expression	LeMillenia, LeAcknowledge, LeHeart Song	diffuse; use in the bath; wear as perfume
Shingles	LeDeeper, LeDeliverance, ravensara, geranium	LeDeeper and ravensara: dilute and use for pain relief and tissue regeneration; use LeDeliverance to fight the virus
Shock, Trauma	LeIQ, LeBelieve, LeCrystal Clear, LeTurmoil, LeLife Force, LeVitallity, LeRevitalize, basil, lavender, black pepper, peppermint, rosemary, calamus, melissa (heart), neroli	hold one of the listed oils under the nose like smelling salts; dilute and apply to the bottoms of the feet

Sinus	LeBreezey, LeAspire, LeDeliverance, bay, cajeput, myrrh, niaouli, peppermint	inhale; diffuse; dilute and apply to sinus areas on the face or on the feet
Skin Health	LeSego Lily, LeBaby Me, LeVallee, LeReconciliation, rosewood, grapefruit, caraway, carrot seed, jasmine, laurel, lemongrass, lime, litsea cubeba, manuka, neroli, orange sweet, rose, sage palmarosa (oily and dry)	dilute in distilled or clear spring water and sponge on skin with clean cotton balls (do not use carrier oils as they will feed any bacteria that may be contributing factors)
Skin and Tissue Regeneration	LeReconciliation, LeVallee, helichrysum, patchouli, lavender, geranium, rosemary	dilute and apply to the area
Skunk Spray odor (on animals)	LePurify	Dump one or two packages of liquid douche directly on the animal where it was sprayed. Add a few drops of LePurify and massage in thoroughly. When dry, shampoo. LePurify (quite a lot of it) added to water to soak fabric that has been sprayed) removes much of the odor.
Sleep Apnea	LeIQ, LeCrystal Clear, LeBreezey, LeAspire, LeGood Nite, LeMillenia	dilute and apply to the sinus areas or to the feet
Slimming and Toning	LePatches, LeSego Lily, basil, grapefruit, lavender, lemongrass, orange, rosemary, sage, thyme	Dilute and apply. I like to apply patches to the places that I am concentrating on losing fat or cellulite. Not miraculous, but helpful
Smoking see addictions		
Snoring	LeBreezey, LeGood-Nite, LeAspire, LeMillenia (use in conjunction with one of the other listed oils)	place a drop or two under the nose at bed-time or diffuse in the bedroom; best results occur when these oils are used alternately, changing every few nights
Sore Throat	LeDeliverance, LeSpiceC, LeEndo Relief, LeBreezey LeAspire	dilute and apply to the throat and the sides of the neck, including the area behind and under the ear
Sprains, Sports injuries	LeWarm Down, LePaine, LePatches, LeTenda Care, LeDeeper, LeMillenia (if any structure is out of place), black pepper, marjoram, sage	dilute in carrier oil and apply to the affected area. The carrier oil should contain arnica if there is any swelling
Spider Bites	LeMela Plus, LePurify, LeMillenia, tea tree	apply a drop, undiluted, to the area

Stains	lemon (pure, uncut with carrier)	place a little on the stain, rub it in and then launder
Stamina	LeEZ Traveler LeRevitalize, LeVitality, LeKadence	inhale; diffuse; dilute & apply to Thymus area; use 1 - 2 drops in the bath (no more)
Strep Throat	LeDeliverance, LeSpiceC, melissa	dilute and apply to the throat
Stress	LeBelieve, LeBenediction, LeFaith, LeHeart Song, LeInner Peace, LeLetting Go, LeMeditation, LeSanctuary, LeSego Lily, LeTomorrow, LeTranquility, LeUnity, LeWeightless, LeWisdom,LeWhispering Hope, sandalwood, allspice, benzoin	inhale; diffuse; wear as perfume; place over the thymus or heart chakra areas; use in a bath or shower
Stretch Marks	LeBaby Me, LeSego Lily, jasmine, myrrh, rosewood	add to carrier oil (or open a Vitamin E capsule, also very effective) and apply all over abdomen and hip area
Stroke	LeVitality	breathe deeply; apply to neck and forehead.
Structural Alignment	LeMillenia, LeWarm Down	apply to the area or to the feet (to save time and effort—and also the alignment seems to remain in place longer)
Suicidal depression	LeHeart Song, LeWhispering Hope, LeAcknowledge, LeAngel, LeLetting Go	diffuse; inhale; wear as a perfume or cologne
Sunburn	see 'burns'	
Sunscreen	helichrysum	dilute with carrier (coconut oil is especially nice) and apply to the skin
Tendons, damaged	***LePatches,*** LeDeeper, LePaine, LeWarm Down, LeTenda Care, birch	dilute and apply regularly to the area until it is completely healed
Thrush	see 'candida'	
Thyroid	LeEndo Relief (Hyper- or Hypo-types), ledum, myrtle, palmarosa	hyper—apply under big toes hypo—apply on top of big toes
Ticks	LePurify or thyme & lavender	1 or 2 drops of LePurify or thyme backs the tick out; then 1 drop of lavender every 5 minutes to prevent infection and swelling
Ticks, repel	rose geranium and palmarosa	mix 2 Tablespoons of vegetable oil with 15 drops of rose geranium and 10 drops palmarosa; add 1 teaspoon of above mixture to 1 cup of water and mist to repel ticks

TMJ	LeMillenia, LeWarm Down, LeTenda Care, LeDeeper, LeMagi, LeMeditation	LeMillenia diluted and applied along the jaw line will help the jaw to realign; LeWarm Down, LeTenda Care, LeDeeper will reduce the pain and inflammation; LeMagi, LeMeditation are for the emotional aspects of the tension that is being held in the jaw
Toe Nail Fungus	LeDeliverance, LeMela Plus, LeSpiceC, LeNo-More	add a few drops to water and soak feet; apply locally to the area (diluting with water rather than a carrier oil is recommended)
Toothache	LePurify, clove, spearmint chamomile Roman	apply on the gums at the location of pain/ problem and along the jawbone
Toxemia	LeVitality, cypress	dilute for massage; diffuse; inhale deeply
Trauma	LeTurmoil, LeLife Force, angelica, peppermint	dilute and apply to the chest and the feet; diffuse; place anywhere on the body
Varicose veins	LeVitality, LeSunburst LeVisibility, copaiba balsam, cypress, lemongrass	dilute for massage or application to area of concern; use in a bath
Vertigo	LeEZ-Traveler, LeInside Out, LeKadence, LeMillenia, calamus, melissa, melissa blend, tangerine	diffused; inhaled; carry with you in an inhaler, place on the wrists or temples
Viral Infection	LeDeliverance, LeDiscernment, LeSpiceC, LeEndo Relief, LeJourney, LeLife Force, thyme, oregano, melissa	dilute and apply to bottoms of feet and to the chest; carry an essential oil inhaler
Vitality	LeEndo Relief, LeEnergy, LeEverlasting, LeRevitalize, LeVitality, LeKadence, peppermint	dilute and apply to the chest or the feet; diffuse
Vitamin absorption	LeEternity, LeEZ-Traveler, calamus, pine needle	inhale; diffuse; dilute for full body massage; use in bath; wear on body as perfume or cologne
Yeast Infection	see Candida	
Warts	LeMela Plus, LeDeliverance, LePurify w/clove, manuka	apply 1-2 drops to wart several times a day, rubbing in well. Each of these has proven successful
Weight loss	LeWeightless, ledum, aniseseed, neroli, celery seed, lemongrass	dilute and apply to the body or just to the bottoms of the feet; the aroma of LeWeightless is often effective to curb food cravings
Worms	see Parasites	
Wrinkles	LeSego Lily, carrot seed, myrrh, rose geranium, frankincense, rosewood, sandalwood, orange sweet	dilute with Almond oil or carrier oil and apply to areas of concern
Zest (for living)	LeEnergy, LeAssurance, LeExhilaration	diffuse; inhale; wear as perfume

Essential Oil Constituents

Essential oils have very complex structures and several unique characteristics. Individual oils have as many as 800 different chemical constituents in their molecular makeup, all put together in such as way as to be readily available to the human body. Of these 800 components that have been identified, research into the healing properties has been done for only about 200. It is known that the others are necessary to the overall healing effect of the oils, but it is not known exactly how or why.

Even though the effects of each separate element are not completely understood, they can be roughly grouped into families according to their dominant characteristics. Essential oils can be subdivided into two distinct groups: the hydrocarbons and the oxygenated compounds.

Hydrocarbons:

This category is made up almost exclusively by the various members of the terpene family. This family group inhibits the accumulation of toxins and helps discharge existing toxins from the liver, kidney and glandular system.

Sesquiterpene have been mentioned briefly before in this text because of their ability to cross the blood/brain barrier and enter the brain tissues, nourishing and balancing as they go. In addition, sesquiterpenes are antiseptic and anti-inflammatory. Their primary action (other than in the brain) is on the liver and glandular system. Research from Germany and Austria indicate that in the presence of essential oils containing sesquiterpenes, there is increased oxygenation around the pineal and pituitary glands.

Sesquiterpenes carry oxygen molecules throughout the body and into the cells. They have the unique capability of deleting faulty information in cellular memory. Our cells often have incorrect perceptions imbedded in their memories. The rooting out of these mis-perceptions often eliminates the root causes of a disease, especially a chronic one, and allows permanent healing to occur.

More than two thousand sesquiterpenes have been isolated from plants to date and their structures and uses vary widely. Whatever their major function, they all are effective immune stimulants.

Farnesene The major characteristic of farnesenes is antiviral and antibacterial activities. Farnesene tends to inhibit the growth of bacteria instead of killing them. This makes essential oils which contain farnesene very effective in rebalancing in the the digestive tract.

Limonene ***is found in 90% of the citrus oils and is strongly antiviral. There are no antibiotics that are antiviral in action; the antiviral activities of essential oils are invaluable!*** A study of the effects of limonenes against the herpes simplex and other viruses has been well-proven.

Pinene is found in large proportions in all of the conifer oils (pine, fir, spruce, juniper) and is strongly antiseptic.

There are many other members of this grouping, each with its own unique characteristics.

Oxygenated Compounds

Esters are found in nearly all essential oils, not as a main ingredient, but as a crucial part of the structure. Physically, esters are anti-fungal. They have a direct calming effect on the central nervous system and can be powerful antispasmodics. Chamomile Roman contains a number of esters that are not found commonly in other essential oils.

Aldehydes are the main chemical features of the oils of melissa, lemongrass, citronella and a lemony form of eucalyptus. All of these oils are very antiseptic (almost caustic, should be diluted well), also calming to the nervous system, anti-inflammatory.

Ketones major function in aromatherapy is easing or increasing the flow of mucous, which is the body's way of dealing with infections and toxins. Simply inhaling the vapors of oils containing Ketones and Phenols can stimulate the coughing up of mucous and phlegm. In addition, oils containing ketones are cytophylactic, meaning they aid in the generation of new cells. This makes them very important in healing burns and wounds of any sort. Ketones are also known for their cleansing and detoxifying properties.

Alcohols are among the most used molecules in aromatherapy. There is an amazing diversity among the alcohols in healing properties and fragrance, and though they are powerful therapeutic agents, they are mild and non-toxic. The usefulness of this group has continually been pointed out in scientific research.

Phenols are responsible for the fragrance of many essential oils and are, usually, strongly stimulating. They are antiseptic, antibacterial, immuno-stimulating, and have strong antioxidant properties; however, they can also be quite caustic and irritating to the skin. They should be used in appropriately low doses and diluted well. Like Ketones, they increase the flow of mucous.

Oxides include the important family member eucalyptol (or cineol) and is almost a class by itself as far as therapeutic properties because it acts as an expectorant when needed.

All pure essential oils have some antibacterial properties because they increase the production of white blood cells, which helps fight infectious diseases. Research (and my personal experience) has shown that people who consistently use pure essential oils have a higher level of resistance to illnesses, colds, flus and diseases than the average person. Further, such individuals, if they do contract an illness, will recover faster than those who do not use essential oils.

Essential Oils by Plant Family

It can be educational and informative to place essential oils in the plant family from which they are derived to study them. Plants are classified according to the structure of their flowers, but this classification goes beyond the flower itself to include leaf and seed structure, similar rhythm (time of year, etc.) and similar chemical composition.

In homeopathy and other philosophies, the physical nature of plants and their interactions with the environment have been noted to correlate with their medicinal properties. A type of therapeutic activity is attributed to each botanical family and the variations within it, and this approach seems to be quite accurate and very informative. It is amazingly consistent with the more traditional systems of herbal and aromatherapies. I have found that careful observation or study of a plant and its environment can tell me much about its medicinal properties and uses.

Classification of essential oils by botanical families tells more about their therapeutic activity than a simple alphabetical listing. Unless you understand botanical families well, however, a botanical listing can be cumbersome and annoying. I will attempt to give you a condensed version here.

Botanical Families:,

For information on the 'elements' mentioned here, refer to Chapter 11

Burseraceae: This family is considered dry fire in the Eastern tradition. The oils in this family are strengthening to all of the meridians. Myrrh has a particular affinity for the metal (#4) element, while frankincense is particularly effective at grounding our energies to the physical, more earthly (element #5) aspects of life. This family includes the essential oils of elemi, frankincense, myrrh, and opoponax. This botanical family grows in desert and tropical areas and in some of the most extreme climates imaginable. The sun's rays burn hot in these areas and these oils act in a drying manner against congestive ailments such as bronchitis, coughs, and pleurisy. They are especially useful in diseases related to over secretion and inflammation. In the desert, life is harsh and elemental. It takes great strength to exist and flourish there. This strength of purpose and character is reflected in the emotional healing qualities of these oils. They are soothing and comforting to the soul and they encourage us to find our own inner strength. For centuries, myrrh and frankincense have been used in religious ceremonies.

Coniferae: Affinity for the Central and Governing Meridian, referred to as the Air Element (#0). In the Eastern tradition they are considered to bring light and inner warmth. Members of this family are cedarwood, cypress, fir, juniper, pine, spruce and thuja. This botanical family is imposing in its simplicity; everything is structured around the central vertical trunk. Conifers are noted for their longevity, as a coniferous forest shelters and protects its creatures and appears immortal and eternal. An outstanding characteristic of conifers is their ability to maintain their foliage through cold winters. This indicates an inner fire and stability which is indicative of their therapeutic uses. Conifer oils are warming, reviving and give a feeling of protection and safety. Their major influence in the body is on the nervous system and they are best taken in through the lungs. Interestingly, conifer oils are often used for arthritis.

Labiatae: Labiatae are considered plants of heat. Every one of them is warming to the body and the spirit. All members of the labiatae family balance yang energy (see Chapter 9). Each member of this family has an affinity for a particular element/meridian or two. This family includes basil, catnip, clary sage, hyssop, lavender, marjoram, melissa, mints, oregano, patchouli, rosemary, sage, and thyme. All members of the labiatae family have some known healing attributes that are being used around the world by different cultures and people. In addition many labiatae are culinary herbs, which indicates their strong affinity for digestive and metabolic processes as well as respiration and blood formation. There are no bland, gloomy or narcotic oils in this family. These plants adapt well to changes in their environment which is indicative of their immuno-stimulant properties. They are often used for conditions of weakness and for bringing increased vitality to organs and body systems. Essential oils from this plant family should be considered for anemia, digestive problems, respiratory problems, diabetes. They are often employed by healers and those who are overly sensitive to the environment and the energy of others.

Compositae: This well-structured and varied family is considered in Eastern thought to strengthen the spiritual aspects of one's goals and the organization of one's life and mission, and the physical structure of the body. Plants in this family include arnica, blue tansy, all of the chamomiles, davanna, helichrysum, Idaho tansy, tagette, tarragon, yarrow, and wormwood. The compositae constitute the largest botanical family and grow all over the world in profuse abundance. Member of this family grow from seashores to mountain tops, from deserts to swamps. They all seem to have a love of open spaces and crave exposure to light. Like the plants themselves, the therapeutic action of this family shows a great diversity; there seems to be a plant and an essential oil with an affinity for every organ or system of the body. It is almost impossible to categorize this large and varied family except to note that no matter what element or organ a particular oil may have the most affinity for, it is the yin side of that element that will be most benefited. The theme of this family, and the action of the essential oils, is the return of perfect balance and harmony to all aspects of the body and the soul.

Umbelliferae (Apiaceae): Plants of the Air Element (#0)—Central and Governing Meridian. This family includes ajowan, angelica, aniseseed, cilantro, coriander, caraway, carrot seed, celery seed, cumin, dill, fennel, galbanum, and parsley. The plants of this species have large, hollow, airy spaces in their stems, seeds and roots. The essential oils created from members of this family have an affinity for the respiratory system, the intestinal areas of the digestive system, and glandular system. They are considered outstanding tissue regenerators. This is especially true of cumin, fennel, celery and parsley, which are all produced from seeds. Each plant as an herbal remedy and each essential oil derived from plants of this family has a special affinity for a particular body organ or system.

Geraniaceae: The geranium species has been cultivated into many sub-species (rose geranium, tangerine, geranium, lemon geranium, etc.) and can be made to produce a wide variety of chemotypes and fragrances. There are even geranium oils that imitate the burning heat of plants containing thymols. These plants are very different from the sweet-smelling rose geranium oil that is marketed commercially. Geraniums show strong adaptability and the expected immuno-stimulant properties that adaptability indicates. These oils are astringent and diuretic, among other properties, and useful for diabetes, kidney stones, wounds, and burn care. In the emotional realm they are used for depression and stress management. Geraniums have a particular affinity for the heart and triple warmer meridians. These two meridians are the yang portions of element #5 and #6. Essential oils of this family include geranium and rose geranium.

Rutaceae with the genus of Citrus: Essential oils produced from this family include bergamot, clementine, grapefruit, lemon, lime, mandarin, neroli, orange, petitgrain, tangerine, zanthoxylum. Most of the large and complex rutaceae species grow in mild tropical areas. They display beautiful abundant flowers which are shaped like symmetrical stars. They have delicious, exhilarating fragrances. Essential oils are produced from the bark, the fruit, and the flower, in different instances. The part of the plant used and the time of year that the plants are harvested greatly affects the therapeutic qualities of the essential oil produced. This makes this family of essential oils very versatile. Varying members of this family are strengthening to different elements and chakras. All of them seem to affect the energy of the solar plexus chakra. The solar plexus chakra radiates a generous, giving light. This light glows, in varying degrees, from each of us. Balance in this chakra makes us radiant, generous, confident, and outgoing, and gives us vibrant physical health. The general therapeutic characteristics of this family are in the maintenance of fluid levels and warmth in the tissues of the body. The oils produced from flowers are cooling, refreshing and sedating; the fruits exert control over liquid processes and secretions. Pettitgrain, distilled from orange bitter leaves and twigs, is sedative to the nervous system and an intellectual stimulant.

Graminae: A large majority of the plants which are considered ground covers or grasses belong to the Graminae family. The graminae species is considered, in both herbal medicine and Eastern tradition, to be the nutritious family. Essential oils included are citronella, gingergrass, lemongrass, litsea cubeba, palmarosa, and vetiver. From the poles to the equator, from the swamps to the deserts, this family shows an amazing adaptability and diversity. Graninae's ability to cover huge areas, spreading very quickly, denotes great strength. This strength lies in its powerful root systems, which form an intricate network that efficiently utilize and incorporate nutrients from the soil of its environment into itself. This family does not spend much energy in the floral process. Its leaves and seeds are a gift to the animal kingdom and essential oils distilled from this family are a gift of grounding, strength, and nutrition to us. The plants of this family, though having few flowers, develop very distinctive fragrances. There is often a scent reminiscent of freshly cut hay. There is also a fresh, green, lemony, slightly rosy fragrance. The subtleties vary from plant to plant and become quite pronounced in the essential oils because of their concentration. Oils in this family are used for stimulation of the digestive system, as diuretics, for disinfection, and for pest and parasite control.

Mints: Mints are a subspecies of the **Labiatae** family and include the essential oils of peppermint in all its varieties, spearmint, catnip, and pennyroyal. The members of the mint family, both as herbs and as essential oils, have the distinction of being both warming and cooling. They can act in the capacity of stimulants and revitalizers or they can be used to produce a calming, even analgesic, effect. In the essential oils and herbals of this family, whether it will act as a stimulant or a nervine depends on the quantities used and the frequency of the applications. Aromatically, a little bit calms and relaxes the nerves, while larger quantities refresh and stimulate. Peppermint is often used by long-haul truck drivers and others to maintain alertness and stay awake. (This really works!) Topically, the mints relieve pain, but they do this in part by increasing circulation and healing to the area while also acting as an analgesic. In Eastern traditions, increasing circulation is a 'warming' application, while relieving pain is considered a 'cooling' function. There are about 20 members of the mint family, only a few of which are being utilized as essential oils at this time. Common uses include confusion, mental and physical fatigue, pain, digestive problems, motion sickness, poor circulation, nerve regeneration and loss of memory.

Myrtaceae: Traditional philosophy and usage claims that this family brings balance to and between all of the meridians/elements and all of the chakras. These plants are powerful healers. The essential oils include allspice, bay, cajeput, clove, eucalyptus, myrtle, nutmeg, niaouli, and tea tree. Plants of this family grow in every tropical region of the world. They have learned to survive and thrive amidst the powerful forces of earth, water and heat. An interesting fact about the plants and trees of this family is that, while there are no mild plants among them, there are also no poisonous plants to be found here. Among this diverse family are plants which have very hard woods, strong leaves, intense flowers, and others that produce strong, sugary fruits and/or pungent spices.

The scope of action of myrtaceae includes metabolism, the energy centers (Chakras), the meridians, and the lungs. They are effective for respiratory diseases, metabolic or energetic imbalances, and helping us to be more resistant to disease. Just as the plants themselves are robust and strong, the aromas of the essential oils are strong and pungent. Each essential oil is unique in fragrance and therapeutic usage. You would hardly suspect from their aroma that they are members of the same species. Eucalyptus is such a potent and versatile oil that it is regarded in Australia, and even other parts of the world, as a cure-all. Eucalyptus is such a strong oil that it actually becomes more antiseptic and therapeutic as it ages.

Zingiberaceae: The not so commonly used oils of cardamom, ginger, and turmeric are members of this family. They have been used for thousands of years in India and China. References to them are found in writings from the middle ages. All members of this family have an impact on the entire body, physically through the organs and systems and energetically through the meridians and chakras. There is, however, a particularly affinity for the digestive system and, like the mints, can be both a stimulant and an analgesic. All essential oils of this family impact the base chakra and the core of our beings. These oils are extremely potent and should always be used sparingly or in a blend with other mild or stabilizing essential oils..

Betulaceae: Birch is the only oil of this family that is produced in quantity. Birch is strongly analgesic, and has excellent diuretic and lymph cleansing and draining properties. Wintergreen oil is quite similar to birch as far as constituents go, although the amounts of the individual components vary a great deal. Birch and wintergreen, although from different species, contain large amounts of methyl salicylate. This ingredient is considered by many ‘experts’ to be toxic. (Please see the General Information section in the description of birch essential oil in Chapter 14 of this booklet for more information about the safety of oils containing methyl salicylate. There are many rumors and falsehoods in print. If the essential oil has been made from actual plants and no chemically produced methyl salicylate has been added, both birch and wintergreen are safe to use).

Rosaceae: Rose essential oil has the highest frequency of any of the oils. Growing conditions and the type of roses used affect the finished essential oil in many ways. Rose essential is often diluted or adulterated because of the expense involved in its production. The essential oil that is the result of this adulteration does not have the expected high frequency of rose and is, of course, not as therapeutic as it should be. It is much better to buy a little bit of pure rose oil, and use it sparingly, than to use an adulterated or diluted version. A single drop of rose oil in a carrier is all that you will need for most applications. The frequency of rose and its amazing volatility makes the aroma alone highly therapeutic. Rose oil is specific to the female reproductive system and the heart chakra, although the high frequency of this oil raises the overall frequency of every body system and function.

Santalaceae: In the world of essential oils, this family is represented by the various species of sandalwood. Sandalwood (*Santalum album)* is considered sacred in India. Sandalwood essential oil contains a high percentage of sesquiterpenes, which cross the blood/brain barrier, carrying oxygen and nutrients to the brain. Sesquiterpene rich essential oils such as sandalwood are also said to go into the DNA of the cell and unlock emotional trauma. Sandalwood is a very 'warm' oil. It is loved by most people because it opens the mind and heart to feelings of contentment and well-being. Breathe sandalwood in deeply and, if it is a good one, you will feel the center of the chest (solar plexus chakra) open immediately and expand emotionally. A wonderful oil! Only patchouli and cedarwood essential oils have a higher percentage of sesquiterpenes than sandalwood oil. Frankincense, which is the best known of the essential oils for its sesquiterpene content and the therapeutic properties that are the result, actually has a much lower percent of sequiterpenes than sandalwood.

Lauraceae: The essential oils distilled from the lauracea family includes cassia, cinnamon, cinnamon berry, howood, laurel, ravensara, rosewood, sugandha kokila, and tamala. The plants of this species are widely divergent but a common theme among them seems to be their anti-fungal properties. Though members of the same botanical family, cinnamon and rosewood are, in more than just aroma, very dissimilar. Cinnamon is one of the oldest spices of which we have recorded use and has been renowned for centuries for its medicinal value. Cinnamon oil is a stimulant to circulatory, cardiac and pulmonary functions. Rosewood, on the other side of the scale in this family, does not have any dramatic curative powers, but its mildness and safety to use make it useful in skin or body care. Rosewood, rather than being slightly caustic to skin and mucous membranes, is valued for its tissue regeneration properties. It is even said to slow the aging process when applied to the skin.

Anonaceae: The only essential oil that I know of from this family is ylang-ylang. Ylang ylang means, literally, 'flower of flowers.' The oil is distilled from the beautiful yellow flowers. This is a very delicate process. When purchasing, you will note that there are many gradients listed. The 'complete' is considered most therapeutic, although some of the other fine grades are very good. Ylang ylang is one of the best oils for balancing the male-female energies of the body but is not considered hormonal in a way that is balancing and harmonious. (See ylang ylang in the single oil descriptions in Chapter 14.)

Valerianaceae: The essential oils of valerian and spikenard represent this family. Oils in this family are calming and strengthening to the nervous system. They have a positive effect on the root and base chakras, making them effective for intestinal and reproductive issues. These two oils help us meet our emotional needs by calming the fears that reside in the root and base chakras. We can see more clearly and accept more openly the kindness, love, and respect of those around us.

Piperaceae: There are over 3,000 species in the pepper family, but only the *Piper nigrum* is used in essential oil production. The differences in green pepper and black pepper essential oil is brought about by the difference in harvest times. One is harvested when the berries are green and the other when the berries have ripened and turned black. Both are stimulating to the system and balance the yang energies, particularly those affecting the heart. *Piper nigrum* addresses the cores issues of feeling sufficiently strong within ourselves to reach out and bless the lives of others.

Ericacea: This family is typically represented by wintergreen, benzoin, and ledum essential oils. There is a newcomer from Nepal, *Rhododendron anthopogon* (commonly called just anthopogon). The theme of this family seems to be resistance to disease and environmental pollutants and increased strength in the entire system. Perhaps this can be attributed to an affinity for the base and crown chakras. It is as though they strengthen the energetic connections between these two chakras, aiding energy flow up and down through the body. Essential oils from this family are high in sesquiterpenes and help break down fat in the liver. They are very supportive of the fire element (meridians #5 and #6).

Fabaceae (also call Leguminosae): The fabaceae is the third largest family of flowering plants on our planet with nearly 20,000 species. Many of these species are nutritionally, therapeutically, and economically important to mankind. There are a great many medicinal plants in this family. There is an astonishing variability in the plants from which essential oils are distilled. The various balsams, fenugreek, and cabreuva are representative of this variety in plant structure and therapeutic uses.

Oleaceae: In the essential oil world this family is represented by the jasmines and osmanthus. This family of plants includes many species that are recognized for their heady fragrances. This family also includes the olive and plants that are renowned for their tough woods.

Verbenaceae: Chaste tree essential oil is a member of this family. The theme of this family is rich personal experiences and relationships. There is a strong focus on the building or rebuilding of nerves and hormone balance.

Acoraceae: Calamus essential oil has been classified as belonging to the Araceae family, but recent studies have led to the conclusion that it should be placed in its own family. Although not all experts agree, many now list calamus as belonging to the Acoraceae family which is composed of a single genus called Acorus. Only *Acorus calamus* and one or two other species of *Acorus* are included in the genus. It is claimed that calamus will keep people young and improve their overall health. This oil is new to the market and it is very strong, so care should be taken with its use.

Lilliceae: This family includes everything from onions and garlic through asparagus and hyacinths. Garlic and onion are the most common essential oils in use from this family.

Orchidaceae: This family is the second largest among flowering plants, but vanilla is the only commonly used essential oil.

Cistaceae: This small family of plants is known for its ability to regrow rapidly after a wildfire has destroyed its natural habitat. This ability is reflected in the ability of cistus essential oil (a member of this plant family) to aid us in rebuilding and reconnecting emotionally after traumatic events or losses.

Clusiaceae: Two common genera of this family are *Hypericum and Caulophyllum.* Some members of these genera live as long as 50 years. This vitality and longevity seem to be such a part of the species that these aspects are found in the essential oil. St. John's Wort is a member of the *Hypericum* portion of this family.

Plant Cycles and Essential Oils

A Brief Overview

Essential oils can be divided according to the part of the plant the oil is made from. This is a very practical distinction because the properties of the oils and what they are used for, both in physical and emotional work, are very different according to the part of the plant used and the season in which that part of the plant is at its most active and strongest.

Each plant begins in the physical (or base sphere) with the seed and then the development of a root system. The plant then produces leaves, which are considered to be the most vital, growing phase of its life cycle. The plant then moves on to the sphere which corresponds to the astral aspect of development with the opening of the flowers. The flowers lead to the production of the fruit, which is the seed of most plants, thus returning the plant to the physical world. Along the way it has produced elements which mankind the whole world over has long recognized as medicinal herbs and pungent spices. The plant has also given us woods, resins, and aromas that heal and make our hearts glad.

Just as the plant's leaf system corresponds to its vital body, so essential oils produced in the leaves seem to have a toning affect on the body and an affinity for the gathering and storing of knowledge. In Chinese medicine, the vital body is represented (and fed and nourished in large part) by the respiratory system. You will find these oils listed as having an affect on the lungs, etc. and on the vital organs.

Essential oils produced in the roots (such as angelica) tend to have a very peaceful and grounding energy, and they have a nourishing, strengthening quality about them. Still surrounded and nourished by the earth they are, at the same time, in a dynamic and vital growth phase. They are usually potent stimulants of the vital functions (particularly digestion) and are often recommended for anemia and other conditions of poor absorption of nutrients.

The flower is the plant's ultimate achievement and in some cultures the intricacy and fragrance of a plant indicates its 'spiritual' development. The plants with the most intense floral creativity rarely produce any significant fruit or seed (rose and neroli are notable exceptions and their functions are also unique). The essential oils found in the flowers occur in extremely small amounts, but their fragrances are typically very intense. Such fragrances tend to have the highest frequencies and can be exhilarating or even mildly intoxicating.

As described above, the oils produced in the seed (fennel, coriander) bring us back to earth where new experiences of growth await us if we are ready and willing to accept them and move forward in our lives. This usually means that we will need to make one dramatic change or another. Seed oils are often used to invigorate and fortify and seem to show a strong affinity with the digestive system. This is particularly true of those seeds that are used as foods or spices.

The fruit of a plant, while usually containing the seed, is very much a separate classification. The production of a fruit is the representation of the plant's ability to take its energy all the way through to fruition, and is very much representative of the "sufficient strength for the day" emotional nature of the essential oils produced from them (citrus fruits, vanilla, clove, etc).

Essential oils made from plants which are considered spices are among the most nutritional plants available, with astonishing high levels of vitamins and, especially, minerals. This has been known by herbalist for centuries. These nutrients are utilized by the body when absorbed through the skin as essential oils are applied. Essential oils made from the spice plants and the plants recognized as herbal remedies nourish, heal and prepare us mentally and physically to accomplish our particular missions in life. Spice oils have flamboyant personality styles, just as you would expect.

Trees and bushes also have the ability to create oils in their wood. Such oils are centering and grounding in nature. Here the creative process is drawn into the heart of the wood and they show a corresponding ability to aid us in becoming firm and full of strength in our own centers. A tree is firmly anchored to the earth, strong and upright, reaching valiantly for heaven, but at the same time is able to bend in the wind of new ideas. A good way to be for all of us. If we become too rigid in our thinking and emotions, we can be easily broken by the storms of life.

Some essential oils are produced from the resins or gums. These essential oils have a strong affinity for the glandular system; they control secretions and demonstrate cosmetic and healing properties (skin care, wounds, ulcers). Emotionally, they deal with issues of right and wrong and the ability to make choices and decisions.

The 9 Groupings in More Depth

(These lists are only partial, based on the most commonly used essential oils)

We will do: 1) a definition of what constitutes this category; 2) a description of the physical aspects of the body and physical ailments that this type of oil supports; 3) an emotional/spiritual picture of the strengths and characteristics these oils promote and help us achieve; 4) a picture of the emotional patterns of a person needing the strengths provided by one or more of these oils; 5) a list of the most commonly used oils in this category.

Roots: Extracted from the roots of plants

Physical: These oils are stimulating and nourishing to the body's vital functions, particularly to the digestive and nervous systems. They are often used to improve conditions of slow absorption of nutrients.

Emotional: People strong in their emotional connections with other people have peace and harmony about them and in their lives. The use of essential oils made from the roots of plants can help us be more firmly grounded in ourselves, allow us to be good-natured yet firm, which will promote serenity and stability around us. We can feel trusting of ourselves and others, be kind and supportive, even mediate quarrels between others if needed. We can learn to be self-confident without being over-bearing and to establish deep relationships with a wide variety of people. The greatest gift of the root oils is in helping us to be observant, humble, teachable, loyal and reliable.

In need of: We can know that we are in need of root essential oils if we are disorganized, neglectful, feel confused or muddled in our thinking processes, are absent-minded, moody, obstinate, apathetic, depressed or just plain emotional.

Oils: angelica, calamus, garlic, ginger, spikenard, turmeric, valerian, vetiver

Leaves: Extracted from the leaves of trees or plants

Physical: These oils' main impact is on the vital organs in either toning or cleansing. These oils have a particular affinity for the respiratory system.

Emotional: In Eastern healing traditions, the vital organs of the body are fed and nourished to a very large extent by the respiratory system, not just the digestive system as is generally thought in our own culture. It is thought that, along with the air that is essential to life, new thoughts and ideas (also essential to life in the eastern view) are drawn into the body with the breath and it is on the breath that old ideas and misconceptions are expelled. Just as the leaf of the plant takes in air and nutrients, these essential oils help our minds to be always taking in new ideas, considering them and making the best parts of them useful in our own lives. Knowledge and learning become sustenance to people who are working to strengthen their 'leaf energy' and they will spend as many waking minutes as possible getting more of it. These essential oils can help us keep the whole picture in mind, even when specializing in a particular area. We can become innovative thinkers with multiple solutions and theories in every situation but hard-working and with enough energy, concentration and confidence to carry out our ideas. People needing 'leaf energy' usually can not handle aggression or conflict. They will be completely drained by it.

In need of: People out of balance in this area and in need of the support these oils can bring, find it hard to keep the whole picture in mind or to admit that the conclusions they have drawn are flawed or lacking in some way. They can become paranoid, hostile, scornful, cynical or just plain exhausted and over-whelmed. They often choose to spend a lot of time alone and can become suspicious and out-of-touch with the world around them. Sometimes they are resentful or exhausted by the demands of family and friends.

Oils: allspice, anthopogon, basil, bay, birch, blue tansy, cajeput, cassia, cinnamon, citronella, clary sage, cypress, davanna, eucalyptus, fir, galbanum, geranium, marjoram, melissa, myrtle, niaouli, oregano, palmarosa, patchouli, peppermint, petitgrain, pine, ravensara, rose geranium, rosemary, sage, spearmint, spruce, tamala, tarragon, tea tree, wintergreen

Florals: Defined as oils and absolutes that are extracted from the flowers or petals of plants or trees

Physical: Floral oils can aid us with a wide variety of physical ailments that, with a little analysis, are clearly based on emotional needs or mis-perceptions. These oils are often helpful for any type of pain that is made worse or seems to be caused by emotional stress or nervous tension. Particularly useful for issues involving the feminine reproductive cycles and the lack of absorption of nutrients

Emotional: People unstable or depleted in floral energy need to have status, to be admired, and to feel that they stand out from the crowd. Physical appearance is important to them. When well balanced they are dynamic, bursting with energy and enthusiasm; totally confident and ambitious but full of love and passion. When out of balance they can appear superficial but, even then, they are very sensitive and soft-hearted, often sensing others moods and trying hard to help. People who are balanced in this sphere bring a lot of happiness to others.

In need of: The floral essential oils are always quite 'heady.' Unless you are in need of them, you will usually find them almost offensive. You can be sure you need one if you are becoming insensitive, manipulative, envious, power and status hungry, are having difficulty loving others and sharing with them, have shallow values or tend to lie to achieve goals or look good. The problem is that you probably won't admit these traits to yourself or seek change.

Oils anthopogon, blue tansy, catnip, chamomile Egyptiona, chamomile German, chamomile Roman, helichrysum, Idaho tansy, jasmine, lavender, melissa, neroli, rose (maroc and otto), tagette, yarrow, ylang ylang.

Seeds: Extracted from the seeds of plants

Physical: The seed of a plant is dormant until placed in the ground and watered, but it possesses within it a potential for growth. Essential oils derived from the seed have an impact on the glands, the digestive organs and anything having to do with growth and development. They often help the body rid itself of accumulated toxins and poisons that are interfering with growth and normal functioning, which make them useful for cleansing and supporting the liver.

Emotional: The potential (while invisible and dormant) of a seed is reflected in its creative and intuitive abilities, particularly as the seeds focus on opportunities for growth. People strong in this energy have a remarkable ability to go through the same mundane experiences day after day and keep finding great joy in each experience. They joyfully spend the time and energy necessary to create a suitable environment for growth and development for themselves and others. People strong in this energy seem to be constantly reinventing themselves by changing job, appearance, or direction. They need beauty and romance in their lives and, like a seed, they can be delicate and sensitive to their environment. Just as many different plants can come from seeds that often look quite similar, there is an endless variety to the characteristics that seed oils can help you strengthen and affirm in your life. It is important to remember, when using essential oils, that the closer we get to God the more of our own individual we will be. It is perfectly acceptable, even a good thing, to be a little different from those around you.

In need of: When you are over-whelmed and feeling despondent, depressed, insecure, self-pitying, disillusioned and worthless, you can find energy and stability by the use of one or more seed oils. You might try one of these oils if you tend to start projects but become dissatisfied with them and throw them away unfinished.

Oils: ajowan, aniseseed, caraway, cardamom, carrot seed, celery seed, coriander, cumin, dill, fennel, fenugreek, manuka, nutmeg, parsley

Fruits: Extracted from the fruit of a plant or tree

Physical: One of the various kinds of fruits (from clove buds to citrus fruits) and the oils extracted from them will have something nourishing for every body system and gland. Some have an affinity for the nervous system, others for the skin and others for circulation or for glandular deficiencies and problems.

Emotional: We all have a need to feel clear, connected and satisfied with ourselves and we usually need to have the respect and approval of those around us. The use of fruit oils helps us to feel kind-hearted, friendly, supportive, and able to take responsibility for ourselves and any project in which we are involved. Just as the fruit of the tree represents the ability of the plant to survive and thrive to fruition, oils from this stage of plant life can help us be finishers, recognized for our diligence and dependability as well as for our joyful, passionate natures.

In need of: Some indicators that you would benefit from an essential oil in this family are being indecisive or just contradictory, being hesitant and cautious, being defensive to the point of unreasonable, being clingy, anxious and oversensitive, or feeling impatient, spiteful, sarcastic and having feelings of inferiority. Your ability to finish projects is limited because of indecision or because of your hurt feelings, which caused you to walk away from something or someone.

Oils: allspice, aniseseed, bergamot, black pepper, chaste tree, cinnamon berry, clementine, clove, grapefruit, green pepper, juniper, lemon, lime, litsea cubeba, mandarin, orange, suganda kokila, tangerine, vanilla, zanthoxylum

Spices: Extracted from various parts of plants or trees and commonly recognized as culinary spices

Physical: Because they are derived from various parts of plants, spice oils are varied in their nature. Two common denominators, however, are that all spices are high in minerals, and that every condition they are recommended for will be an extreme state. Conditions that are hypo-this or hyper-that, a severe infection of highly resistant bacteria, complete collapse, extreme fatigue, and volatile emotions are just a few examples of physical conditions the spice oils might be helpful with. There is nothing bland or mediocre to be found here.

Emotional: The balance the spice oils can bring to our lives is amazing. We can love life, be animated, happy, warm-hearted, spontaneous, dynamic and self-assured. The spice oils in a blend are there to help us become energetic, productive and practical and they do this by increasing cellular oxygen levels. The spice oils have a stimulating and toning effect on our bodies and minds, and, interestingly, enhance the action and power of other oils in any blend in which they are placed, making them a great example of synergy. Spice oils also illustrate the principle of natural remedies returning the body to a state of homeostasis, or balance, because they often act as both a stimulant when energy levels are low and as a sedative during times when our bodies and minds are stressed and need to rest and relax.

In need of: People in need of spice oils have become unbalanced either by burnout (running too fast, too far, and having too much fun) or by the frustration of not achieving their goals and desires, which were usually unrealistic in the first place. If you find yourself being any degree of demanding, resentful, rude, abusive, insulting or you have a tendency to treat others like servants designed to meet your needs, you might consider working on these traits and using the spice oils to help you. Behaving much like a child when our 'wants' are not met, hysteria, panic attacks and depression are other common symptoms.

Oils: aniseseed, basil, black pepper, caraway, cardamom, cinnamon, clove, coriander, cumin, dill, lemongrass, ginger, marjoram, nutmeg, oregano, rosemary, tarragon, turmeric

Herbs: Oils extracted from plants generally thought of as medicinal herbs

Physical: I find that with the herbal essential oils, as with the herbs themselves, I have a favorite one or two for just about every body system or gland. Herbal essential oils are nutritious and this nutrition is absorbed and used by the body whenever they are applied to the skin. Herbs seem to be concentrated vitamins in highly absorbable form while the herbs and oils that are considered spices are stronger in mineral content.

Emotional: The herbal personality is that of the healer who has a two-fold mission of providing unconditional love and care for as many others as possible, and needing to find that same love and caring for themselves. If you find yourself over-whelmed by the needs of others, no longer consider it a joy to serve or you resent being needed by other people there are probably nutrition deficiencies robbing you of energy.

In need of: When over-whelmed, people needing herbal essential oils can become resentful, but they are usually unable to say 'no' or stop taking on everybody else's troubles. They even tend to 'smother' people with their concern and worry and they are unable to let their children grow up or leave home with gracefulness. They tend to get too intimate and intrusive in other people's lives and get insulted when they feel themselves excluded from even the most intimate details of that person's life. If you find yourself forgetting to say thank you to those around you, but need to be thanked for every little thing that you do for others, herbal oils are for you. Perhaps you have even been known to use guilt as tools of manipulation (shame on you!)

Oils: basil, clary sage, geranium, hyssop, marjoram, melissa, myrtle, peppermint, spearmint, oregano, rosemary, sage, thyme both red and white, blue yarrow, green yarrow

Woods: Extracted from twigs, wood chippings, or shavings of trees

Physical: The essential oils in this category, especially the conifers, have strongly to do with maintaining firmness and strength in our own centers. Any physical ailments on which they have an effect will almost always be driven, at least in part, by a wavering and lack of faith in our own core beliefs and in our ability to live by them. With this being said, they are often useful for glandular system disharmonies and the skin afflictions that result from them. This fact should tell us something about the emotional drivers of glandular problems. Of particular note in this family is sandalwood, which can help us tap into our own inner strength when facing our difficult challenges. Wood oils are also useful for heart irregularities that have their roots in the inability to handle stress or tension.

Emotional: Wood oils aid us in being strong, independent, bold and forthright. People strong in this energy stand for justice and courage and have a great capacity for hard work. They are usually warm-hearted people with a lot of tolerance and compassion for the mistakes that others have made although they, themselves, are moral, self-confident, motivated, perceptive, faithful and steadfast.

In need of: Out of balance wood characteristics include the following: tendencies to dominate; becoming dictatorial and threatening; being very unyielding, meaning they expect their opinions to be accepted by others and their methods of doing things to be considered correct and to be acted on immediately by others. At times the wonderful characteristics of balance in wood energy becomes argumentative, egotistical, harsh, vengeful, and severe to the point of meanness. There is often a wood oil somewhere in a blend; its inclusion brings the blend together, adding a sweetness and structure that would otherwise be missing.

Oils: cabreuva, camphor, cedarwood, cypress, galbanum, hinoki, howood, pine, ravensara, rosewood, sandalwood, spruce, cinnamon

Resins: Extracted from the resin or balsam which exudes from the bark of some trees and shrubs

Physical: In a very strong corollary to the way resins exude from the plant, these essential oils have an affinity for secretions, pus filled and inflamed infections, catarrhal conditions, ulcers, and inflammations of any sort. They are also helpful for maintaining or returning elasticity to the skin. Frankincense and myrrh are of particular note in this group of essential oils.

Emotional: If your energy is strong in this area you will be driven, in the best sense of the word, by high ideals. Morality, truth, justice and purity of thought are things you constantly and consciously seek. Your values, principles, and ethics are part of everything you do and you understand that there are principles that underlay every decision of our lives. Deep spirituality is a personal goal but you are usually realistic and tolerant in your dealing with others.

In need of: If these strong personalities make a moral mistake they are devastated and find it difficult to forgive themselves. They are often harshly critical of themselves and can get caught up and immobilized by guilt. When out of balance you will see traits such as being self-righteous, dogmatic, intolerant and very, very angry. The disappointment they feel with themselves or others can lead to discouragement, which is followed closely by nervousness and depression. It feels to them as though it is them, single-handed with no help or hope in sight, against all of the evil forces of the universe!

Oils: benzoin, copaiba balsam, elemi, frankincense, myrrh, opoponax

A Very Brief Explanation of Yin and Yang

Most of us have been raised in the western approach to health care which deals primarily with the state of the physical body. In western thought, disease is too often considered an isolated entity residing or beginning in one bodily organ or another.

Oriental philosophies view human beings as a series of subtle bodies, and disease as a disturbance in the *energy* of one or more of them. These philosophies maintain that healing is a process that must be accomplished throughout these subtle layers, meaning throughout the entire person—body, mind, spirit, soul, etc. Regardless of where in the physical body the symptoms are manifesting, it is understood that the entire body/mind/spirit complex is ill.

Western medicine is often considered to be scientific and logical, while the deeply philosophical eastern thinking sometimes seems, to those of us conditioned to western thought, to be metaphysical and even bizarre. Closer examination, however, reveals the underlying principles to be logical, sound, valid and easily observed all around us in nature. Difficulties in understanding, when they arise, seem to be the result of terminology. We in the western world have no appropriate words to describe eastern thinking; we end up using their words and struggling to come to terms with the layers of meaning that are embodied by them.

Two such words are yin and yang. An adequate explanation of these two words would take several pages; a very short paragraph will be provided here.

Basically, yang refers to the energizing force that streams down from Heaven above, while yin refers to the receptive, creative, material world of earth. Yang is creative, forceful and enthusiatic, while yin is quieter and more contemplative. Yin and yang can be seen in every function and aspect of living. We can observe yin and yang in the change of the seasons, the cycle of night and day, the growth of plants, and in the functions of our own bodies. Every function of any living thing manifests these two opposing forces. An understanding of the way yin and yang relate and manifest in the body, creating symptoms of sickness or health, as they slide in and out of balanced states is an asset to any branch of the healing arts.

To know which oils balance the energies of yin or yang most effectively gives another dimension to your understanding, application and use of essential oils. Many oils, especially ones comprised of several different single oils, seem to affect both energies for the better. The strengthening of one aspect allows a corresponding strengthening of the other, making the entire system stronger.

The following is a list of essential oils considered strongly yang or yin.

Yang: basil, bay, benzoin, bergamot, black pepper, caraway, cardamom, cedarwood, clary sage, elemi, frankincense, hyssop, jasmine, juniper berry, lavender, marjoram, melissa, myrrrh, neroli, oregano, patchouli, peppermint, rosemary, sage, sandalwood, thyme. Many of these are members of the labiatae family (see Chapter 9).

Yin: blue tansy, chamomile, cypress, eucalyptus, geranium, palmarosa, rose, rose geranium, vetiver, ylang ylang

Balances yin and yang : vetiver

Moderates yin: clary sage

A Brief Over-view of the Meridian System
and
Some Suggested Essential Oils for Each Meridian

In Oriental medicine the subtle energy that moves throughout the body is considered of prime importance. Blockages in this flow are believed to occur long before the physical problem that will be the result if the blockage is not dealt with and removed. Meridians (sometimes called channels, vessels, or elements) is the term chosen to describe the overall distribution system of this energy. It must be understood, however, that energy frequently moves between these meridians and back and forth among the chakras also.

Each of these meridians (with the exception of 0, which is considered to be Mind and Air) is associated with a season and with the emotional patterns appropriate to that season. These emotional characteristics have been drawn from the observation of nature in the earth and human nature over the centuries.

Most of us seem to live quite strongly within one rhythm, or season, while being greatly influenced by the seasons preceding and following it in the Chinese Creative Cycle. Our own basic rhythm is made up of the strengths and weakness within our primary rhythm, mixed with a unique combination of the abundance or depletion of the qualities of the others. This is a fascinating, but complicated, topic and too lengthy for in-depth consideration here.

Although we seem to live our lives in our particular rhythm or blend of rhythms, we also move through all five of the seasons many times during the cycles that make up a lifetime. Both your core rhythm and the season through which you are passing at the moment profoundly influence the way you respond to your world and the people in it.

Understanding your rhythms can help you to understand your vulnerabilities and your responses to people and situations. A study of the emotional patterns of the meridians can help us identify our faults and our strengths, understand the amazing things we are capable of accomplishing, and point out to us the things in our core personalities that we should be on our guard against. Behaviors that exhibit the out-of-balance patterns of these seasons are usually not serving us well or making us happy and should be identified and abandoned.

Understanding our children and the people around us can also be helpful, but only if we can contemplate them with love and compassion, while managing to mind our own business and not use our new-found understanding in any manipulative or controlling manner.

Professional aromatherapists use personality classifications to help determine which oils from the wide range available will be most beneficial to a person. Of course, it is not ever just one personality type that fits us at any point in our lives, but several layered one on top of another. Sometimes a particular characteristic only becomes apparent in certain stressful situations and when dealing with, or associating with, certain people.

As shown in the previous chapter, the properties of essential oils are very much a part of the plant family they come from, the part of the plant they are extracted from, and the season in which it is harvested. Each oil, or combination of oils, has very strong characteristics and affinities for certain personality imbalances as well as physical problems.

Each meridian (rhythm or personality type) is prone to certain types of imbalances, and can be brought back into balance most quickly in certain ways and with the use of the essential oils which have an affinity for or a balancing effect on those problems. The next few pages will give you a brief over-view of each meridian and suggest essential oils that are useful in balancing and strengthening them.

When you achieve a deep harmony between a particular person and a particular essential oil, physical, mental and emotional problems can clear up very quickly. Choosing oils based only on personality type, without any regard for physical ailments, often brings about very dramatic results. This illustrates that certain types of personalities are prone to certain types of physical illnesses. This phenomenon is often seen, and used successfully, in homeopathic treatment programs. It is effective in working with essential oils, also.

It is interesting to ponder on and consider what it is that we inherit from our ancestors. Is it just the shape of our nose or the color of our hair or do we also inherit a tendency to certain personality traits and a vulnerability to certain types of illnesses? Will an oil that has been successful for you also be successful for your children? Is your husband partial to particular oils that you are not fond of and are some of your children fond of your favorites and some fond of his favorites? Is there a correlation between the oils that work for your spouse and children and their various personality types?

The goal of this type of study is to help us achieve as many of the abundant characteristics of all the groups as we possibly can. For example, one person might eventually have the enthusiasm shown by the florals, the good natured equilibrium of the fruit group, the practicality and caring skills demonstrated by the herbal world, the intuition and vision that is common among the leaf group, the wisdom and maturity of the resinous oils, the peace making qualities of the roots, the joy and vitality of the spices, and the courage of the woods. A person with all this qualities would be a pretty wonderful and well-balanced individual, wouldn't they. This life, and the perfection we are seeking, is a journey of a thousand miles that begins with the baby steps we are taking today as we meet our challenges in the best ways that we can.

0 - Air/Mind

Governing Vessel

Moving forward on life's path with faith and confidence or
embarrassment, reluctance to move forward at all

Controls the peripheral nervous system, which has two main divisions: the *somatic* nervous system and the *autonomic* nervous system.

The *somatic* nervous system has two separate functions. The first is to collect information from the outside world using the sensory organs and the second is to transmit this information to the central nervous system and on to the skeletal muscles. The second is the *autonomic* nervous system, which is concerned with those functions over which we *do not consider ourselves* as having *conscious* control such as the heartbeat, the function of the kidneys, the flow of hormones, etc.

Emotionally, the peripheral nervous system represents our perception of the world around us, our place in it, and our ability to stay firmly on the path that we believe is right for us. When we are out of balance or weak in this meridian we are vulnerable to self-doubt and becoming overly controlled by other people's opinions of what we should do and who we should be.

Blends: [Le]Believe, [Le]Benediction, [Le]Focus, [e]Good-Nite, [Le]Letting Go, [Le]Meditation, [Le]Millenia, [Le]Sanctuary, [Le]Vitality
Singles: frankincense, mandarin, vanilla, coriander, pine, spruce, clary sage, marjoram, lavender, clove, niaouli

Central Vessel

Firmness; balance between logic and emotion; considerate of, but not unduly influenced by, other people's energies or opinions
feelings of shame, shyness

Controls the central nervous system whose core processing units are the brain and the spinal cord. This meridian is closely attuned to both your left-brained analytical side and the more right-brained creative side. When weakened in this meridian you are at the mercy of your own widely fluctuating emotions and are more vulnerable to the energies (particularly the negative ones) of others. Your ability to analyze and act appropriately on facts becomes erratic or inhibited.

Blends: [Le]Believe, [Le]Acknowledge, [Le]Benediction, [Le]Meditation, [Le]Millenia, [Le]Sanctuary
Singles: cedarwood, cypress, rose, rosewood, angelica, fennel, sandalwood, cardamom, fennel, celery seed, clove, frankincense, lavender, niaouli

Governing Vessel — **Moving forward on life's path with faith and confidence**
Embarrassment, reluctance to move forward

Central Vessel — **Firmness; consideration; balance between logic and emotions**
Feeling of shame, shyness

Blends

LeMillenia — the easiest way to balance all meridians at once; always brings feelings of courage, self-confidence; helps us move forward with calmness and purpose; use in combination with the most appropriate blend or single listed below for these meridians

LeLetting Go — letting go of the desire to please others instead of walking our own way; letting go of past mistakes while still learning from them

LeFocus — helps us see more clearly the negative thought patterns and self-defeating behaviors that unduly influence our decision; helps to clear the clouds of confusion in our minds because of the many different voices and choices that we have every day

LeBelieve — confidence that we are just as smart, just as lucky, and just as blessed by Heaven as anyone else; confidence that we will be in the right place, at the right time, and able to do the right thing

LeVitality — increases stamina and nervous system function; strengthens our belief in ourselves; decreases self-doubt and moderates the influence of other people's opinions

LeAcknowledge — enthusiasm for new things and new ideas; an expectation that things will work out well for us, bringing us joy and abundance; a dose of reality with a focus on the positive

LeBenediction — protection from other people's negativity and opinions

LeMeditation — targets decision making ability, including communication with Heaven; this is a good oil for use when pondering spiritual things or thinking about the direction of one's life

LeSanctuary — self-awareness and spiritual judgement

Singles

frankincense — communication with the Creator; improved attitude and judgement

mandarin — moderates irritability; helps us make decisions based on rationality instead of irritation

vanilla — helps to ease anger and frustration; helps us to feel warm and welcome in our world

cedarwood — enhance spiritual communication while remaining firmly in the present and concerned about things in our physical and material world

cypress — considered in many cultures to be symbolic of life after death; centering and an aid in helping us decide, and live by, the things of eternity

rose — highest frequency oil; best choice for emotional crisis or extreme debility and fatigue

rosewood — feelings of peace and gentleness; helps us find a balance between giving and receiving

angelica — aid the liver in discharging anger and toxins so that decisions can be rationally made

coriander — for emotional/mood swings during convalescence from an illness or following a particularly traumatic time

fennel — fennel supports the liver and balances hormones, making it useful for emotional stability

pine/spruce — conifers are noted for their ability to maintain their needles in times of cold; there is a definite corollary between this stability and their ability to aid us in remaining constant even when under a great deal of stress or when life is being a trifle hostile or difficult

niaouli — helps us see the bigger picture of our lives and find the things we were born to do

sandalwood — the energy of sandalwood vibrates between the crown chakra and the base chakra along the governing and central meridians. Sandalwood brings harmony to the entire complex.

1 - Wood/Season of Spring & Wind (The Pioneer)

Gallbladder **Feelings of love and adoration or *feelings of rage***
Liver **Happy and cheerful or *angry and annoyed***

If Spring is your primary rhythm, your disposition is to push forth with your roots firm and your territory clearly marked. The sound of your voice is often choppy, almost a shout. This element embodies the power, energy, confidence and enthusiasm of new growth. A wood phase involves the transformation of energy into matter and ideas into genuine productivity and accomplishment. Wind is considered an element of change, bringing in new ideas and totally rearranging old patterns.

A balanced *Liver* meridian allows our lives to flow more smoothly as we are able to 'take things in our stride.' Through its management of the blood, the liver nourishes our muscles and tissues, regulates menstruation and strengthens our heart and mind. Of course, the liver absorbs what cannot be digested, physically, emotionally and spiritually.

The Gallbladder, which is closely associated with the *Gallbladder* meridian is the only yang organ that is an organ of storage. When the gallbladder is compromised, fats can accumulate in the bloodstream or tissues. The gallbladder also controls that part of the energy system that governs choice.

People balanced and clear in their wood meridian are able to take a strong stand. seek challenge and push to their limits. They enjoy and do well under pressure and like to be first ,best and only. They are bold and decisive and act immediately on their hunches with a clear and inspiring vision. They are organized. Their goals are sound. They show good judgement and make wise decisions.

The 'terrible twos' are the first cycle of Spring's rhythm

Symptoms of imbalance:
Self-confidence sometimes becomes arrogance and their assertiveness can become inflexible and self-indulgent. In their self-righteousness, they judge those who do not agree with them harshly and vocally. When they lose their vision they become discouraged, angry and indecisive under stress.

Physical complaints: Stiff neck, frequently caused or aggravated by wind and weather. The stress in their liver creates headaches, migraines, high blood pressure and nerve inflammations

Balance is restored by:
Expressing themselves creatively; yoga and other forms of flexibility and stretching exercises; learning to back down from arguments and retreat from or use judgement in adventures

Age usually mellows the characteristics of Spring into wisdom, a healthy determination and they acquire the ability to work better with others.

Gall Bladder

Blends: LeBelieve, LeConnection, LeKadence, LeMillenia, LePurify, LeReconciliation, LeSanctuary, LeWhispering Hope, LeWisdom

Singles: helichrysum, mandarin, orange bitter, bergamot, fennel, lavender, lemon, sandalwood, carrot seed, chamomile German, clove, frankincense, lime, melissa, orange sweet, peppermint, yarrow

Liver

Blends: LeAcknowledge, LeTranquility, LeUnity, LeAspire, LeAngel, LeLetting Go, LeMillenia, LeReconciliation

Singles: lemon, petitgrain, copaiba balsam, vanilla, nutmeg, spruce, rosemary, lavender, orange bitter, orange sweet, peppermint, lime, melissa, yarrow

Gallbladder	**Feelings of love and adoration or *feelings of rage***
Liver	**Happy and cheerful or *angry, and annoyed***

Blends

LeMillenia	the easiest way to balance all meridians at once; always brings feeling of courage, self-confidence and a desire to move forward with both calmness and purpose;
LeBelieve	release negativity at the cellular level; promote feelings of self-worth and contentment; confidence in your ability to do the right things and be in the right place in the future
LeConnection	sage has an affinity for the pelvic area chakras and organs while spruce has to do with the solar plexus and receiving divine inspiration. This blend connects those two areas giving us a great inner strength
LeWhispering Hope	a synergistic blend that encompasses several plant cycles and plant families; frustration at other people's choices and at the impossibility of stepping in and 'doing it for them', when you can only sit and wait.
LeTranquility	fuller understanding of all parts of a situation; inner strength and decisiveness
LeUnity	contains several of the single oils specific to these meridians; balances all of the chakras; promotes unity within ourselves and with those around us
LeAngel	release both the anger and the toxic build-up that is stored in the liver, especially connected to traumatic or negative childhood experiences and abuse
LeLetting Go	letting go of anger and frustration and the rebelliousness that sometimes accompanies these feelings; aids the gallbladder and liver in letting go of past resentments and anger

Singles

helichrysum	calm acceptance of change; emotional blockages from some type of abuse; self-confidence to make choices; relief from emotional and mental fatigue; physically healing to tissues
mandarin	for those who are dwelling in the past; calming to those who are easily over-stimulated or excited; aids in relationships with children and the very elderly; anxiety; depression
orange, of bitter	very little information available but is being used recently (since MaHuang ran afoul the FDA) as an ingredient in weight loss formulas and as a gallbladder stimulant
bergamot	promotes 'young at heart' qualities; helps build confidence and ability to concentrate; helps the inner despair and depression that is often covered by outward cheerfulness
fennel	inner courage and confidence to stand by decisions already made; break down walls that have been built around emotions; stabilizes hormones and the absorption of nutrients that are sometimes the cause of deep depressions and sudden mood swings
lavender	called the 'grandmother' of essential oils because of its ability to care and nurture us through a variety of physical and psychological imbalances; balance between masculine and feminine traits; calming; protection from outside energies and influences
lemon	handling life's problems calmly, with a bit of joy and a lot of energy; creates an attitude of 'I can do it'; lemon can be both sweet and sour—both sensitive to others and critical of them; a good oil for those who start projects but have difficulty completing them
sandalwood	desire to ponder and then act on solutions to problems; curb manipulative or controlling tendencies; create an attitude of forgiveness
petitgrain	orange family; helps overcome pessimism and insomnia due to anger (often with feelings of betrayal); stabilize from mental fatigue, confusion and irrationality
rosemary	use for loss of memory, learning difficulties, indecisiveness, mental fatigue
vanilla	soothing to the spirit; promotes feelings of confidence and ability to listen to the Spirit

2 - Water/Season of Winter The Philosopher

Kidney **Trust in self and in the future, feelings of faith or *feelings of fear, trembling***

Bladder **Authoritative, sure, in-tune or *timid, with lack of back-bone or self-will***

In winter, life appears to have ceased when in reality it is growing and changing though out of sight and underground. The season of Winter is about beginnings; childlike enthusiasm but with periods of deep introspection where energies are directed inward. Water people tend to 'go with the flow' and seek the path of least resistance. They would rather adapt than try to change a situation, but when feeling safe they are playful and spontaneous (like a small child). ***This aspect is very rarely seen in most of them as they rarely feel that safe.*** Water people can be articulate and self-sufficient. They spend a lifetime seeking understanding, truth, the meaning of life, and finding their own spiritual strengths. They are particularly good at envisioning a project and getting it under way, but their energy sometimes runs out before the project is completed. They withdraw into themselves, seeking quiet and alone (much like a hibernating bear) to restore themselves.

Symptoms of imbalance:
The negative side of water is fear! Fear is what Water people feel when they have over-extended themselves or been pushed beyond their comfort zone or imagined limitations. Confronted with a situation they feel they have no control over or lack the skills to cope with, Water people respond with fear and its attendant health problems and energy disturbances.

The energies of Winter/Water people may be limited (since this season has little light and light is energy). They are usually more vulnerable to illness and fatigue than most. Their energy is easily depleted; they frequently fall into the stress patterns of their rhythm. On the other hand, a little time alone usually brings back their energy and optimism just as quickly. Winter/Water people sometimes think they need special care and attention (surviving in winter seems difficult to them) and they are often unable to recognize how their actions affect other people, focusing only on what others are doing to them. Can be difficult to live with because they must be showered with love in order to feel loved. *Water* meridian people tend to adapt to other people's ideas and will; they are only truly themselves when alone. When they are under stress their natural courage becomes fear, particularly fear of moving forward or making a commitment. They are sometimes paralyzed by dangers, either real and imagined, doesn't matter much which, since they usually can't perceive the difference.

Physical complaints include hardening of the arteries, heart problems, bladder infections, black circles under the eyes, deterioration of teeth and gums, back ache, chilliness, loss of libido.

In maturity a Winter person's tendency to be fearful tempers into a wise and discerning caution that includes great faith in life, God, and other people. They usually develop an astonishing ability to listen to the Spirit.

Balance restored by:
Water (Winter) people's energies can be seriously depleted by the excess energies of Fire and Earth people. Time alone to study, think, reflect or just putter around is essential to Water people.

Bladder

Blends: LeBelieve, LeBenediction, LeMagi, LeMillenia, LeSanctuary

Singles: lavender, palmarosa, rosewood, yarrow, sandalwood, chamomile, frankincense, neroli, thyme, tea tree

Kidney

Blends: LeBelieve, LeFaith, LeMillenia, LeSolitude, LeEZ-Traveler, LeSanctuary, LeSolitude, LeWhispering Hope

Singles: juniper, bergamot, coriander, lemon, neroli, cedarwood, franincense, lavender, tea tree, thyme

Kidney	**Feelings of faith, trusting in self and in the future or *great fear, trembling***
Bladder	**Authoritative, in-tune or *timid with lack of backbone or self-will***

Blends

LeBelieve	replace the overwhelming and pervasive fear of everything with confidence that we have the ability to do what is needed and be where we need to be at the appropriate time
LeBenediction	protects against the 'energy drains' to which *Winter* meridian people are so susceptible
LeMagi	particularly helpful for fear of being alone or being left alone; helps to clarify intuition and the ability to receive divine inspiration; offsets the despair of this meridian
LeMillenia	fear and courage are opposing states—the *Water* meridian is about fears and lack of courage and faith. Millenia is the #1 oil for moving forward with confidence, courage and faith.
LeSanctuary	feelings of protection and safety; trust in one's intuition, wisdom and good-judgement
LeFaith	feelings of peace and hopefulness instead of fear and trembling; issues to do with abandonment; confidence instead or worry
LeSolitude	this meridian needs peace and quiet to regenerate and rebuild. This blend is like a little dose of solitude when there simply isn't time for any of the real thing.
LeEZ-Traveler	calms the nervous stomach that so often accompanies a state of fearfulness; adds a bit of humor and gladness just to be alive

Singles

lavender	faith and confidence even in times of hardship or great unease and distress; calming
palmarosa	feelings of security and recovery from nervous exhaustion; affinity for cardiovascular system, thyroid gland and the heart chakra
yarrow	in Chinese folklore this herb, and its essential oil, are said to bring about the meeting of Heaven and Earth, allowing us to have both the vision of our head in the clouds and the stability of our feet firmly planted on earth
sandalwood	inner calm even when knowing that there are difficult challenges ahead; developing communication and management skills
juniper	developing a reverence for sacred things and the ability to be directed by inspiration and religious beliefs; delight in new experiences, rather than dread them; antidote for uneasiness and unnamed fears
bergamot	for those times when the weight of other people's distress is bearing you down and the cheerful face you would like to present to the world is sagging badly
coriander	self-doubt and fear of failure; lack of usual zest and passion for life; overly cautious and concerned about ability to make decisions
lemon	the constant fearfulness of this meridian can lead to a great deal of resentment, even grudges, toward the people and situations that are 'perceived' as causing all the problems. Lemon adds a zestful dose of reality here
neroli	helps with cynicism and despair and the feeling that 'nothing changes, nothing ever will'; for those who are becoming fearful, withdrawn and timid because the world out there feels like a really scary, ***cold*** place
cedarwood	quiets the mind and lets us come to a decision, then gives us the backbone to carry it through

3 - Metal/Season is Late Fall The Alchemist

Large Intestine **Feelings of confidence and self-worth or *feelings of guilt***

Lung **Humility, feeling of tolerance or *pride and intolerance***

This rhythm seems to be stretched between Heaven and Earth and is called 'the Alchemist' because of the ability to find truth from every day experiences and restore order from chaos. These people maintain personal standards and see clearly what needs to happen for the best in any situation.

Balanced Metal people are almost always high achievers. They maintain standards of excellence for themselves yet they manage to be sympathetic to the problems of those around them. They are neat, orderly, meticulous; logical, analytical and reflective. They are only accepting of authority if the person in authority is more competent than they are (which is something they rarely see). They enjoy moderation in all things and are reluctant to express opinions but, somehow, make excellent leaders anyway. An amazing thing to watch. They often exhibit great depths of kindness, honesty and integrity.

This is the cycle of coming death—the final death and all the little 'deaths' that change and moving on in life brings to each of us. Autumn is a season of closure but there need not be the grief of regret for the past. Rather this season should be about release and letting go. Resolve is the gift that comes after grief and should bring to us the recognition that we have the choice to move forward, taking with us the many blessings and lessons that we have learned from loss and the changes that have occurred in our lives.

This is the energy we often feel when we experience a death, a breakup with a friend, or other loss

Symptoms of imbalance:
Metal people are vulnerable to becoming overly serious, sinking into depression, and becoming dry and too restrained. They sometimes appear, or even are, aloof, and often try to cram more into each day than it can contain. The type of depression that out -of-balance metal people are prone to comes from the pressure they put on themselves to reach perfection. They often look forward to things in the future while ignoring things that need their attention today. They 'freeze in place' while they obsessively evaluate and re-evaluate a situation, looking for the right solution. Sometimes they struggle with patience, especially when others fail to 'live by the rules.'

Physical complaints: stiff joints and muscles; dry hair and skin; sensitive to climate and climate changes; poor circulation; acne; respiratory problems; cough

Maturity sometimes brings sadness for opportunities missed and for what must be left behind. There is also an understanding and a deep peace and acceptance of maturity and death. Metal people become wise and often become teachers who pass their knowledge along to others.

Balance restored by:
Metal is associated with dryness. Many of the imbalances of *Metal* people can be corrected with water—taking a drink or going for a swim or a soak.

Large Intestine

Blends: LeMillenia, LeWisdom, LeSanctuary

Singles: basil, cedarwood, cypress, sandalwood, elemi, myrrh, clove, fennel, frankincense, lavender, tea tree, bergamot, thyme, yarrow

Lung

Blends: LeBelieve, LeAspire, LeMillenia, LeTrust, LeSanctuary

Singles: peppermint, eucalyptus, frankincense, lavender, pine, birch, cajeput, clove, fennel,myrrh, bergamot, cardamom, tea tree, thyme, yarrow

Large Intestine **Feeling of confidence and self-worth or *feelings of guilt***
Lung **Humility and tolerance or *pride and intolerance***

Blends

LcMillenia	in this situation, this blend seems to be balancing the moisture and fluids in the body as well as finding an equilibrium between being organized, neat, orderly, meticulous, logical and analytical and being obsessively focused on perfection in themselves and in others; tolerance for other people's lack of neatness and orderliness
LcWisdom	in this cycle of impending change and/or death, LcWisdom helps us to maintain a firm presence in today and not become distraught over the pressures to be perfect or to be ready for tomorrow; helps one in overcoming resistance to change
LcSanctuary	helps us to see clearly our own strengths and weakness; aids us in developing wisdom and good judgement; makes it easier for us to replace fear with confidence, and guilt with forgiveness

Singles

basil	a good oil for burnout and exhaustion; helps to restore powers of concentration and feelings of joy; tempers a tendency to be too blunt or too insistent on 'doing it my way'
cedarwood	helps with tendencies to be dogmatic or self-righteous; move on from obsessively evaluating and re-evaluating everything to the point of doing nothing; helps to moderate obsessive tendencies
cypress	for those who have become unbending or fixed in their attitudes and ideas or have a tendency to pride or arrogance; loosening of the purse strings and opening themselves to spending on things that are not absolute necessities
sandalwood	help 'dryer' personalities open to the pleasures and relaxations available in this life; acceptance of others; tempering of ego-centricities
frankincense	relieve feelings of bitterness, skepticism and cynicism; promotes a return of drive, forcefulness and the will to live; relief of anxiety attacks brought on by stress; this meridian is about forceful, alive, remarkably gifted people and frankincense is about returning to normal stability and effectiveness when stress has forced them over the edge to an imbalanced state
lavender	as always, promotes feelings of calm and a return of psychological harmony and balance, particularly a return to kindness and generosity from a place of judgement
pine	specific for moving on from regrets and self-judgement; relief from feeling that they are carrying the whole world on their shoulders every day; establishing a healthy respect for one's own needs and desires
yarrow	helps us keep heaven's view of who we can be in our minds and hearts, even while we are struggling with who we are in the here and now.
cardamom	allows us to see the endless possibilities and opportunities that are before us; reminds us of the abundance and blessings in our lives; helps us understand that we are of worth with many fine qualities

4 - Earth/Late Summer The Peacemaker

Stomach **Contentment, appreciation for what is or *disappointment, greed, never has enough***

Spleen **Happy anticipation of the future or *anxiety about the future, lack of faith and hope***

This is a season of transition between the extremes of summer and winter—and symbolizes the strength to stay stable while nurturing the changes that are happening around them or within them. Justice and fairness are important to earth people but they can be supportive and compassionate when others are struggling. They are able to bring a fresh perspective to the most mundane of situations and almost always give people a feeling of safety. Both their balanced and imbalanced states include putting the needs of others before their own, and being involved, or too involved, in other people's lives. They are loyal and always accessible to friends and relatives.

Because Earth holds within it all of the other elements, this meridian reflects the whole of the meridian cycles more than the other meridians do. Earth's wood facets control the shifts between yin and yang, or the masculine/feminine sides of our nature. Earth's fire elements create a balance which is the management of opposing forces. Energy out of balance creates heat but balanced energy produces a calm and peaceful atmosphere. Earth's wood attributes are about accumulating the nutrients and resources needed for growth and development later. This part of the *Earth* meridian is where money issues and imbalances occur. An interesting aspect of this meridian is the metal aspect in that when Earth has nourished others (which it is constantly doing) these resources are then lost to the Earth person. All things related to reproduction and birth, with the natural result of the child growing away and leaving the mother, are Earth element functions.

Any cycle of your life that is bringing change can fall into this category

Symptoms of Imbalance:
obsessive worry; lack of concentration; putting the needs of others too far ahead of own needs; over-protective or controlling; able to see other's mistakes and how to fix them but fail to see or grow from their own; will stay with a bad situation (marriage, dull job, etc) too long, co-dependence out of sympathy; accepts other people's assessments of themselves and their lives; relies too much on the skill and judgement of other people

Physical complaints: nausea, vomiting; canker sores; eating disorders, diabetes, menstrual pain

With maturity, exaggerated compassion ripens into a wise and balanced compassion along with a healthy sense of one's own worth.

Balance restored by:
Walking barefoot on the earth; lying on the earth; spending time alone or meditating; learning to value self and set boundaries for others.

Stomach

Blends: LeInside-Out, LeVision, LeBountiful, LeMillenia, LeSanctuary

Singles: fennel, ginger, patchouli, pine, dill, sage, hyssop, yarrow, ylang ylang, caraway, clove, coriander, frankincense, lavender, marjoram, myrh, neroli

Spleen

Blends: LeBelieve, LeEndo Relief, LeRevitalize, LeMillenia, LeSanctuary

Singles: anthopogon, lemongrass, orange sweet, chamomile German, chamomile Roman, tangerine, clary sage, cypress, eucalyptus, geranium, lavender, marjoram, cedar wood, grapefruit, rose, frankincense, myrrh, neroli, benzoin, cardamom, caraway, peppermint

Stomach **Contentment and appreciation for what is in one's life or**
disappointment, greed, feeling that there is never enough

Spleen **Happy anticipation of the future or**
anxiety about future, lack of faith and hope

Blends

LeInside-Out imbalance in these two meridians almost always brings about the types of obsessive worry that creates nausea, vomiting and eating disorders

LeVision ability to see and grow from mistakes and mis-perceptions; move past over-reliance on other people's opinions of them and their lives; learn to rely on own judgement and skill

LeBountiful this meridian is where money issues have residence and this blend can help ease the feeling that there is never enough for everybody to have what they need that creates greed and lack of faith in the future

LeMillenia clarity of mind about what is and what is not necessary for happiness and contentment

LeEndo Relief the endocrine system is easily thrown out of balance and depleted of energy—use this blend for strengthening the various organs and re-establishing the boundaries between ourselves and others; allows us to be both tactful and firm about our boundaries

LeRevitalize this meridian is especially prone to depletion from serving and doing for others. This blend helps to replenish inner stores of strength; also increases mental alertness and alleviates mental fatigue

Singles

fennel believed to bestow strength and courage; establishes a balance between appropriate service to others and service to the point of exhaustion and burnout; a stomach herb and oil

ginger another good stomach tonic herb but more appropriate to the usually fiery and dynamic soul who has lost all drive and has become confused, apathetic and without direction; for a particular type of profound sadness that is not depression but rather the opposite of warmth and connection with others

patchouli usually well-grounded, strong personalities, the person in need of patchouli is unaccustomed to paying attention to his health and has ignored it to the point of collapse, mentally and physically from 'burning the candle on both ends' for too long

pine relief from trying to fix everyone's problems day in and day out; help establish a healthy respect for one's own needs and desires, including the need to rest and rejuvenate

dill affinity for the pancreas; helps control glucose and insulin levels and keep energy on a even plane—no spikes that are followed by lows; calming to the autonomic nervous system

sage deeply supportive of all pelvic organs and functions

lemongrass aids those who too often put other's need before their own; depletion when all of our internal resources have been given away or squandered; deep compassion

sweet orange encourages escape from patterns of emotional and physical abuse; helps to reestablish optimism and a sense of humor when they have become lost

chamomile the deep, emotionally strong blue chamomile personality, when out of balance, is prone German to dark moods, periods of indifference, and outbursts directed at those nearest to them— use this oil, or a blend it contains, to subdue these tendencies

clary sage for those with a tendency, when tired, to be hypersensitive and find fault with others; also for those whose pattern has been to chose the wrong friends and companions

5 - 6 Fire/Season of Summer The Wizard

This season has four meridians associated with it, the first two of which are protective in nature

Triple Warmer	**Protection of the physical body**
	Feelings of lightness and hope or *feelings of heaviness and depression*
Pericardium	**Protector of the heart and emotions**
	Open & peaceful in relationships or *withdrawal into anger and hurt*

The ***Triple Warmer*** is closely associated with the immune system and protects the entire body from external threats. It gauges everything from the temperature of the room to the safety of the building that we are entering or standing in. Triple Warmer governs those 'feelings' or 'inspirations' that we get concerning external events such as what is happening with our children or to the economy or in politics.

This meridian is responsible for the distribution of water in the cells and tissues of the body. It energetically connects all the organs to each other and distributes energy among them. Some suggest that the Triple Warmer has a correspondence to the connective tissue that wraps every organ, every vessel, and every muscle, tendon, and nerve in the body. This connective tissue has been shown to conduct bioelectricity.

Because the heart, of necessity, must be open and able to feel both joy and sorrow, the body has provided a strong defense for it. It is called by several different names in different cultures; here we will call it the ***pericardium*** because the physical pericardium is the sack that surrounds and protects the heart.

The heart protector, or pericardium, considers its job to be to protect the heart from unexpected hurt and violation. It evaluates every person, remark, or action for potential to harm the heart. An important part of this function is providing us with an evaluation about the trustworthiness of the people around us. The pericardium allows us to be open only with those who have demonstrated themselves to be responsible and gentle. Apology and forgiveness are Heart activities but it is the *Heart Protector* meridian that signals us that we need to apologize or that it will be safe to accept another's apology. The *Heart Protector* meridian, or *Pericardium* (as it is sometimes called), also keeps us from being overwhelmed by the thousands of signals that other people are sending out about themselves all the time.

When in balance these two meridians help us feel hope and a lightness of spirit and body. We can delight in physical and emotional intimacy and feel safe enough to be open and vulnerable with close loved ones.

Symptoms of imbalance:

If there is too much energy in this meridian, there is often unrealistic expectations of others that are rarely met and when their joy and enthusiasm for a project fail to bring about the desired results they sink into hopelessness and despair. On the other hand, deficiency in this area can lead to withdrawal into anger and hurt, deceit and mistrust in relationships, depression and despair because people cannot be 'trusted' or because of a feeling that relationships always 'go sour.'

Triple Warmer

Blends: LeBelieve, LeBountiful, LeMillenia, LeReconciliation, LeSanctuary, LeTurmoil, LeWisdom
Singles: eucalyptus, frankincense, lavender, jasmine, melissa, sandalwood, aniseseed, anthopogon, clove, coriander, grapefruit, neroli, tea tree

Pericardium

Blends: LeAngel, LeBelieve, LeBountiful, LeDreams, LeKadence, LeMillenia, LeReconciliation,
Singles: black pepper, frankincense, ylang-ylang, basil, clove, lavender, melissa, neroli, tea tree, anthopogon, coriander

Triple Warmer **Protection of the physical body**
Feelings of lightness and hope or
feelings of heaviness and depression

Pericardium **Protector of the heart and emotions**
Open & peaceful in relationships or
withdrawal into anger and hurt

Blends

LeBelieve balances the need to protect, that is characteristic of this meridian, with trust in the future and forgiveness of the past

LeMillenia maintains or re-establishes the integrity of the connective tissues that wrap, connect and protect every organ and emotion; courage to pick oneself up, make amends and move on when mistakes have been made

LeTurmoil treatment for shock and trauma to body or soul; remedy for both the wounded warrior and the wounded healer; helps us view trials from the perspective of learning

LeWisdom recovery from the losses sustained in spite of Triple Warmer's valiant efforts to protect us from every emotional or physical trauma

LeAngel aids in the release of traumatic memories and the anger and helplessness felt when Triple Warmer was unable to protect us because we were simply too young and vulnerable to change the situation

LeBountiful immune stimulant; promotes feelings of abundance and protection; strengthens the energy fields that surround us, bringing abundance and joy into our lives

LeDreams an over-active heart protector (pericardium) meridian can lead to bad dreams and insomnia, especially in children or fear things they cannot see in the dark; use this oil to release pent-up emotions, resentments and fears from the sub-conscious

Singles

eucalyptus while doing its job of watching out for things that might hurt the emotional heart, the heart protector sometimes stores resentments and remembrances of slights and insults; these need to be released calmly, without an explosion of temper or hostility

frankincense return to a state of generosity, warm-heartedness and equanimity from one of bitterness and recrimination; recovery from anxiety attacks and stress related behavior patterns

black pepper increase cellular oxygenation; help maintain stamina and energy; find empathy and compassion for others; more realistic expectations of others

ylang ylang insecurity; dare-devil tendencies; temper tantrums thrown with the intent of getting their own way; sudden loss of interest in work, appearance or family members

anthopogon pulls us into a mood of remembering, but with the blessing of a focus on the good times and the good in people; helps us find perspective and forgiveness in our relationships

neroli changes a negative outlook and brings us renewed hope; neroli is one of the best oils for people who are timid or who have withdrawn from people because they have been hurt emotionally; it can help alleviate feelings of "nothing changes, nothing ever will" when things really are changing and that emotion no longer fits the situation

grapefruit addresses the emotional issues of self-worth and discontent with one's body; alleviates the depression that is often the result of aiming too high in your expectations of yourself and others; frustration often leads to blame and grapefruit alleviates these feelings

Small Intestine **Feelings of great joy or *feelings of deep sorrow***
Heart **Feelings of love and forgiveness, with miracles in your life or *anger and judgement***

Summer meridian people enjoy the present and bask in its warmth. Their voice is often full of laughter and they have a characteristic up and down movement to their walk, with their arms rising and falling. Called 'The Wizard' because this is the dynamic personality that is often a catalyst for miracles. Just as in cooking, fire alters the properties of anything to which it is applied—hopefully, improving them. Fire is the stage of peak power and maximum activity and productivity.

The ***Small Intestine,*** as an energetic meridian, separates truth from untruth. It sorts beliefs and precepts, discerning which to hold onto in our hearts and which to discard as unworthy or untrue.

When the heart and small intestine meridians are working properly, S*ummer* people are warm, empathetic, joyful and exuberant. They have a great deal of charisma, relish excitement, love drama and sentiment (chick-flicks.) They are animated, enthusiastic, organized, liking to categorize and consolidate things into piles. The most extroverted of the rhythms and also the most principle driven. They are often faithful throughout life to a particular belief system, holding every aspect of their lives to its standard and measure.

Adolescence is the first major cycle of summer's rhythm

Desire is one of the marks of a Fire phase and teenagers are absolutely driven by their desires: for independence, for someone who understands them, for peace and social justice, for love, for knowledge, and especially for freedom and for the understanding of all the mysteries of life.

Symptoms of imbalance:
Fire is explosive; there is little room for error because they are already at maximum, right to the edge, 'playing with fire.' They rarely recognize dangerous or negative situations. Fire must 'burn something up' to keep itself going. Out of balance *Fire* people can draw energy from those around them, to the detriment of others. They often burn themselves out because they are over-committed.

Physical complaints: blood pressure problems; heart disease; insomnia; night sweats; Pollyanna optimism often followed by the despair of burnout.

Balance restored by:
Exercise; expressing himself at great length to others; playing, having fun; being creative; learning to set priorities and limits

Maturity should bring compassion, patience with others, stability and the outstanding characteristic of deep love for their spouse and family. Balanced people with these meridian strengths are often able to look at all sides of a situation quickly and accurately. They have deep faith and communicate easily with the Spirit. They possess the absolute knowledge that God exists.

Small Intestine **Joy/Sorrow**
Blends: LeBelieve, LeInner Peace, LeMillenia, LeUnity, LeReconciliation, LeSego Lily
Singles: Peppermint, Rosemary, Ginger, anthopogon, clove, coriander, frankincense, lavender, melissa, tea tree

Heart **Love-Patience/Anger-Resentment**
Blends: LeBelieve, LeBeloved LeDiscernment, LeHeart Song, LeMillenia, LeKadence, LeReconciliation, LeWisdom, LeSanctuary
Singles: thyme, frankincense, rosemary, myrtle, spruce, cedarwood, hyssop, clove, lavender, anthopogon, coriander

Small Intestine **Feelings of great joy or** ***feelings of deep sorrow***
Heart **Feelings of love and forgiveness or** ***feelings of anger and judgement***

Blends

LeBelieve	the perfect blend for replacing negative feelings with love, forgiveness, peace and understanding; returns the heart to a state of joyous anticipation of the rest of life
LeInner Peace	promotes harmony between ourselves and others; helps us stay focused on the direction we would like our life to be going in; like LeBenediction, LeInner Peace protects our minds and bodies from attacks upon and depletion of our energy resources
LeMillenia	always a good choice for restoring joy, faith, courage and perspective to our lives and energy and well-being to our bodies
LeUnity	affinity for and strengthening to every chakra; promotes emotional balance and spiritual growth
LeBeloved	a beautiful oil for healing relationships—even our relationship to God; helps us to respond to others generously from our 'whole' heart
LeDiscernment	helps us discover the path that is most likely to bring us happiness and contentment; promotes faith in the future and helps us achieve our goals and dreams
LeHeart Song	a very effective, high-frequency blend for reminding us that we are loved and cherished by many; a remedy for deep sorrow and depression; use with LeUnity to overcome blockages to loving and being loved in return
LeSego Lily	A simple, delightful smelling blend. LeSego Lily smells nice enough to wear as perfume anywhere. It promotes feelings of being loved and appreciated and inspires us to show love and appreciation for others
LeWisdom	The high floral notes of ylang ylang and neroli, which help connect us to our spiritual center and divine source, are blended with the grounding and protecting forces of spruce. This mixture is then modulated by the optimism of orange sweet and the clarity, strength and direction of lemon. This blend is amazing for helping us move from anger and judgement to love and forgiveness

Singles

thyme	not often used in emotional work, but effective for protecting the heart
frankincense	has a specific place for those needing a new way to look at an old situation; helpful when there is intellectual or physical exhaustion and a lack of direction
rosemary	balanced rosemary people are vibrant, happy, sensitive, industrious people. Use this oil to revive these qualities when they have become lost due to perceived hurts or injustices. Rosemary people rarely suffer from or become imbalanced because of overwork, because they have aa great capacity to organize and they move quickly from project to project
ginger	appropriate to the usually fiery and dynamic soul who has lost all drive and has become confused, apathetic and without direction; for a particular type of profound sadness that is not depression but rather the opposite of warmth and connection with others
peppermint	specific to those who struggle between highs and lows, sadness and happiness until the ever-widening mood swings settle into lethargy, intolerance and frustration; before the apathy sets in, people needing peppermint were almost fearless, loving bright colors, able to think quickly and always alert to the opportunities of life
anthopogon	remembering the good times and the good in people
coriander	helps us find contentment in situations that are routine or predictable; helps us overcome any fear of failure that we may have

Essential Oils for Specific Chakras:

Root (or Base) Chakra : Balanced-Harmonious/Victim Mentality

Blends: LeBelieve, LeConnection, LeMillenia, LeMeditation, LeMoonlight, LeUnity, LePatches, LeVitality, LeAngel, LeSanctuary

Singles: cedarwood, black pepper, chamomile Egyptian (absolute), cinnamon, clove, fir siberica, frankincense, myrrh, sandalwood, tea tree, thyme, ginger, frankincense, lavender

Sacral (or Navel) Chakra: Serenity-Self Awareness/Martyr-Loss of self to others

Blends: LeAcknowledge, LeBelieve, LeMoonlight, LeSanctuary, LeUnity, LePatches, LeWisdom, LeAngel, LeMillenia

Singles: cedarwood, clary sage, cinnamon bark and berry, fennel, ylang ylang, coriander, zanthoxylum, tamala, nutmeg, tea tree, orange sweet, oregano, patchouli, sage, sandalwood, frankincense

Solar Plexus Chakra: Self worth-Confidence/Low self esteem-Easily manipulated

Blends: LeAssurance, LeBelieve, LeConnection, LeCrystal Clear, LeMagi, LeAngel, LeEnergy, LePatches, LeUnity, LeMillenia, LeSanctuary

Singles: cedarwood, sandalwood, cypress, lavender, rosemary, palmarosa, clove, fir balsam, geranium, fir siberica, frankincense, rose geranium, lemon, lemongrass, spruce, black pepper, chamomile German, blue tansy

Heart Chakra: Love-Compassion/Resentment-Judgement

Blends: LeAcknowledge, LeBelieve, LeBeloved, LeBaby Me, LeDiscernment, LeEnergy, LeFaith, LeMillenia LeHeart Song, LeInner Peace, LeKadence, LeMoonlight, LePatches, LeSego Lily, LeSolitude, LeUnity, LeExpressions, LeAngel, LeSanctuary, LeReconciliation, LeWake-Up

Singles: cedarwood, rose, frankincense, myrtle, palmarosa, rose geranium, fir balsam, fir siberica, geranium, grapefruit, sandalwood, ylang ylang, jasmine, lavender, anthopogon, bergamot, chamomile German

Throat Chakra: Sincerity-Clear Communication/Suppression of Feelings

Blends: LeAcknowledge, LeAngel, LeBelieve, LeBenediction, LeDreams, LeExpressions, LeFaith, LeUnity, LeGood-Nite, LeHeart Song, LeKadence, LeMeditation, LePatches, LeSanctuary, LeUnity, LeWisdom, LeMillenia

Singles: cedarwood, helichrysum, myrrh, sage, cypress, fir siberica, frankincense, peppermint, petitgrain, rosewood, sandalwood, basil, chamomile Egyptian, chamomile German, chamomile Roman

Brow Chakra: Intuitive (balanced analytical & creative)/Over Intellectualization

Blends: LeAngel, LeBelieve, LeCrystal Clear, LeDiscernment, LeDreams, LeHeart Song, LeKadence, LeMeditation, LeMillenia, LePatches, LeSanctuary, LeUnity

Singles: cedarwood, rose geranium, juniper, angelica, melissa, ravensara, spruce, fir siberica, sandalwood, litsea cubeba, pine needle, tea tree, frankincense

Crown Chakra: Balance in all Chakras
Light, Compassion & Spirituality/Proud, Arrogant, Self-Important

Blends: LeAngel, LEBelieve, LeBenediction, LeDiscernment, LeDreams, LeHeart Song, LeMagi, LeMeditation, LeMillenia, LePatches, LeReconciliation, LeSanctuary, LeUnity, LeVitality, LeWisdom

Singles: cedarwood, jasmine, pine, melissa, neroli, spikenard, anthopogon, fir siberica, frankincense, lavender, sandalwood

LeUnity, LeMillenia, LeBelieve, LePatches, LeSanctuary, and LeAngel bring all the chakras and meridians into balance. LePatches seems to heal the broken places in both the chakras and meridians.

Essential Oils For Various Emotions

(Based on anecdotal experience and traditional usage)

The cells of our bodies are all participants in a very sophisticated communication network. Interleukins, interferons, and lymphokines are types of messenger cells whose communications manage our immune systems. Interleukin 2 has been identified as the messenger cells that our bodies use to instruct the immune system on how to recognize cancer cells and other enemies of our physical well being. Without sufficient and well-functioning interleukin 2 cells, our phagocytes, B-cells, and T-cells, which would normally attack and kill abnormal cells like cancers, will misjudge them as friendly and allow them to live and multiply.

Interleukin 2 levels are reduced with overproduction of cortisol, a necessary steroid hormone that regulates many bodily functions. Having the right amount of cortisol is healthy, but too much can lead to sickness and even death.

A variety of emotional and spiritual factors have been shown to result in the overproduction of cortisol and the reduction of interleukin 2. These emotions include chronic anger, fear, anxiety, bitterness, and resentment. Negative attitudes such as lack of forgiveness, desire for revenge, repressed rage, a poor self image, inability to deal with a significant loss or trauma, and unrelieved stress around any issue can set up conditions favorable to the growth of cancer cells.

With a properly functioning immune system, it is impossible for cancer to take hold and grow. We have been given a certain amount of control over our immune systems by how we think, feel, and live. The molecular and cellular activities in our bodies may be chemical in nature, but much of the control of that chemistry is ultimately in the spiritual nature of our lifestyles.

Because of the ability of essential oils to help us release emotions, they can be of great assistance in getting to whatever emotional or spiritual roots our diseases and discomforts have. Do essential oils change our personalities or even our emotions? Of course not. But they seem to mitigate some of the power of these emotions and give us a little extra space in which to look more realistically or more creatively at our lives. Solutions seem to present themselves in the pause provided by the aroma of the oil. I can't explain it to you. I can only say that I have experienced it myself and seen it in others.

Ability to Let Go: LeBelieve, LeLetting Go, LeTranquility, coriander, lemon, peppermint, pine

Abandonment (fear of): LeFaith, lavender

Abundance: LeBountiful, LeAcknowledge LeUnity, cardamom, myrrh, patchouli

Abuse (all/any): LeAngel, LeBeloved, LeAbuse

Acceptance (of love): LeAngel, LeBelieve, LeBeloved ,LeTrust, LeFaith, pine, rose, chamomile Roman, melissa

Acceptance (of self): LeBelieve, LeBeloved, LeInner Peace, LeFaith, LeLetting Go, peppermint, cypress, helichrysum, petitgrain

Acceptance (of change): LeBelieve, LeBeloved, LeFaith, LeInner Peace, LeTranquility, grapefruit, helichrysum, geranium, lemon

Alertness: LeIQ, LeCrystal Clear, grapefruit, lavender, thyme, bergamot, black pepper, cinnamon, coriander, eucalyptus, juniper, lime, peppermint, petigrain, pine, rosemary

Alone (fear of being): LeGood-Nite, LeInner Peace, LeMagi, LeWhispering Hope

Anger: LeAngel, LeExpressions, LeInsight, LeLetting Go, LeRevitalize, LeTranquility, LeTrust, LeTurmoil, LeUnity, LeWisdom

Anxiety: LeAngel, LeAssurance, LeEZ-Traveler, LeGood-Nite, LeHeart Song, LeTranquility, LeTrust, LeSego Lily, LeSolitude, LeVision

Apathy: LeAssurance, LeBelieve , LeIQ, LeVision

Appreciation: LeMoonlight, LeConnection, LeTrust, LeReconciliation, LeUnity, LeSego Lily (feeling appreciated)

Arrogance: LeDiscernment, LeReconciliation, LeVision, LeTrust, LeLetting Go

Assertion: LeMillenia, LeVitality, jasmine, fennel, basil, cedarwood, cypress, frankincense, ginger, patchouli, bergamot, ylang ylang, black pepper, coriander, lime, litsea cubeba

Awareness (self): LeSanctuary, grapefruit, lemon, jasmine, lavender, rosemary, helichrysum.

Awareness: (spiritual): LeBelieve, LeInner Peace, LeSanctuary, LeVision, LeReconciliation, chamomile Roman, neroli, frankincense, juniper, rose

Baby Blues: LeBaby Me, LeReconciliation

Balanced (emotionally): LeConnection, LeHeart Song, LeTranquility, LeBelieve, LeReconciliation, LeUnity, lavender, lemon, rose, cedarwood, orange sweet, mandarin, sandalwood

Benevolence: LeBountiful, LeGrateful Heart, LeReconciliation, cinnamon, benzoin, patchouli, lavender.

Bonding: LeBaby Me, LeMoonlight

Calming (general): LeBelieve, LeEZ-Traveler, LeGood-Nite, LeTranquility, LeHeart Song, LeInsight, LeMeditation, LePaine, lavender, melissa and melissa blend

Calmness: LeBelieve,LeGood-Nite, LeUnity, LeAssurance, LeSanctuary, LeSego Lily, LeTomorrow, chamomile German, chamomile Roman, clary sage, rose, helichrysum, lemon, mandarin, marjoram, neroli, ylang ylang, frankincense

Cellular Memory: LeInsight, LeLetting Go.

Changes (going through): LeMillenia, LeTomorrow, cypress, cedarwood, rosemary, lemon

Clarity: LeMeditation, LeMillenia, LeUnity, basil, fennel, grapefruit, lavender, lemon, rosemary

Clarity (of thought): LeCrystal Clear, lemon, rosemary, basil, clove, petitgrain

Co-dependency: LeTrust, LeReconciliation, sandalwood

Comforting: LeBelieve, LeBaby Me, LeGood-Nite, LeInner Peace, LeMagi, LeSanctuary, cedarwood, chamomile Roman, cypress, frankincense, geranium, marjoram, rose, lavender, sandalwood, melissa

Communication: LeConnection, LeTrust, LeReconciliation, LeUnity, geranium, chamomile German, grapefruit, peppermint, lemon

Compassionate: LeBelieve, LeMeditation, LeTrust, LeUnity, LeGrateful Heart, chamomile German, chamomile Roman, lavender, rose, neroli, pine, cypress, melissa

Competence: LeBaby Me

Concentration: LeCrystal Clear,Le Focus, LeIQ, LeWake-Up, peppermint, rosemary, cedarwood, eucalyptus, lemon, thyme

Confidence: LeBeloved, LeMillenia, LeWisdom, LeBreezey, LeExhilaration, LeTranquility, LeWhispering Hope, bergamot, cedarwood, clary sage, coriander,

cypress, fennel, ginger, grapefruit, jasmine, ylang ylang, marjoram, pine, petitgrain, rose, rosemary

Conflict (fear of conflict): LeEZ-Traveler, LeMillenia.

Confusion: LeCrystal Clear, LeFocus, LeIQ, ginger, rosemary, benzoin, cinnamon, clove, marjoram, lavender

Consoling: LeBelieve, LeMillenia, LeSanctuary, chamomile Roman, cypress, benzoin, melissa, melissa blend, rose, geranium

Contentment: LeBelieve, LeSanctuary, LeTranquility, cypress, rose, lavender, neroli, bergamot,

orange sweet, sandalwood, patchouli, ylang ylang, chamomile Roman, clove

Cooperation: LeBelieve, LeBeloved, LeUnity, chamomile Roman, grapefruit, rose, jasmine, ylang ylang

Coping: (inability to) LeBeloved, LeEZ-Traveler, LeMillenia

Courage: LeEZ-Traveler, LeMillenia, LeExhilaration, frankincense, marjoram, cedarwood, orange sweet, thyme

Decisiveness: LeConnection, LeMillenia, LeVision, LeWake-Up, LeEnergy, basil, thyme, cedarwood, patchouli, peppermint

Dependence: (fear of) LeBountiful, LeTrust, LeReconciliation, peppermint

Depression: LeBelieve. LeBeloved, LeHeart Song, LeTurmoil, LeAcknowledge, LeBaby Me, LeUnity, LeMeditation, LeTranquility, LeLetting Go, LeSego Lily, LeSolitude, LeGrateful Heart, LeMy-graine, mandarin, rose, bergamot, orange sweet, ylang ylang, rose, geranium, lavender, chamomile Roman, lemon, jasmine, neroli, sandalwood, marjoram, frankincense, ravensara, rosewood

Dreams: LeDreams, LeExhillaration, LeGood-Nite, helichrysum, cedarwood

Emotional baggage (releasing): LeLetting Go, LeTrust, LeBelieve, LeInner Peace, LeReconciliation, LeTomorrow, LeUnity, LeVision, LeWhispering Hope, LeWisdom

Empathetic: LeGrateful Heart, LeUnity, LeReconciliation, chamomile Roman, lavender, melissa and melissa blend

Energizing: LeBountiful, LeEnergy, LeRevitalize, LeVitality, LeWake-Up, orange sweet, pine,

thyme, basil, peppermint, rosemary, cinnamon, eucalyptus, grapefruit, helichrysum

Energy Work: LeBenediction, LeMagi

Energy Protection: LeBenediction

Enthusiasm: LeMillenia, LeVitality, LeWake-Up, orange sweet, jasmine, lemon, grapefruit,

ylang ylang, coriander, geranium, melissa and melissa blend

Exhaustion: (Physical) LeAspire, LeEnergy, LeEndo Relief, LeWake-Up

Expressing Needs: LeBenediction, LeMillenia,

Faith: LeBelieve, LeFaith, LeSanctuary, LeDiscernment, frankincense, spikenard, juniper, coriander,

chamomile Roman, neroli

Fear: LeAssurance, LeFaith (abandoment, poverty), LeMagi, LeWisdom

Flexibility: LeInsight, LeMillenia, LeTomorrow, geranium, lavender, clary sage, lemon, myrtle, ylang ylang

Forgiving: LeBelieve, LeTrust, LeTomorrow, pine, rose, neroli, chamomile Roman, spikenard

Fortitude: LeBeloved, LeEZ-Traveler, LeMillenia, cedarwood, frankincense, rosemary, thyme

Frustration: LeAcknowledge, LeDiscernment, LeTranquility, LeLetting Go, LeWisdom

Future (looking forward to with joy): LeTomorrow, LeTrust, LeWhispering Hope, LeExpressions, LeFaith, LeMillenia, LeVision, LeWake-Up, LeVitality, LeKadence

Generosity: LeBelieve, LeBountiful, LeReconciliation, LeTrust, grapefruit, benzoin, nutmeg, cinnamon, sandalwood, melissa and melissa blend, lavender, geranium

Gratitude: LeBenediction, LeFaith, LeGrateful, Heart

Grief: LeBelieve, LeHeart Song, LeTrust, LeBaby Me, LeWhispering Hope, LeWisdom, LeLetting Go, LeSanctuary, LeMagi, LeMillenia, LeBenediction, LeReconciliation, LeTurmoil, lavender, chamomile Roman, rose, rose geranium, palarosa, orange sweet, clementine, anthopogon,

Healing (desire to): LeFaith, LeReconciliation, LeMillenia, LePatches

Humility: LeFaith, LeTrust, LeUnity, juniper, pine, chamomile Roman & chamomile German, melissa and melissa blend, neroli

Independence: LeLetting Go, LeMillenia, LeWake-Up, geranium, clary sage, lemon, grapefruit, peppermint

Inner Strength: LeBelieve, LeBeloved, LeEZ-Traveler, LeMillenia, LeTranquility, LeUnity, LeVision helichrysum, geranium, chamomile Roman, melissa

Intuition: LeBelieve, LeInsight, LeSanctuary, LeVision, LeInsight, LeMagi, jasmine, neroli

Irritability: LeWisdom, LeLetting Go, LeWoman Wise, LeBenediction, LeConnection, LeUnity, LeReconciliation, LeExpressions, LeInner Peace, LeInsight, LeLetting Go, LeMillenia, LeMoonlight, LeTranquility

Jealousy: LeUnity, LeLetting Go, LeKadence, LeTrust

Joy: LeUnity, LeWhispering Hope, LeTomorrow, bergamot, lemon, neroli, orange sweet, rose, sandalwood, frankincense, ylang ylang, chamomile Roman, grapefruit, jasmine, helichrysum

Journaling: LeConnection

Judging, Judgemental: LeUnity, LeLetting Go, LeKadence, LeTrust

Leadership: LeDiscernment, LeUnity, LeIQ, LeTomorrow

Limbic System: LeDiscernment, LeMillenia

Loneliness: LeBelieve, LeBenediction, LeGood-Nite, LeMagi, LeReconciliation,

Love Oneself: LeBelieve

Loved (feeling): LeAngel, LeSego Lily

Meditation: LeConnection, LeDreams, LeMeditation

Memories (traumatic): LeAngel, LeReconciliation

Memory: (improve) LeCrystal Clear, Le IQ, LeWake-Up, coriander, lemon, rosemary, peppermint

Mood: LeBeloved, LeBountiful, LeEverlasting, LeTenda Care

Mood Swings: LeAngel, LeBalance, LeBeloved, LeBountiful, LeHeart Song,LeTomorrow, LeWoman Wise

Motivating: LeAssurance, LeBelieve, LeMeditation, coriander, lavender, clove, rosemary, grapefruit, lemon, pine, cypress, bergamot, black pepper

Negative Emotions (cellular level): LeBelieve, LeLetting Go LeDiscernment, LeEverlasting, LeFocus (patterns), LeReconciliation

Nightmares: LeDreams

Non-acceptance of a pregnancy: LeWhispering Hope

Optimism: LeBelieve, LeEnergy, LeMillenia, LeEverlasting, LeWhispering Hope, coriander, jasmine, petitgrain

Organized: LeInsight, LeTurmoil, LeConnection, LeMillenia, chamomile German, cedarwood, peppermint, lemon

Overwhelmed: LeWhispering Hope

Quarrelsome: LeUnity

Parent/Child Relationships: LeBaby Me, LeReconciliation,

Patience: LeTranquility, LeUnity, LeTranquility, chamomile German, cypress, pine, helichrysum, rose

Peace (in the home or office): LeUnity

Peaceful: LeBelieve, LeGood-Nite, LeTranquility, LeTrust, LeUnity, LeReconciliation, LeSanctuary, LeSego Lily, LeSolitude, LeWhispering Hope, mandarin, melissa, sandalwood, neroli, chamomile German, chamomile Roman

Perspective: LeReconciliation, LeBountifu, LeDiscernment, LeExpressions, LeFaith, LeGrateful Heart, LeHoliday Spirit, LeLetting Go, LeMillenia, LeTranquility, LeVision

Pride: LeDiscernment, LeReconciliation, LeLetting Go, LeUnity

Problem solving: LeExhillaration

Procrastination: LeBelieve, LeAssurance, LeAcknowledge

Rebellion: LeLetting Go, LeTranquility, birch

Relationships: LeBeloved, LeExpressions, LeHoliday Spirit, LeReconciliation, LeMoonlight (romantic)

Relaxation: LeEverlasting, LeGrateful Heart, LeSunburst, LeBaby Me, LeDreams, LeExpressions, LeHeart Song, LeGrateful Heart, LeInner Peace, LeInsight, LeLetting Go, LeSanctuary, LeSego Lily, LeSolitude, LeTranquility, LeUnity, LeWhispering Hope

Release Emotions: LeBelieve, LeReconciliation,

Resentment: LeLetting Go, LeReconciliation,

Safe: LeAngel, LeLetting Go, LeSanctuary

Security: LeBountiful, LeHoliday Spirit, LeReconciliation, LeLetting Go, LeWhispering Hope,

Self confidence: LeAssurance, LeFaith, LeVision

Self-esteem: LeBelieve, LeMagi, LeSanctuary, LeInner Peace, LeMagi, sandalwood, ylang ylang, rose, vetiver, jasmine, bergamot, geranium, cedarwood

Self-forgiveness: LeBelieve, LeLetting Go, LeSolitude, chamomile Roman, frankincense, geranium

Self-worth: LeBelieve, LeBeloved, LeBreezey, LeMillenia, LeFaith, LeVision, juniper, rose, mandarin, orange sweet, patchouli

Serenity: LeBelieve, LeLetting Go, LeSolitude, chamomile Roman, sandalwood

Soothing: LeBelieve, LeBaby Me, LeInner Peace, LeMagi, LeSanctuary, LeSolitude, LeTranquility, LeWhispering Hope, LeUnity, chamomile German, chamomile Roman, jasmine, patchouli

Stamina: LeVitality, LeWake-Up, LeRevitalize, black pepper, cinnamon

Stubborness: LeUnity,, LeReconciliation, LeLetting Go, LeVision

Studying: LeCrystal Clear, LeFocus, LeIQ, rosemary, laurel, peppermint

If restless, easily distracted: frankincense, geranium

Forgets what was read: pine, lemon, rosemary

Sympathetic: LeBelieve, LeTrust, LeUnity, LeReconciliation, mandarin, orange sweet, geranium, rose, rosewood

Tenacity: LeBelieve, LeMillenia, pine

Tenderness: LeBelieve, LeGrateful Heart, LeUnity, rose, mandarin, benzoin

Thankfulness: LeBountiful

Tolerant: LeBelieve, LeGrateful Heart, LeLetting Go, LeTrust, LeReconciliation, thyme, peppermint, frankincense, clary sage, lavender, marjoram

Trauma: LeHeart Song, LeTurmoil, LeRevitalize LeAssurance, LeTrust, LeLetting Go, LeLife Force, LeMillenia, LeSanctuary, LeWhispering Hope, LeTurmoil

Traumatic Memories: LeAngel, LeReconciliation,

Trust: LeBelieve, LeBeloved, LeTrust, LeLetting Go, LeDiscernment, LeSanctuary, basil, cypress, lavender

Understanding: LeBelieve, LeTranquility, LeUnity, chamomile Roman, chamomile German, cypress, neroli, pine

Uplifting: LeHeart Song, LeMillenia, LeSanctuary, LeTomorrow, clary sage, grapefruit, jasmine, juniper, mandarin, orange sweet, petitgrain, ylang ylang

Vitality: LeRevitalize, LeVitality, juniper, peppermint

Victim: (consciousness): LeFocus, LeReconciliation

Willpower: LeEz-Traveler, LeVision, cypress

Wisdom: LeSanctuary, LeTomorrow, LeWisdom, LeReconciliation, frankincense, rose, cypress, sandalwood

Worry: LeBelieve, LeBountiful, LeEZ-Traveler, LeFaith, LeKadence

Essential Oils
for Women, Pregnancy, Childbirth and Children of All Ages

Women have always played a central role in the care and nurture of others. Caring for the sick was one of the most important domestic skills that was passed from one generation of women to the next. Caring for others seems to be an innate gift of femininity that can bless our lives and the lives of those around us. It is our role as women to create new life and then to protect and bless those lives in every way that we can. It seems to come naturally to most women to put the needs of others first, even at the expense of their own health. There is much to be learned in the world of essential oils about service and honoring oneself and the balance between the two. The fact is that a woman must care for herself if she is to have the strength and energy to give as much as she wants to the others that are so dear to her.

Many of the normal functions of a woman's body, such as menstruation and pregnancy, have been treated for too long as abnormal or just plain dirty/evil. This is changing in our time as more women learn about how their bodies and minds work and take responsibility for their own physical and emotional health.

Nevertheless, and not withstanding that these are normal functions, they can take a heavy toll on a woman's energy and general health. The bearing of and caring for children, while enormously rewarding, is an enormous task. The demands of our fast-paced society, in which many women juggle family life and work, while often times rewarding and exciting, only adds to the daily stress. As women, we sometimes add to our own stress by negative feelings about our physical selves and overemphasizing the importance of the outer self while ignoring our own inner beauty and wisdom.

Essential oils, like other aspects of natural health care, can make a significant difference in the lives of modern women and their families in caring for both emotional, spiritual and physical needs.

Out of balance hormones can affect every aspect of a woman's existence. They affect her reserves of physical energy, general sense of well-being, emotional and spiritual state, efficiency and ability to concentrate and even the kind of wife and mother that she will be.

Puberty—moving into womanhood

Adolescence is a time of great physical change as well as a period of intense intellectual and emotional development. The young woman is often struggling to find her own personal balance between independence and staying safely close to her support systems. She is trying to find a balance between her parent's advice, her own inner voice, and the clamor of her peer group.

Energetically, this is the cycle of *Spring* energy and a comparison with the 'terrible twos' is not that far off the mark. Many of the same essential oils that are recommended in Chapter 11 page 5 are appropriate here, with the addition of those that are specifically appropriate to hormone balance and the emerging attitudes and attributes of womanhood.

A balanced gallbladder and liver meridian system is essential here but, often, the diet of the teen-age girl is far less than adequate to her needs. As an incentive to your teen-age daughter to eat better, you might point out that a compromised gallbladder causes fats to accumulate in the bloodstream and in the tissues—usually exactly where they don't want extra fat.

The out-of-balance emotional aspects of this phase include the things that all parents dread—sudden swings from a delightful little girl to an angry, annoyed, rebellious, sassy, weepy, over-sensitive 'almost woman.'

Recommended essential oils:

Emotional	LeBelieve, LeMillenia, LeWhispering Hope, LeTranquility, LeUnity, LeAngel, LeLetting Go, LeAcknowledge, orange sweet, sandalwood, vanilla
Hormone	LeWoman Wise and/or LeEndo Relief, frequently, on the feet in the area around the ankles or in the bath
Skin	usually the result of poor diet and the widely fluctuating moods that result from hormones out of balance; clay foot soaks with an appropriate essential oil is usually very helpful

Additional oils to use during the period itself or at various times throughout the month:

LeBaby Me, LeMy-graine, ylang ylang

These can be used around the ankles, areas of particular glands on both body and feet, lower back, abdomen and along the spine

Often women will tell me that they were happy and healthy as children, but have never really been well since puberty and the 'kicking in' of their hormones. This is so sad. The proper diet and the use of essential oils and herbal remedies has changed this for many women.

Some artificial sweeteners inhibit the body's production of estrogen which contributes to many of the hormone related problems of women today. There are also many hormones injected into and fed to the cattle and chickens that we eat and the cows which produce our milk supply.

Menstruation

All things related to reproduction and birth are part of the Earth element/meridian phase. Many of the Earth's natural processes are cyclical in nature. Our physical femininity is a reflection of our connection to 'Mother Earth.' Menstruation is only one of these cycles in our lives. Our attitude towards ourselves as women and towards our monthly cycle has more of an effect on the comfort and ease with which we move through it than is often supposed.

The essential oils recommended in the next several sections for hormone imbalance related problems are often the same ones that are contra-indicated for pregnancy. The time should always be taken to study and ponder on the use of these oils during the child-bearing years.

Amenorrhea is the absence of menstruation. Agents to assist are called emmenagogues.
Recommended emmenagogue essential oils:

LeWoman Wise, basil, clary sage, hyssop, lavender, marjoram, rose, rosemary, sage

Menorrhagia is abnormally heavy or extended menstrual flow. It may refer to irregular bleeding that occurs at odd times throughout the month. This is occasionally a sign of something serious, so if it doesn't clear up quickly, consider the advice of a health care professional.

Suggested essential oils:

LeMillenia, cypress, geranium, chamomile, Roman, bioplasma homeopathic and cayenne tincture

Dysmenorrhea is the term given to painful periods and the symptoms of PMS
Recommended essential oils:

LeWoman Wise, LeEndo Relief, clary sage followed by basil, cypress, jasmine, lavender, marjoram, peppermint, chamomile Roman, rosemary, sage, yarrow

During the Period	LeWoman Wise and clary sage rubbed around the ankles or on the abdomen for balancing the hormones and LeDeeper massaged into the abdomen or onto the back for pain and cramping

Some symptoms of PMS and suggested essential oils:

Headache
LeLetting Go, LeMy-graine, LeWoman Wise, clary sage
General aches and pains and backache
LeDeeper, LePaine
Constipation/diarrhea
LeInside Out
Nausea, vomiting
LeEZ Traveler, LeInside Out, orange sweet
Hypoglycemia
LeRevitalize, LeEndo Relief, LeGrateful Heart, LeWake Up, dill, ylang ylang
Tension, mood swings, panic attacks
LeBeloved, LeHeart Song, LeUnity, LeTranquility

Pre-conception

A child's pattern of health begins with the egg and sperm that contain the genetic blueprint for the child's entire future. I wish that there was a way to impress upon every teenager that, for the sake of their future children, they cannot afford to damage their health with poor eating habits during these critical years.

The four months prior to conception are vital for the development of the sperm and egg that will eventually become a baby. Both ova and sperm can suffer from the effects of poor nutrition, toxic metals, environmental chemicals, viruses, and some drugs before conception has even taken place.

Most women who are pregnant don't realize it until they are six to eight weeks pregnant. Much of the crucial development of the baby's nerves, organs and bone structures has already taken place by this time. A nutritional deficiency that is causing little or no symptoms in the mother can be critical for the rapidly developing embryo.

Essential oils are highly concentrated plant material and, as such, contain a wide variety of nutrients which are absorbed into the body through the skin. The regular use of essential oils can help to fill nutritional needs and give a woman planning to conceive an additional margin of safety.

The use of hormone balancing oils such as LeWoman Wise and LeEndo Relief can also make a major difference to the pregnancy and to the developing baby.

Fertility, Infertility and Conception

Fertility requires good general health and well-balanced hormones in both the man and the woman.
Recommended essential oils:
LeEndo Relief for general endocrine and glandular health, LeVitality for circulatory and vein health, LeWoman Wise for hormone balance in the woman and LeBalance for hormone balance in the man.

Miscarriage and the Prevention of Miscarriage

Miscarriage is far more common than generally supposed. It is estimated that 1 in 2 very early pregnancies miscarry and appear to be only a delayed or extra heavy period and that 1 in 6 women who have a positive pregnancy test suffer miscarriage. It is also estimated that with proper care and the use of natural remedies, over half of 'threatened miscarriages' can be successfully brought to a full term.

Some women have spotting or even light periods regularly throughout their pregnancies. This does not necessarily indicate an impending miscarriage. However, at the first sign of bleeding, especially if it is accompanied by cramping or softening of the cervix, measures should be taken.

LeMillenia to tighten the uterus and cervix, realign everything structurally and energetically; false unicorn and lobelia, not oils, but herbal remedies, taken in either tincture or capsule form. The ratio should be 3 parts false unicorn to 1 part lobelia. This combination taken as soon as spotting begins has saved many a pregnancy. The reason is a protective covering over the ovum called the corpus luteum which fails to dissolve promptly after fertilization. If it does not dissolve, the ovum is unable to implant in the uterine wall and the hormone changes that are triggered by the developing embryo fail to occur. The uterus empties and a miscarriage has occurred.

Following a Miscarriage

LeMillenia causes the uterus to fold and return rapidly to a pre-pregnant state. This is the best way to deal with any excess bleeding. LeMillenia also helps the woman look forward and cope with the myriad of emotions that miscarriages create. LeHeart Song and LeWhispering Hope can also be helpful.

Return to a lifestyle that includes a good diet, exercise and a program for overall hormone balance.

Pregnancy

Many of the blended essential oils listed below contain oils which, by themselves, are contra-indicated for pregnancy. Because they are part of a blend and the recommendations are for only a drop or two at a time, they are generally considered safe. Caution and common sense on your part are expected; if you feel that the oil is likely to or is causing any problem, however slight, quit using it immediately!

Minor (and not so minor) Ailments of Pregnancy:
The oils that may be needed during a pregnancy or during a labor and delivery are as individual as every mother. The ones listed below are personal favorites or ones that have worked well for several women in the past.

Morning Sickness/ Nausea

Orange, sweet—place a drop behind each ear; put a few drops on a cotton ball in a small plastic bag, carry with you and sniff throughout the day. Peppermint—it is the aroma that helps, so place a few drops on a cotton ball much the same as directed with the orange oil above; geranium—is for hormone balance and relaxation. Massage a few drops diluted with almond oil on the feet or place 2 - 3 drops in the tub and enjoy a quiet and relaxing bath. ^Le^Inside Out—on the abdomen or feet; jasmine or rosewood—diffuse; wear on the body or sniff it as needed.

Ambivalence or non-acceptance of the pregnancy

^Le^Acknowledge—acceptance and ability to connect with the developing child; ^Le^Whispering Hope—particulary when feelings are deep despair, almost suicidal; ^Le^Heart Song—depression, lack of joy and anticipation.

Fear Surrounding Pregnancy or Delivery

^Le^Tomorrow or ^Le^Trust—place on sternum, wrists or diffuse for the aroma

Stretched or Striated Abdominal Wall (and elsewhere) Muscles

^Le^Baby Me—dilute with a carrier oil (vitamin E or something with jojoba works well) and apply to the affected areas; increase the nutritional value of the foods being eaten and supplement with a natural Vitamin E; mild exercise to strengthen these muscles and a faithful exercise program when the pregnancy is complete.

Stretch Marks

^Le^Baby Me—dilute with a carrier oil (vitamin E or something with jojoba, apricot or avocado works well) and apply to the affected areas; increase the nutritional value of the foods being eaten and supplement with a good Vitamin E.

Anemia

The use of ^Le^Millenia or ^Le^Eternity often helps the body uptake nutrients in a more efficient manner.

Constipation

Constipation is the natural consequence of hormones that relax the muscles (of which the intestine is one) so that the stretching that needs to be done can be accomplished. Solutions: always obey nature's urges immediately; drink lots of water; eat correctly to get proper nutrition for muscle and skin elasticity; use *^Le^Inside-Out* applied to the abdominal area and the bottoms of the feet.

Leg Cramps

Often an indication of poor absorption of calcium; poor calcium absorption is sometimes a factor in the prevalence of false labor contractions in the later stage of pregnancy; ^Le^Warm Down massaged into the calf muscles helps relieve these cramps.

Spider Veins or Varicose Veins

Helichrysum—regenerates damaged tissue and dissolves clots and pooled blood in and around the vein; cypress layered with helichrysum—to heal while improving circulation; ^Le^Vitality—to improve circulation; ^Le^Warm Down—dilute and massage into leg muscles to relieve pain and heavy sensation; ^Le^Visibility—specific for the small, spidery veins.

When large, swollen veins are present, always massage <u>above</u> the vein and movie upward.

Xyphoid Process Pain
The xyphoid process is the triangular bit of bone at the base of the sternum. Often the pressure of the full uterus pushing upward displaces this bone and causes varying degrees of pain. ***LeBaby Me***—dilute and apply topically to the area.

Misalignment or Mal-presentation of the Baby
LeMillenia—dilute and apply over the abdomen and back. This needs to be done in the final 3 weeks before term, but not during the labor itself. LeMillenia, during labor will keep the cervix from opening and even cause it to close to quite an extent.

Toxemia and/or High blood Pressure
LeVitality—if related to heart and circulation and there are high levels of protein in the urine; lavender, rose, LeHeart Song—for relaxation, stress and general fears.
This is a serious condition and can cause death or impairment in both mother and child if left unchecked. If the oils do not make a significant difference very quickly, seek professional help.

Pre-term Labor
Lavender—for relaxation; clary sage—this one is also used post-term to get labor going, demonstrating natural remedy's ability to 'balance' and return the system to a normal state.

Avoiding an Episiotomy or Tear
LeBaby Me—massaged with olive, or vitamin E oil, onto the perineum in the weeks prior to delivery.

Labor and Delivery

Early labor
The following 5 oils can be diluted and applied, usually to the ankle, the bottoms of the feet, or the abdomen. They may also be diffused or sniffed for a moment or two. Clary sage—aids cervical dilation; marjoram—relaxes muscles, easing the pain of contractions while allowing them to work more efficiently; geranium—stimulates circulation, eases breathing, regulates pulse and blood pressure; fennel—for pain relief; nutmeg—supports adrenals & nervous system, helping with fatigue and blood sugar levels.

The following 6 oils can be placed on the body but are most often diffused or sniffed by the mother. I usually prefer to have the woman smell an oil because sometimes an oil that is needed and smells good one minute is offensive, or even nauseating, a few minutes later when the need for it has passed.
Lavender—relaxes muscles and skeletal structure, takes the edge off pain; jasmine—for lack of progress, stalling out of labor, emotional support; rose—diffused at a birth can greatly improve everyone's emotions and confidence and ability to focus; rosewood—for lack of progress, fear or tension; chamomile German—this oil is relaxing, uplifting, calming; LeWisdom—for the mother who seems to lack concentration and focus or seems to be concerned with and focused on things other than the labor and the coming baby.

Transition Stage
LeWhispering Hope, LeUnity—these oils are best just sniffed because this stage is usually short and something else will be needed in a moment or two.

Post-Partum

Retained Placenta

Basil—rub on abdomen; angelica or jasmine—sniffed. Often the best thing to do is get the mother up and have her move around a little bit.

Hemorrhage

Ylang ylang, helichrysum—dilute and rub on the abdomen to cause the uterus to clamp down; geranium—aids contraction of uterus, pulls together stretched and dilated tissues, heals endometrium, constricts abdominal blood vessels; LeMillenia—helps fold and firm the uterus, realign hips and pelvic structure. This one is amazing. Use only after the placenta has delivered as it works very quickly and can close the cervix and prevent proper discharge of the placental tissue.

Post-Partum Depression (Baby Blues)

LeHeart Song, LeTranquility, LeTrust, LeUnity, geranium, jasmine. These oils can be diluted and applied to the body, 2 or 3 drops placed in the tub for a relaxing bath, diffused or sniffed.

Nursing & Breast Care

Clary sage—to bring in milk; fennel or basil—to increase milk supply; peppermint with cold compress—to decrease milk supply. *Caution: fennel should not be used for more than 10 days as it will excessively increase flow through the urinary tract.*

Chamomile German, LeBaby Me—sore or cracked nipples
Be sure to wash the breast thoroughly before nursing the baby whenever essential oils are applied.

Breast Infections (Mastitis)—comes on swiftly and can be devastating to breast tissue; there is a really good herbal poultice that has proven itself many times. Use good herbals to fight the infection and help cope with the attendant fever, headache and chills.

Babies and Children

When working with babies and children, always dilute especially well and use only a very small amount. More will not be better; often a small amount of an oil is soothing and calming but a larger amount will cause agitation and fussiness. Premature babies have such delicate and almost transparent skin, that it is best to avoid the use of essential oils until the skin has achieved more maturity.

Many of the blends mentioned here contain oils that are often considered too strong for babies and children. You must use these at your own risk, understanding that because they are blends there is not a high percentage of contra-indicated oils in them. If you chose to use them, please always dilute extremely well and use only a drop or two of the diluted mixture. Never apply an oil undiluted to an infant or small child and certainly keep your essential oils out of the reach of children!

Colic

LeInside Out, LeTranquility, bergamot, mandarin, chamomile Roman, rosemary, ylang ylang—dilute and apply to stomach and back

Constipation
Ginger, mandarin, orange sweet or rosemary; dilute one of the oils and massage stomach and feet

Cradle Cap
[Le]Delicate—dilute with almond oil, apply to the head, after a few moments use a soft bristled brush to remove the crusts.

Diaper Rash
[Le]Baby Me, 1 drop lavender and 1 drop chamomile Roman mixed with carrier oil

Dry Skin
Rosewood or sandalwood, well diluted and applied

Earache
Lavender, tea tree, chamomile Roman, thyme or garlic (Dilute all of them very well, especially the garlic as it can burn the ear if too strong or was not stirred thoroughly.) Place a diluted drop or two on a piece of cotton ball and place in the ear; rub a little bit of diluted oil behind the ear.

Fever
Lavender—dilute with carrier oil and massage the baby—cover the back of neck, feet, behind the ears, etc. *(The right homeopathic can also be very useful here.)*

Jaundice
Geranium, lemon, lime, mandarin, or rosemary—dilute and apply on the liver area of the feet or on the baby's abdomen.

Teeth Grinding
Lavender, [Le]Tranquility—rub on feet or diffuse.

The 'Golden Years'

Menopause
[Le]Endo Relief, [Le]Balance, angelica, cypress, orange sweet, chamomile Roman, rose, nutmeg, rosemary, sage—apply diluted oils to ankles, lower back and pelvis.

Osteoporosis
(Considered a disease related to calcium absorption; more properly understood as beginning with hormone imbalance—consider all the oils listed above for menopause.) [Le]Warm Down seems to aid calcium absorption; [Le]Paine, [Le]Tranquility, [Le]Deeper, birch, chamomile Roman, chamomile German, hyssop, lemon, nutmeg, pine, spruce, rosemary, wintergreen—dilute and use as a massage oil or put 2 - 3 drops in the tub; rub on feet.

Bone Spurs
[Le]Aspire—using arnica oil as the carrier, massage into the area several times a day; will relieve the pain and, eventually, dissolve the spurs. At the same time, work should be done to improve the sources of calcium consumed and to improve the body's absorption of calcium.

Single Oils

There are many wonderful single oils that promote healing. However, in my opinion, essential oils can be utilized more effectively as part of a well-done blend where each essential oil is only a percentage of the entire blend. This allows you to take advantage of all the wonderful properties of the single oil with less chance of problems and contra-indications. Combining different essential oils together also allows the blend to contain essential oils which both moderate and support each other. The use of good blends raises the effectiveness of essential oils to entirely new levels. It also makes it most unlikely that you will ever create any kind of a problem from the over-use of a particular oil. (See comments on synergy, Chapter 15, page 1.)

The claims made in this document are based on traditional uses, current literature, anecdotal experiences, and many years of personal experience with essential oils. These claims have not been evaluated by the FDA, nor are they meant to diagnose or treat any ailment or condition. They are provided here as a public service and for your information only.

Ajowan

(Tracyspermum copticum)

Ingredient In

LeEternity , LeTurmoil

Therapeutic Properties

digestive, anti-emetic/anti-diarrheal, anti-infectious, antibacterial, antiviral, anti-fungal, anti-parasitic, antiseptic, tonic, stimulant, antispasmodic

Affinity For

digestive system   circulatory system

Resonance	**Plant Family**	**Part of Plant Used**
physical, mental	Umbelliferae	seeds

Application

Ajowan should always be diluted well when applied to the body; application can be on the feet or any area of the body needing assistance.

Aromatic Considerations

Ajowan is reminiscent of thyme in both aroma and action.

Emotional/Spiritual Aspects

Ajowan is predominantly an oil for physical complaints. Ajowan also assists with mental and physical exhaustion. It can be calming and moderately sedating under certain circumstances.

Physical Aspects

Ajowan essential oil contains over 50% thymol, making it very effective against bacteria, viruses, fungi, and parasites. The high thymol content also makes it extremely potent and quite caustic. Ajowan is an excellent aid to digestion. It often helps relieve nausea, flatulence, and the cramping pains that accompany these conditions.

Although antispasmodic and sedating under certain conditions, ajowan makes an excellent circulatory stimulant. Ajowan is helpful for fatigue, weakness, and to assist recovery after illness or accident. It also assists with mental or physical exhaustion, especially when the exhaustion is accompanied by great listlessness. Ajowan has been used in India (for a very long time) in the treatment of toothaches; clove oil also works great for a toothache but tastes better.

General Information

Ajowan is considered a fair substitute for cumin therapeutically, although the aromas are vastly different.

Cautions

Ajowan has a very high thymol content. It is best used as a small percent of a synergistically blended essential oil, especially for application to the skin. Pregnant women should certainly avoid its use as a single.

Allspice

(Pimenta dioica)

Ingredient In

LeEternity , LeKadence, LeVitality

Therapeutic Properties

anesthetic, analgesic, antioxidant, antiseptic, carminative, muscle relaxant, rebefacient, stimulant, and tonic

Affinity For

digestive system, respiratory system, circulatory system, muscles

Resonance	**Plant Family**	**Part of Plant Used**
physical, mental, emotional	Myrtaceae	leaves, fruit

Application

Always dilute allspice with a carrier oil. Allspice should be applied to the chest for respiratory ailments, the abdomen for digestive disorders, and on any area of the body where increased circulation is needed.

Aromatic Considerations

Allspice has a warm and spicy aroma with a bit of sharpness. The aroma of allspice is warming and stimulating. When added to blends, it provides a distinctive aromatic layer.

Emotional/Spiritual Aspects

Allspice is used to treat depression, nervous exhaustion, tension, stress, and neuralgia where the symptoms are worsened by emotional stresses.

Physical Aspects

Allspice offers a wide range of therapeutic properties. It is of benefit to the digestive system, as are most oils made from plants traditionally used as spices. Allspice supports respiratory function. It has outstanding analgesic, anesthetic, and muscle relaxant properties. These properties make it beneficial for injuries, arthritis, and muscle cramps.

General Information

Familiar to cooks, allspice tastes like a combination of cloves, cinnamon, and black pepper, but it is actually a single distinctive plant. Allspice produces a small berry-like pepper. The essential oil is made from the leaves and the fruit.

Cautions

Allspice, used as a single essential oil, should be diluted well. It can be irritating to delicate membranes and cause skin irritation if used undiluted. Allspice is wonderful in a blend. It blends particularly well with ginger, geranium, lavender, orange, patchouli, and ylang ylang.

Angelica

(Angelica archangelica)

Ingredient In

LeBenediction, LeConnection, LeEverlasting, LeInner Peace, LeMagi, LeMoonlight, LeTrust, LeUnity, LeVision

Therapeutic Properties

anti-coagulant, antiviral, calming, expectorant, sedative, stomachic, tonic

Affinity For

liver, respiration, central vessel meridian, digestion, hormone balance, brow chakra

Resonance	**Plant Family**	**Part of Plant Used**
physical, emotional	Umbelliferae	root

Application

Angelica can be applied to the feet or on any area of the body.

Aromatic Considerations

The aroma of angelica is not pleasant by itself, so it is rarely diffused except as part of a blend.

Physical/Emotional/Spiritual Aspects

Angelica is often called the 'oil of angels.' The physical and emotional aspects of this oil cannot be easily separated, even in a description. Angelica, either by itself or as part of a blend formula, seems to weaken the power of traumatic memories and events. The event still happened and the memory is still there, but the devastating effects on the body and mind are greatly minimized. Angelica has this effect on the mind because it releases toxins and congestion from the liver. The liver, according to Eastern tradition, is the seat of anger and rage. The letting go of these emotions allows the liver to let go of physical toxicity as well. Physically, a toxic liver produces headaches, muscle aches, fatigue, dry hair and skin, poor circulation, and respiratory problems. A liver clogged by toxic emotions creates feelings of displacement, annoyance, resentment, anger, and discontentment.

Additional Physical Aspects

The use of angelica is also appropriate for anorexia, bruises, colds, colic, coughs, flatulence, indigestion, menopause, pre-menstrual tension, and arthritis.

Cautions

Angelica should be avoided if diabetic or pregnant. Areas of the skin to which angelica has been applied should not be exposed to direct sunlight for a few hours.

Aniseseed

(Pimpinella anisum)

Ingredient In

LeEternity , LeKadence, LeTurmoil , LeVitality

Therapeutic Properties

antispasmodic, estrogenic, bronchial dilator, diuretic, expectorant, invigorating, stimulating, carminitive, galactagogue, stomachic, heart tonic, and stimulant

Affinity For

digestion
circulation
lungs
cardiovascular system
hormones
triple warmer/pericardium meridian

Resonance
physical, mental, emotional

Plant Family
Umbelliferae

Part of Plant Used
seed (fruit)

Application

Aniseseed can be diffused, diluted and applied anywhere on the body or used as a massage oil.

Aromatic Considerations

Aniseseed has a very sweet, licorice-like aroma. Nice diffused, if you like the smell of black licorice.

Emotional/Spiritual Aspects

The triple warmer meridian is responsible for the protection of the body. The triple warmer also communicates information about our physical bodies to our mind and emotions. Aniseseed brings light, life, and perspective to this meridian. The result is love and acceptance of our naturally imperfect physical bodies. This more balanced perspective has a dramatic impact on eating disorders, weight loss, and sexual dysfunction.

Physical Aspects

Like fennel, aniseseed has estrogenic properties, but its effects are somewhat stronger. Aniseseed is antispasmodic, making it effective for menstrual pain and stomach cramps. Because it is both a bronchial dilator and expectorant, aniseseed is used for asthma and respiratory conditions that include phlegm and mucous. Herbal forms of aniseseed have been used traditionally in many countries to speed labor along and encourage milk production.

General Information

Aniseseed contains a natural substance that forms crystals if the oil is chilled. If this occurs, just warm the bottle slightly.

Cautions

Because aniseseed is estrogenic, it should be avoided during pregnancy. Aniseseed is also phototoxic; avoid direct sunlight on skin to which this oil has been recently applied.

Anthopogon

(Rhododendron anthopogon)

Ingredient In

[Le]Reconciliation

Therapeutic Properties

anti-inflammatory, antibacterial, anti-fungal, antiviral, balsamic, depurative, hepatic, immunostimulant, nervine, restorative, sedative, tonic, anti-neuralgic, decongestant, nervous system tonic

Affinity For

immune system
digestive system
ligaments, bones
liver
hair
skin
all four fire meridians
heart and crown chakras
spleen meridian

Resonance

physical, emotional

Plant Family

Ericaceae

Part of Plant Used

flowers, leaves

Aromatic Considerations

Anthopogon has a unique and very appealing fragrance which hangs in the air, becoming softer and more lovely as time passes. It is described as being fresh, green and balsamic with undertones of vanilla and conifers. I would simply describe it as delightful. It creates a feeling of openness, love, and connection, especially to family members and old friends.

Application

Anthopogon should be diffused, worn as a perfume, or diluted and applied anywhere on the body.

Emotional/Spiritual Aspects

Anthopogon essential oil is very warming emotionally. It pulls one immediately into a mood of remembering, but with the blessing of a focus on the good times and the good in people. This oil is especially good for people whose lives have carried them far away from home and heritage. Anthopogon, and blends to which it has been added, are important and amazing oils for loss or bereavement of any kind.

Physical Aspects

Perhaps anthopogon's most important characteristic in the physical realm is on the immune system. It has been used in Nepal for various types of blood disorders and systemic infections for a very long time. The Department of Pharmaceutical Sciences at the University of Padova in Italy has done extensive research as well as gas chromatography and mass spectrometry on this essential oil. Their results, published in a renowned scholarly scientific journal which targets important new discoveries, claim that anthopogon essential oil reduced cancer cell growth in all types of cells tested, using varying treatment protocols and varying concentrations of essential oil. The cancers anthopogon was tested against were ovarian, cervical, and colon—certainly three of the deadliest and fastest moving cancers known. The research team speculated that the high *pinene* content was responsible, at least in part, for this action. ***This is truly important new research!***

Anthopogon was also shown effective against candida, e-coli, and several other strains of bacteria. Anthopogon is a stimulant essential oil, with a particular affinity for the liver and digestive system. It can stimulate appetite during illness or convalescence. This oil is useful for gouty arthritic conditions. It is strongly anti-inflammatory when applied to fibrous tissues, ligaments, and joints.

In Nepal, where anthopogon has been used for many years, it is considered a symbol of balance in the fire meridian. Anthopogon's therapeutic properties certainly indicate that it affects this meridian in all of its aspects; physically, mentally, and emotionally. It relieves headaches, backaches, and joint and muscle pains that were brought about by excesses of some kind (over-the-top activity or consumption of food and drink). This oil is of great benefit to people whose illnesses are aggravated by windy or stormy conditions.

General Information

Anthopogon is the national symbol of Nepal, where it is used in meditation and healing.

Cautions

There are no known contra-indications for this essential oil.

Basil

(Ocimum basilicum)

Ingredient In

Le Crystal Clear, LeDandy, LeJourney, LeWarm Down, LeWeightless

Therapeutic Properties

antispasmodic, restorative (stimulant for nerves and adrenal cortex), general stimulant, emmenagogue, digestive tonic, intestinal antiseptic, carminative, antibiotic

Affinity For

cardiovascular system	muscles	pericardium meridian
respiratory system	bones	large intestine meridian
hormone balance	deficient yang energy	throat chakra

Resonance	**Plant Family**	**Part of Plant Used**
physical, emotional	Labiatae	stems, leaves, flowers

Application

Basil should be diluted well. It may be applied to any area of concern or on the feet.

Aromatic Considerations

Basil is strongly antiseptic when diffused. Basil helps open the mind to ideas, possibilities, and opportunities. Basil helps us to act with integrity, from our hearts, in a straightforward manner.

Emotional/Spiritual Aspects

Emotionally, basil is both stimulating and soothing. It energizes the mind while, at the same time, relieves doubts and fears and lightens our burdens. Basil moderates a tendency to be too blunt, outspoken, or independent. Basil is used in treatments for depression, hysteria, nervous tension, and mental fatigue.

Physical Aspects

Basil stimulates the adrenal cortex and strengthens the nerves, making it beneficial for mental fatigue, headaches, insomnia, fainting, loss of the sense of smell, memory loss, and poor concentration. Basil strengthens the digestive function, being of particular use with hiccups, flatulence, indigestion, and vomiting. Basil has strong antispasmodic and expectorant properties. It calms muscle spasms from injury or fatigue and alleviates coughs. The antispasmodic properties quiet dry coughs. The expectorant properties keep mucus from building up in the lungs.

Basil is also analgesic, providing pain relief when applied to the body. Basil is excellent applied undiluted to insect bites and stings and, in Indian (Eastern) medical lore, is listed as a remedy for snake bite. Many people like basil, either diluted and applied to the chest, or inhaled, in the treatment of chronic colds, earaches, and mucus. The hormonal properties of basil, being yang moving toward yin, have a specific affinity for prostate problems in men.

General Information

The action of basil on the system resembles both peppermint and thyme in many ways. In a bath, even a drop or two produces an interesting sensation of tiny pin pricks as it increases circulation to the capillaries just under the skin.

Cautions

Basil should be avoided if pregnant or epileptic. Undiluted, basil may irritate sensitive skin.

Bay

(Pimenta racemosa)

(occasionally referred to as Pimenta acris or Myrcia acris)

Ingredient In

LeBenediction, LeMariah

Therapeutic Properties

stimulant, expectorant, antiseptic, antibiotic, antispasmodic, emmenagogue, febrifuge, insecticide, sedative, neuralgic

Affinity For

digestion	respiration	yang energy
lymph drainage	circulation	

Resonance	**Plant Family**	**Part of Plant Used**
physical, emotional, mental	Myrtaceae	leaves

Application

Bay, diluted well, may be applied to the feet or any area of the body.

Aromatic Considerations

Bay has a sweet, spicy, balsamic aroma. It diffuses well, but care should be taken when inhaling. Bay is pungent and may burn the delicate lining of the nostrils.

Emotional/Spiritual Aspects

Bay essential oil is for those times when you are feeling lost, alone, or not strong enough to face every day events. Bay produces layers of emotions, most of them centering around feelings of safety and protection. The aroma of bay makes you feel as though you have just been wrapped in the arms of a loving and protective father. The anchor of this complex oil is trust in yourself, and in your own emotional and spiritual strength and resilience.

Physical Aspects

Bay, *Pimenta racemosa,* is a close cousin to allspice. As bay increases circulation, it creates a sensation of heat—much like commercial sports rubs. This increase in circulation brings relief to muscle spasms, sprains, arthritis, and neuralgia. Bay is commonly used as an ingredient in massage oils to stimulate lymph drainage and blood circulation. Bay oil has also been used traditionally to bring relief from digestive complaints. It is an expectorant and mucolytic for the lungs and sinuses. Bay leaf is also said to improve memory and relieve headaches that are related to poor circulation in the neck and shoulders. Bay is a very strong antiseptic, antibiotic, antiviral essential oil.

General Information

Bay is not the same plant or essential oil as laurel (Laurus nobilis), although they are often confused. See 'Laurel' for further information on these two species of essential oils.

Cautions

Bay should be used in small amounts and always be well diluted. It is one of the stronger essential oils and may cause skin and mucus membrane irritation.

Benzoin

(Styrax tonkinesis)

Ingredient In

Le Dreams, LeHoliday Spirit, LeEverlasting

Therapeutic Properties

antispasmodic, antidepressant, calmative, aphrodisiac

Affinity For

cytophylactic (promotes cell regeneration)	yang energy	spleen meridian
circulation	earth energy	

Resonance	**Plant Family**	**Part of Plant Used**
physical, emotional	Ericaceae	resin

Application

Benzoin is particularly suited for diffusing or inhaling. It can be applied anywhere on the body including the feet.

Aromatic Considerations

The aroma of benzoin is slightly woody with a strong vanilla scent. Diffused, benzoin can aid recovery from extreme stress or deep depression.

Emotional/Spiritual Aspects

Benzoin is useful for persons who feel unloved (or undeserving of love), even when surrounded by family and friends who love them deeply. Benzoin creates soft, warm, fuzzy feelings in the heart. It is like coming home at last from far away. This oil, even as a small percentage of a blend, helps one feel reassured and deeply supported. Insufficient energy in the spleen meridian results in over-thinking and excessive worry. Benzoin raises this energy and soothes anxiety that is aggravated by exhaustion.

Physical Aspects

Benzoin is a powerful antimicrobial. It has a pronounced effect on congestion, literally 'melting away' blockages in the lungs, lymphatic vessels, and intestines. Benzoin is used by Far Eastern physicians to treat respiratory and urinary disorders that are *cold and damp* in nature. Benzoin is a circulatory stimulant. It has a particular affinity for the tiny capillaries that feed the skin. Benzoin is thick and viscous, and is often used as a fixative to stabilize the aroma of oils and perfumes made from more volatile ingredients.

General Information

Benzoin is sometimes known as onycha oil. According to David Stewart, PhD, in The Chemistry of Essential Oils Made Simple, alcohol tincture of benzoin was used for more than 200 years in hospitals as the primary antiseptic. The medical profession then began using antiseptics derived from petroleum products because they were less expensive. It has become obvious during the last several years that bacteria are becoming resistant to these antiseptics. Bacteria does not become resistant to benzoin, therefore, many hospitals are returning to the use of this natural antiseptic. The use of benzoin, since it does not create resistant strains of bacteria, does not contribute to the worldwide problem of 'super-bugs.'

Bergamot

(Citrus bergamia)

Ingredient In

LeBaby Me, LeBeloved, LeDreams, LeEverlasting, LeFaith, LeHeart Song, LeRevitalize

Therapeutic Properties

anti-inflammatory, analgesic, antiseptic, antispasmodic, disinfectant

Affinity For

digestive system
endocrine system
hormone balance
metal element
wood element
water element
yang energy
heart chakra

Resonance

emotional, physical

Plant Family

Rutaceae

Part of Plant Used

fruit

Application

It is *always* recommended to dilute bergamot well. Well diluted bergamot becomes soothing and emollient; not diluted sufficiently, it can be irritating to skin.

Aromatic Considerations

Bergamot is a sweet smelling citrus oil, with a warm floral scent that is unusual among the citrus oils. Bergamot, diffused, is said to repair the aura and make one feel 'young at heart.'

Emotional/Spiritual Aspects

Because bergamot has a special affinity for the liver meridian, it encourages the release of anger and pain that is being held back or held deeply in the body. A person needing bergamot is usually a good listener. They are described by friends and family as cheerful and supportive. Often this cheerfulness is a mask, hiding anger, despair, or depression. It is as though they are carrying the burden of every sad story they have listened to on their own shoulders. They are very angry, but since the stories are not their own they feel they cannot tell them to anyone. The anger they feel becomes repressed and turns inward. The ability of bergamot to relieve anger, nervous depression, anxiety, and hysteria has been well documented in Europe. Bergamot can help us find peace when our heart hurts for other's distress.

Bergamot is excellent in any emotional crisis and in convalescing from an illness. Bergamot raises the spirits and brings light into our lives and lightness to dark and weary days. It is often used in treatments for eating disorders.

Physical Aspects

Bergamot has a great many applications for physical healing. Bergamot is used for urinary tract infections, sore throat, cold sores, bronchitis, and varicose veins. In Italy, bergamot is commonly used in the treatment of intestinal parasites. It is also used in treatments for candida overgrowth and thrush. Bergamot has been shown effective against tuberculosis bacilli. Like all essential oils, bergamot is antimicrobial. It is particularly destructive of bacteria that live in the mouth.

Cautions

Bergamot should be diluted well and used sparingly. Repeated use of bergamot can result in extreme contact sensitization.

Bergamot contains bergaptene, which is phototoxic. You should avoid direct sunlight on skin to which bergamot has been applied. This caution applies to more than just an uncomfortable sunburn. Damage to the nuclei of cells has been documented when skin to which bergamot was applied was exposed to ultra-violet light. This photo-toxicity lasts up to 12 hours after the oil has been applied. Using bergamot in a blend does not eliminate its photo-toxicity. *There is no problem using this oil as long as you apply it to areas of the body that will not be exposed to ultra-violet light (sunlight or a tanning bed).*

There are bergamot essential oils available that have had the constituents that create photo-toxicity removed. However, these oils lack both aroma and certain therapeutic qualities.

Birch

(Betula lenta)

Ingredient In

LeBreezey, LeDeeper, LeEZ-Traveler, LeMagi, LePaine

Therapeutic Properties

anti-inflammatory, analgesic, antiseptic, antispasmodic, disinfectant

Affinity For

muscles and joints, nerves
nerves
urinary system
lymphatic system
lung meridian

Resonance

physical, emotional

Plant Family

Betulaceae

Part of Plant Used

leaves

Application

Birch should be applied, well diluted, to areas of pain or inflammation.

Aromatic Considerations

Birch has a pleasant aroma. It awakens the senses, increasing awareness and alertness.

Emotional/Spiritual Aspects

Sometimes we get into a frame of mind where we are very much afraid of the truth. We are sure that we will not be able to handle the truth if it is forced upon us. We spend a lot of mental and emotional energy hiding from the truth. Birch essential oil is very eye opening. It shatters our illusions and brings us up against reality. This sounds harsh, but honesty in looking at oneself is a compelling and liberating force. The most important truth we can learn in this life is the truth about our own motivations and triggers. This truth will truly set us free and birch essential oil can help us grasp it and keep hold of it.

Physical Aspects

Birch essential oil has analgesic and anti-inflammatory properties. It is useful for arthritis, muscle and bone pain, tendonitis, osteoporosis, and any inflammatory condition. Birch is also a treatment for bladder infections, recurring cystitis, gout, edema, and kidney stones. Birch helps with eczema and other skin disorders. One of its outstanding uses is reducing fevers.

General Information

One of the key compounds in birch (and wintergreen) essential oil is methyl salicylate. In birch oil, this compound makes up 85-90% of the oil. Methyl salicylate is an aspirin-like compound which has much the same effect on muscles and nerves as cortisone, but as a constituent of an essential oil it *does not* have the side-effects of cortisone.

Methyl salicylate is easily and cheaply produced in laboratories, but the man-made substitute has very toxic side effects. This is not true of birch essential oil—in spite of what you may have heard or read. The 10-15% of other compounds that occur naturally in birch oil balances the methyl salicylate and keep it from being toxic. This 'balancing act' of naturally occurring compounds is common in the natural world. *(The lack of balancing components is why drugs have side effects and herbs do not!!)* Research done by 'aromatherapists' of the British school of thought was conducted using perfume grade essential oils (in other words, synthetic laboratory produced oils diluted in carrier oil). This research has been given extensive coverage in print. Of course, these synthetic oils proved toxic—even when well-diluted. The research has no relevance to the safety or efficacy of pure therapeutic grade essential oils.

Therapeutic grade birch essential oil is safe to use; synthetic reproductions are not! Essential oils are concentrated. In most applications they should be diluted. This is true of birch essential oil.

I visited a web site where it was explained that birch oil aggravated a toxic condition established by medications which contained large amounts of methyl salicylate. This aggravation was sited as a reason to not use birch essential oil at all. The fact that the reaction was set up by the synthetic compound was totally ignored and brushed aside as irrelevant. It was assumed that the the toxic reaction would have been the same with pure birch oil. Although the natural and the man-made compounds have the same name, they are not the same! A study of simple chemistry shows this clearly. (See Dr. David Stewart's book The Chemistry of Essential Oils Made Simple, p221.) The methyl salicylate in the birch oil continued to aggravate the condition because the natural compounds meant to balance it were insufficient for a battle against the synthetic compound in the medications and the natural compound in the birch oil at the same time. More simply put, the 'balancing' substances in the birch were sufficient for the birch; they were wholly inadequate to deal with the deliberate over-dose the drug created.

Why do we use essential oils? Because they are naturally occurring substances, balanced by nature and nature's Creator. They heal quickly, without the side effects of the clones we call drugs. Never forget, all drugs have side effects!!

Cautions

There are some people who are very sensitive to even natural methyl salicylate. There is someone who is allergic to everything, I suspect. Starting slowly with any essential oil is a good thing.

Black Pepper

(Piper nigrum)

Ingredient In

LeEnergy

Therapeutic Properties

analgesic, antiseptic, aphrodisiac, anti-catarrhal, expectorant, tonic, febrifuge, digestive, rubefacient, diuretic, laxative

Affinity For

nerves	circulation	pericardium meridian
digestion	endocrine system	root and solar plexus chakras
		yang energy

Resonance	**Plant Family**	**Part of Plant Used**
physical, emotional, mental	Piperaceae	fruit

Application

Black pepper should always be carefully diluted. It is beneficial when applied to the feet and to areas of pain or poor circulation.

Aromatic Considerations

Black pepper essential oil should be diffused carefully because it is quite pungent. Black pepper contains a significant amount of sesquiterpenes. There are more sesquiterpenes in black pepper than there are in frankincense. (See Chapter 2, page 10 of this book—Blood/Brain Barrier.)

Emotional/Spiritual Aspects

The responsibility of the pericardium meridian is to protect the heart and emotions. Black pepper has an energizing effect on this meridian, stimulating our inner defenses. This inner strength gives us protection from negative energy, and keeps our energy intact and strong. Black pepper helps us keep our perspective clear, even when those around us are mired in negativity and predicting 'the worst' possible scenarios. Black pepper can help us be more realistic in our expectations of others, and more empathetic to their struggles and pain.

Physical Aspects

Black pepper gives a boost to the immune system. It helps maintain stamina and energy because it increases cellular oxygen levels. Black pepper is analgesic, anti-inflammatory, and antispasmodic. It is a good oil to use for improving muscle tone and recovering from sprains or sports injuries. Black pepper strengthens the nervous system and stimulates the endocrine glands.

Cautions

Black pepper can cause mild irritation to sensitive skin. This is definitely a 'warming' oil.

Blue Tansy

(Tanacetum annuum)

Ingredient In

LeAngel, LeDreams, LeLetting Go, LeLife Force, LeMillenia, LeRevitalize, LeTranquility

Therapeutic Properties

analgesic, anti-inflammatory, nervine, antibacterial, anti-histamine, hypotensive

Affinity For

nerves	muscles	solar plexus chakra	yin energy

Resonance	**Plant Family**	**Part of Plant Used**
emotional, physical	Compositae	leaves, flowers

Application

Dilute and apply to the feet or body. This oil should be used sparingly alone, or used as part of a blend.

Aromatic Considerations

Blue tansy is a sweet smelling and very relaxing oil.

Emotional/Spiritual Aspects

Blue tansy, like other oils containing chamazulene, regulates the flow of vital energy throughout the body. As the flow of energy in the body travels more freely, a feeling of peaceful solitude is created in our minds and heart. We are better able to handle stress, and feel less threatened and overwhelmed. We feel more gratitude for our health and our families. Blue tansy increases our creativity, productivity, and desire for achievement on many levels.

Physical Aspects

Blue tansy adds pain relieving and anti-inflammatory properties to blends. Blue tansy relieves nervous tension and is used, very diluted, for itchy skin conditions. Oils containing chamazulene are stimulating to the thymus gland and raise blood pressure that is abnormally low.

General Information

A high chamazulene content gives blue tansy its vivid, deep blue color. This is the same constituent that gives chamomile German its distinctive color. Essential oils containing chamazulene should be a deep and vivid blue. Yellow, brown, or muddy aspects indicate that the oil is of inferior quality. The oil has been over processed, or it has been exposed to excessive amounts of light and air. Chamazulene is a compound created naturally during the distillation process. Since absolutes are not distilled, they will not have the deep blue color. Chamomile Egyptian is an absolute of an oil which is blue and contains chamazulene when distilled.

Cautions

Blue tansy is better used as part of a blend.

Cabreuva

(Myocarpus fastigiatus)

Ingredient In

LeFaith, LeIQ, LeRevitalize, LeSolitude

Therapeutic Properties

antiseptic, cicatrizant (heals wounds), aphrodisiac, cortico-steriod

Affinity For

muscles
tissue repair

Resonance	**Plant Family**	**Part of Plant Used**
physical	Fabaceae	wood

Application

Cabrueva should be diluted and applied on the feet or directly on the body.

Aromatic Considerations

Cabreuva has a delicate woody/floral scent.

Emotional/Spiritual Aspects

Cabreuva quiets the mind and helps us move from useless worry to productive planning. It can help us find the vision to see solutions to our problems and the inner strength to carry out our plans.

Physical Aspects

Cabreuva has been used since ancient times to heal wounds and ulcerative sores, and to treat cuts and scars. It is considered strongly antiseptic. Cabreuva is sometimes used for arthritis because of an action similar to corticosteriods.

General Information

Cabreuva essential oil was, in the past, included in European pharmacopoeias as a medicine.

Cautions

Cabreuva oil is very mild. There are no known contra-indications.

Cajeput

(Melaleuca cajuputi)

Ingredient In

LeMela Plus

Therapeutic Properties

mild analgesic, anti-inflammatory, antispasmodic, expectorant, antiseptic, antiviral

Affinity For

respiratory system
cellular integrity
lung meridian
digestive system

Resonance	**Plant Family**	**Part of Plant Used**
physical, emotional	Myrtaceae	leaves

Application

Dilute and apply to the feet or the body.

Aromatic Considerations

Cajeput is a form of tea tree. If you like the aroma, cajeput can be diffused to kill odors and air borne bacteria.

Emotional/Spiritual Aspects

The emotional aspects of cajeput are helpful for people who are stuck in a situation they are afraid to leave but also find impossible to stay in. Cajeput encourages swift and decisive action and minimizes tendencies to look back and second guess ourselves.

Physical Aspects

Cajeput is one of the best of the cytophylactic essential oils. This means that it has amazing tissue regenerating properties. This action of cajeput makes it useful for skin problems such as excessive oil or acne. As a *melaleuca*, cajeput is very antimicrobial. It is extremely effective against all types of infections in the body, whether in the kidney, colon, lungs, throat, or any other body system. Cajeput is listed as effective when used for arthritis, stiff joints and muscles, bronchitis and pneumonia, sinusitis and hay fever.

Cautions

Cajeput and tea tree are two oils that are often adulterated with synthetic oils. The synthetic oils can cause blistering and skin eruptions. Pure *melaleuca (tea tree)* family essential oils are extremely strong. Always dilute them well. NEVER take them internally! These oils can cause vomiting and internal bleeding. They are excellent oils, but use with reasonable caution!

Calamus

(Acorus calamus)

Ingredient In

^Le^Journey, ^Le^No-More

Therapeutic Properties

nervine, anti-inflammatory, antispasmodic, general tonic

Affinity For

digestive system mental acuity

Resonance	**Plant Family**	**Part of Plant Used**
physical, mental	Acoraceae	root

Application

Always dilute well when applying to the body.

Aromatic Considerations

Calamus has a warm, spicy scent with a hint of cinnamon. Diffused it may stimulate the mind and memory.

Physical Aspects

Calamus is used for a wide range of symptoms pertaining to the head such as vertigo, headache, shock, memory loss, and epilepsy because it increases cerebral circulation. Calamus is also soothing and anti-inflammatory to the intestinal tract. It increases appetite and absorption of nutrients. Calamus, applied to the stomach and abdomen, arrests the growth of unfriendly bacteria in the digestive system.

General Information

A fluid extract of calamus is an official medicinal preparation still listed in the United States Pharmacopoeia and is used in herbal medicine as an aromatic bitter.

Cautions

Calamus has been used for many years in herbal preparations, but it is fairly new to the essential oil world. The constituents it contains make calamus very effective as a disinfectant, but it is too strong for use on children except in the most dire circumstances. Calamus should also be avoided by pregnant women. Always use straight calamus with caution and common sense.

Caraway

(Carum carvi)

Ingredient In

[Le] Inside-Out, [Le]Life Force

Therapeutic Properties

nervine, digestive, carminative, diuretic, expectorant, cytophylactic, emmenagogue, galactagogue, vermifuge, anti-histaminic, antispasmodic, antiseptic, tonic

Affinity For

digestive system
respiratory system
spleen, pancreas
stomach/spleen meridians
yang energy

Resonance
physical

Plant Family
Umbelliferae

Part of Plant Used
seeds

Application

Caraway should be diluted well and applied to the feet or the body.

Aromatic Considerations

The aroma of caraway is stimulating to the mind, but calming to the nerves.

Emotional/Spiritual Aspects

Emotionally, caraway is of benefit to those who were raised in uncaring or emotionally unstable environments. Often abused or neglected children grow into adults that avoid commitment in relationships. They fear any form of stability, doubting that such a thing could be real or doubting their ability to be constant and consistent themselves. Often, they doubt their own worthiness for such a relationship. Caraway reinforces the earth meridian's steadfast constancy and need to nurture others.

Physical Aspects

Caraway is particularly useful for digestive complaints. Caraway alleviates intestinal spasms and encourages peristalsis. It is used to clean wounds. Caraway rebuilds damaged tissues and relieves the pain of bruising. Caraway is often included in formulas for skin and scalp conditions. As a respiratory oil, it is excellent for clearing infections and mucous from the lungs and the bronchials. Caraway is said to increase milk production and quality in nursing mothers.

Cautions

Like most essential oils, caraway should be diluted when applied to the skin.

Cardamom

(Elettaria cardamomum)

Ingredient In

[Le]Inside-Out

Therapeutic Properties

antiseptic, antispasmodic, antibacterial, aphrodisiac, carminative, cephalic, digestive, diuretic, laxative, nerve tonic, expectorant, immune stimulant, supportive, sustaining, tonic

Affinity For

brain and nervous system
digestion
spleen, pancreas
reproductive system
yang energy
central vessel meridian
spleen meridian
lung meridian

Resonance
physical

Plant Family
Zingiberaceae

Part of Plant Used
seeds

Application

Cardamom, diluted well, can be applied over the stomach, abdomen, chest, or solar plexus areas. Cardamom is excellent, used sparingly, in a bath.

Aromatic Considerations

A cardamom oil of good quality is warm, sweet, and spicy, with no harsh over-tones and no hint of eucalyptus aroma. Diffused, cardamom alleviates mental fatigue and nervous exhaustion.

Emotional/Spiritual Aspects

Because cardamom is strongly associated with the earth element, it can remind us of the abundance and blessings of our lives. Cardamom strengthens our ability to see the opportunities before us and gives us the energy to pursue them. It allows us to give generously and live openly and with enthusiasm.

Physical Aspects

Cardamom essential oil has been in use for a long time. It was recommended by Hippocrates as a remedy for flatulent dyspepsia. It is still listed in the British Pharmacopoeia for stomach cramps and gas pains. Cardamom is useful for nausea, even in pregnancy. It is a well-known remedy for sexual dysfunction. Cardamom draws energy upward to the head, increasing concentration and helping us to relax and unwind when we are worried or tense.

General Information

Cardamom is in the ginger family. It has many of the same properties, but is less of an irritant. It is excellent as a massage oil. Cardamom increases circulation, relaxes muscles, and soothes the skin.

Cautions

There are no contra-indications for cardamom, but it should be diluted for application to the skin.

Carrot Seed

(Daucus carota)

Ingredient In

LeVallee, LeRevitalize

Therapeutic Properties

hepatic, nervous system and cardiovascular tonic, diuretic, vermifuge

Affinity For

skin	cardiovascular system	gall bladder meridian
intestinal tract	nervous system	liver meridian
liver	digestive system	

Resonance	Plant Family	Part of Plant Used
physical, emotional	Umbelliferae	seeds

Application

Carrot seed should be used, diluted, directly on the areas of concern.

Aromatic Considerations

When diffused, carrot seed can strengthen our sense of inner fortitude and will power.

Emotional/Spiritual Aspects

Carrot seed oil helps fortify those who are feeling weak, inefficient, or disorganized. This oil is well suited to impractical dreamers. Carrot seed can give focus and energy to those who procrastinate projects because we don't want to put forth the necessary hard work or mental effort.

Physical Aspects

Carrot seed is a powerful liver detoxifier and blood cleanser. It is particularly useful in bowel inflammations. Carrot seed is of benefit for digestive problems such as constipation, diarrhea, and gas.

Carrot seed contains carotene and vitamin A. These nutrients strengthen eyesight and help with anemia. They also make carrot seed a very good oil for skin health and healing. Carrot seed should be considered for burns, psoriasis and eczema, open sores, ulcers, and boils. Carrot seed applied to the hands regularly may lighten or prevent age spots.

Cassia

(Cinnamomum cassia)

Ingredient In

LeBountiful, LeJourney

Therapeutic Properties

stimulant, antiseptic, antibiotic, antiviral, anti-putrescent, analgesic, anti-diarrheal, anti-microbial, anti-emetic, carminative

Affinity For

circulatory system immune system

Resonance	**Plant Family**	**Part of Plant Used**
physical, emotional	Lauraceae	leaves, bark

Application

Cassia should be diluted with particular care.

Aromatic Considerations

Cassia has a warm, spicy aroma, like cinnamon. Cassia, diffused or inhaled, reduces drowsiness and lessens irritability.

Emotional/Spiritual Aspects

Cassia is a good oil for those who display few emotions. It can be stimulating and relaxing to those who are rigid and inflexible in their thinking and, consequently, rigid and inflexible in their bodies. Cassia can help us see new solutions to old problems, or look at old relationships in new ways.

Physical Aspect

Cassia, like other *Cinnamomum* family members, is a powerful oxygenator. Cassia has a stimulating effect on the whole body, but its action is gently insistent. As a cardiovascular tonic, this oil is excellent. Cassia oil is strongly antimicrobial; virus spores, bacteria, and fungi cannot live in its presence. The anti-inflammatory properties of this oil are helpful with arthritis and other aches and pains. Studies have shown that cassia stimulates T-lymphocyte activity and immuno-globulin production by the B-cells of the immune system. Increased activity of these key elements of the immune system strengthens resistance to disease.

Cautions

Cassia should be avoided, except in blends, when pregnant or nursing. It is too strong to be used in the bath. Care should be taken to dilute especially well when using with children or those with sensitive skin.

Catnip

(Nepeta cataria)

Ingredient In

Le Away, LeMela Plus

Therapeutic Properties

bug repellent, antispasmodic, astringent, anti-inflammatory, nervine, sedative, anesthetic, carminative, diaphoretic

Affinity For

digestive system urinary tract circulatory system

Resonance	**Plant Family**	**Part of Plant Used**
physical	Labiatae	flowers

Application

Catnip, or an insect repellent containing catnip, should be diluted and applied as a spray. Mix 1/4 to 1/2 teaspoon essential oil with 1 cup isopropyl alcohol and 1 cup water in a spray bottle. Spray clothes and extremities, being sure to avoid getting any in your eyes. Essential oils do not disperse well in water or alcohol so you will need to shake your mixture before each use. Miracle II Neutralizer is a good medium to use in place of alcohol and water. Do not apply insect repellent oils with a carrier oil. The carrier oil attracts the bugs you are trying to repel.

Aromatic Considerations

Catnip has a strong, harsh, earthy aroma with a subdued mint undertone.

Emotional/Spiritual Aspects

All essential oils affect the emotions but there is nothing studied and recorded about the emotional aspects of catnip essential oil.

Physical Aspects

Catnip is primarily known for its insect repellent properties. It has also been shown to be effective in deterring underground insects such as termites. Catnip oil is antispasmodic. It is effective in treatments for all forms of cramps. It is useful in relaxing tight or strained muscles. Catnip balances the flow of bile throughout the digestive system, making it a very good remedy for anyone suffering with abdominal pain caused by gas in the stomach or intestines. Catnip oil also promotes urination and helps the body to maintain proper water balance in the cells and tissues. Catnip is stimulating and toning to the entire system, but like many herbal remedies and essential oils, it also acts as a sedative. Natural remedies return the system to a state of balance, whether it is stimulation or sedation that is needed. Catnip has astringent properties which aids in tightening loose muscles and skin. Swished in the mouth, catnip can stimulate the gums to keep the teeth tightly in place.

General Information

One of the constituents of catnip, nepatalactone, has been shown in laboratory studies to be 10 times more effective at repelling insects than DEET.

Cautions

Catnip may cause irritation to sensitive skin. Be sure to follow dilution directions and use reasonable caution and common sense. Use very diluted with infants and small children.

Cedarwood

(Cedrus deodora)

Ingredient In

LeAngel, LeConnection, LeBelieve, LeAway, LeExhilaration, LeGood-night, LeIQ, LeKadence LeMoonlight, LeRefresh-Mint, LeSanctuary

Therapeutic Properties

antiseptic, tonic, anti-fungal, anti-seborrheac, regenerative, astringent, diuretic, expectorant, fungicidal, stimulant to circulatory system, but sedative to nervous system—this is a rare and powerful combination

Affinity For

urinary tract
spleen, pancreas
skin and scalp
lymphatic system
kidney meridian
spleen meridian
central vessel meridian
heart meridian
chakras and subtle bodies

Resonance

physical, emotional

Plant Family

Coniferae

Part of Plant Used

bark

Application

Dilute and apply to the feet or to the body.

Aromatic Considerations

Cedarwood is an excellent oil for meditation and clarity of mind. It reduces tension and promotes restful sleep. The aroma of cedarwood can help us realize when we are being self-righteous, rigid, or dogmatic in our opinions.

Emotional/Spiritual Aspects

Cedarwood was used traditionally by the Indian tribes of America to enhance spiritual communication. Like all conifer oils, cedarwood enhances feelings of security and protection. It helps us to feel, and return, the love of heaven. The aroma of cedarwood calms anger and relieves nervous tension. It quiets the mind that is going over and over the same details, analyzing and then analyzing again. Steadiness, integrity, and emotional stability are some of the great gifts of cedarwood oil.

Cedarwood strengthens the energy of the kidney meridian. Strength in this meridian gives us the will to stand firm when we have made a decision, even against persistent opposition. Cedarwood can give us strength in times of crisis as we stand strong, refusing to lose confidence or faith. This is an excellent oil to bolster us when we are going into strange or unfamiliar situations. Cedarwood oil has been shown effective in the treatment of ADHD because it stabilizes beta/theta waves.

Physical Aspects

Because it is mucolytic (dissolves mucous), cedarwood is useful for chest infections, asthma, and coughs. It it also soothing and healing to the skin and, especially, to the scalp. Cedarwood is often used for dandruff, hair loss, and psoriasis.

Cedarwood encourages lymphatic drainage and stimulates the breakdown of fat in the tissues. Mildly diuretic, cedarwood is used for cellulite and water retention. Decongestant, astringent, and anti-infectious, cedarwood is useful for respiratory and urinary tract infections. Cedarwood is of benefit in any physical complaint where the underlying condition is coldness and dampness, physically or energetically.

The wood of the cedar tree is valued for making cabinets and storage chests because the aroma of the wood repels moths and other insects. Because its odor and taste are pleasant, cedarwood is valued as an insect repellent to be used around spices and other food items.

General Information

Cedarwood oil is very powerful at breaking up catarrh. This action of cedarwood oil is a fine example of the connections between the physical body and the more subtle (or energy) aspects of our systems. Just as surely as cedarwood will break up catarrh and phlegm in the physical body, it will remove the congestion and clutter that is clogging our minds and spirits.

Cautions

Cedarwood should be avoided by pregnant women.

Celery Seed

(Apium graveolens)

Therapeutic Properties

Antioxident, antiseptic (urinary), antispasmodic, aperitif, digestive, diuretic, carminative, emmenagogue, galactagogue, hepatic, nervine, sedative, stomachic, hepatic, uterine stimulant,tonic

Affinity For

digestive system
endocrine system
lymphatic drainage
central vessel meridian
central nervous system

Resonance	**Plant Family**	**Part of Plant Used**
physical, emotional	Umbelliferae	seed

Aromatic Considerations

Celery seed essential oil smells like celery but it has a surprisingly warm, earthy and spicy aroma. Diffused, celery seed can help with headaches, insomnia, and mental fatigue. This essential oil can be helpful when stress and fear are holding us back from acting decisively. Celery seed is very nice diffused with frankincense or sandalwood.

Application

Celery seed should always be diluted well before applying to the skin.

Emotional/Spiritual Aspects

The aroma of celery seed, by bringing balance to our central vessel meridian, can bring us back to a sense of our own strength. Celery seed brings us home to our own center, where our reality and our peace can be found. Celery seed acts on the central nervous system, whose core processing units are the brain and the spinal cord. Celery seed, acting on this system, can stabilize mood swings and protect us from the negative energies of other people. Celery seed can aid in analyzing facts and making appropriate decisions.

Physical Aspects

Celery seed increases the elimination of uric acid and is useful in bringing relief from arthritis, gout, neuralgia, water retention, and edema. Celery helps to release toxins from the blood and aids in liver decongestion and jaundice. Massaging celery seed oil onto the lower back and along the sciatic nerve (or using it in the tub) can reduce painful swelling. Celery seed's calming effect on the digestive system makes it useful for bloating and indigestion. Celery seed is used in weight loss programs because it suppresses hunger cravings and calms anxiety.

Cautions

Celery seed essential oil should probably be avoided during pregnancy or if you have high blood pressure.

Chamomile, Egyptian (absolute)

(Matricaria recutita, also called Chamomilla matricaria)

Ingredient In

LeBalance

Therapeutic Properties

The therapeutic uses of the absolute and the distilled oil (explained below under General Information) are similar in many respects. The absolute seems to have a more pronounced effect on hormone balance, but lacks the chamazulene that is a product of distillation. Chamomile Egyptian is calming, analgesic, antispasmodic, antibiotic, emmenagogue, hepatic, and a vulnerary.

Affinity For

hormones
emotions
nerves
root chakra
throat chakra
yin energy
bladder meridian

Resonance

physical, emotional

Plant Family

Compositae

Part of Plant Used

flowers

Application

Chamomile Egyptian can be applied to the base of the neck, on the temples, and over the liver. Absolutes are very concentrated and should be diluted particularly well.

Aromatic Considerations

Chamomile Egyptian absolute has a somewhat different aroma—more 'grassy' and herbaceous and less floral—than the distilled essential oil made from the same species that is known as chamomile German. Chamomile Egyptian absolute is a dark sage green, rather than deep blue. Sage green (and viscous) is appropriate for the chamomile *absolute* but, in the distilled essential oil, the depth of the blue color is an indication of the quality and therapeutic value.

Emotional/Spiritual/Physical Aspects

The properties and uses of this oil are very similar to chamomile German which is discussed in more detail in the next section. Absolutes need to be evaluated in small quantities to be appreciated. You cannot just open the bottle and take a whiff with an absolute.

General Information

Chamomile Egyptian is an absolute made from the same species as the distilled oil marketed as chamomile German. Absolutes are extracted by a complex process using solvents such as alcohol or hexane. The solvent is then effectively removed. Solvent extraction usually results in a more concentrated and complex fragrance than would be obtained by steam distillation. In fact, many plants processed this way cannot be steam distilled due to the small quantity of essential oil in the part of the plant used. This is not true of this chamomile. The steam distilled oil (chamomile German) is a very concentrated and complex essential oil.

Chamomile, German

(Matricaria recutita)

Ingredient In

[Le] Dreams ,[Le]My-Graine, [Le]Millenia, [Le]Solitude, [Le]Tranquility, [Le]Refresh-Mint, [Le]Vision

Therapeutic Properties

calmative, analgesic, antispasmodic, antibiotic, anti-inflammatory, emmenagogue, hepatic, vulnerary

Affinity For

reproductive system
digestive system
nervous system
gall bladder meridian
spleen meridian
bladder meridian
yin energy
throat, heart and solar plexus chakras

Resonance

physical, emotional

Plant Family

Compositae

Part of Plant Used

flowers

Application

Chamomile German can be applied to the base of the neck, on the temples, and over the liver.

Aromatic Considerations

The aroma of the German (blue) variety is deeper, headier, and more floral than the light colored chamomile Roman. The aroma of this chamomile calms and soothes feelings of anger and frustration.

Emotional/Spiritual Aspects

One of the most important actions of chamomile German is on the solar plexus. The solar plexus is the major nerve center that lies mid-way between the gut instinct area of the abdomen and the empathetic region of the heart. The solar plexus also lies at the cross roads between the left and right sides of our energetic bodies. This location puts the solar plexus in charge of balancing our need to be in control with our need to gently nurture. A build-up of energy and tension in the solar plexus intensifies our emotional needs. If we feel that our needs are not being met, we can become frustrated and irritable. We may react by trying harder to control the people around us, manipulating them into meeting our perceived needs. The aroma of chamomile German can release the tension that is building up in the solar plexus area.

Chamomile German increases honest, compassionate communication. It is of benefit to people who have periods of indifference to family and friends, followed by irritable outbursts directed at those nearest and dearest to them. Chamomile German seems to 'unclutter' the mind, allowing us to get organized and then 'unclutter' our lives. This species of chamomile is about learning to let go and trust the unfolding of events in our lives. It helps us remember that when life isn't working out as we planned, it may be working to a better plan.

Physical Aspects

The latin name for the chamomile family, *Matricaria,* means 'caring for the womb' and emphasizes the centuries-old use of this herb for female complaints. Chamomile German is excellent for digestive problems, especially if there is an emotional component to them.

Chamomile German is a necessary ingredient in blends used to treat ADHD in children and anxiety attacks in adolescents and adults. This oil has an outstanding history in the treatment of headaches, insomnia, and nervous tension.

Chamomile German should be tried for severe skin ulcerations or infections, dermatitis, and excema. For those with sensitive skin, application of this oil over a period of time can strengthen the skin's protective barrier.

General Information

Azulene, the component in chamomile German and a few other essential oils, is created by the steam distillation process. Heating plant material sometimes creates compounds that are not found in the fresh plant. These compounds, of which azulene is the best known, have unique therapeutic properties. Azulene is strongly anti-inflammatory and analgesic. The azulene created when blue tansy is heated is largely responsible for the 'realigning' properties of [Le]Millenia.

Cautions

Chamomile German should be used with caution if pregnant.

Chamomile, Roman

(Chamaemelum nobile)

Ingredient In

LeAssurance, LeBaby Me, LeEZ-Traveler, LeRefresh-Mint, LeRevitalize, LeVision, LeWhispering Hope

Therapeutic Properties

calmative, analgesic, antibiotic, febrifuge, anti-inflammatory, immune

Affinity For

reproductive system
digestive system
nervous system
spleen meridian
bladder meridian
yin energy
throat chakra

Resonance

physical, emotional

Plant Family

Compositae

Part of Plant Used

flowers

Application

Chamomile Roman can be applied to the base of the neck, on the temples, and over the liver. It can be added to shampoo or conditioner to cover gray in lighter hair colors.

Aromatic Considerations

The aroma of chamomile Roman, in my opinion, is the most relaxing scent in the entire essential oil world. Chamomile Roman is powerfully soothing. The soothing action of this oil applies to both physical and emotional conditions alike. Diffused, this oil creates an atmosphere of peace and patience.

Emotional/Spiritual Aspects

Chamomile Roman smooths the flow of the *chi* energy throughout the body. It is this regulation of vital energy that makes chamomile Roman so powerfully soothing to both physical and emotional conditions. In fact, so powerfully does this oil unravel the negative emotions behind physical ailments, that it is sometimes hard to tell if it is working at an emotional or a physical level. Chamomile Roman is of great benefit in the treatment of chronic headaches, insomnia, nervous indigestion and nausea, and irritable bowel syndrome—to name just a few.

The smoothing out of the vital energy prevents the build-up of energetic heat, which manifests in the body as inflammation. This chamomile is particularly beneficial for alleviating neuritis, cystitis, rheumatoid arthritis and earache.

One of the outstanding uses of chamomile Roman essential oil is for babies with colic, babies who startle awake and then cry for a long time, and infants that are just plain fussy and want to be held and comforted most of the day and night.

Physical Aspects

This variety of chamomile, though containing less deep blue azulene, has anti-inflammatory properties. It is of benefit when applied to aching muscles and joints. Because it is so mild and soothing, chamomile Roman is wonderful in the tub or used in a compress. This oil is very soothing for menstrual cramps, nausea, PMS, tension, and nerves.

Chamomile Roman cleanses the blood and reduces allergic reactions. Allergy sufferers can find a great deal of relief by carrying an inhaler or just a few drops of this oil on a tissue or cotton ball. Chamomile Roman is an antihistamine and soothing to inflamed tissues.

General Information

The plant from which chamomile Roman is distilled is very tender and delicate. It must be harvested at precisely the right moment in its growth cycle. To accomplish this, growers concerned with quality do a test distillation every few days as the plant matures. They have the distillation analyzed using gas chromatography. This insures the therapeutic quality of the essential oil.

Cautions

Chamomile Roman is, occasionally, found on lists that claim it should to be used with caution during pregnancy. I think, perhaps, those lists are being a little too cautious. This is a very mild essential oil.

Chaste Tree

(Vitex agnus castus)

Ingredient In

[Le]Balance

Affinity For

female reproductive system
nervous system

Resonance	**Plant Family**	**Part of Plant Used**
physical, emotional	Verbenaceae	fruit

Application

Chaste tree should be diluted and applied to the abdomen or feet.

Aromatic Considerations

Chaste tree is not recommended for diffusion.

Emotional/Spiritual/Physical Aspects

There is a lot of literature about the herbal uses for chaste tree, but very little documented usage of the essential oil. Claims have been made that chaste tree essential oil enhances the production of progesterone, bringing balance to female hormones. It may ease menstrual discomforts such as cramps, irritability, headaches, depression and breast swelling. Chaste tree also works well for reducing the symptoms of menopause. Preliminary trials suggest effectiveness in treatment of infertility and irregular menstrual cycles.

Chaste tree, in herbal form, is used for polycystic ovarian syndrome, uterine fibroids, infertility, and miscarriages due to luteal phase defects. (This type of miscarriage is described briefly on page 4 of Chapter 13 in this book.) Essential oils have the same therapeutic properties as the plants from which they are made. The therapeutic properties are more concentrated in the essential oil, often making them even more effective than in the herbal form.

General Information

The Vitex agnus castus variety of chaste tree is native to the Mediterranean area (Turkey), while Vitex negundo is found in Asia and Africa. Studies are being conducted at Ege University in Izmir, Turkey, on the use of Vitex oil for reversing the symptoms of Parkinson's disease. In the book by Connie and Alan Higley, Reference Guide for Essential Oils, the Higleys seem to be indicating that the Vitex studied for Parkinson's is Vitex negundo.

Vitex (both neguno and agnes) appears to be a natural source of L-dopa. L-dopa stimulates production of the neuro-transmitter L-dopamine in the brain. The lack of L-dopamine production is a factor in Parkinson's disease. Several Vitex varieties are now being looked at around the world as natural sources of L-dopa. The essential oils of both plants contain sesquiterpenes. Sesquiterpenes cross the blood/brain barrier, carrying the L-dopa and other therapeutic properties of the essential oil along with them.

The synthetic pharmaceutical products currently in use cannot do this, which makes them very ineffective. Not being able to get medications to cross the blood/brain barrier has been frustrating the medical community for years. Perhaps, natural substances will prove their superiority in medical applications once again.

Cautions

Chaste tree is strongly contra-indicated for pregnancy, except possibly to prevent early miscarriage in women with problems in the luteal phase of the pregnancy (mentioned above). There is just not enough information or studies done on this topic, yet—that I can find. It is well known, however, that chaste tree has a dramatic effect on hormones. That is enough of a reason to leave this essential oil completely alone during a pregnancy.

Cilantro

(Coriandrum sativum)

Ingredient In

LeInside-Out

Therapeutic Properties

analgesic, antioxidant, antispasmodic, digestive, carminative, revitalizing, stimulant, stomachic

Affinity For

digestive system
nerves
endocrine system
circulation
meridians: earth, fire, air, water

Resonance

physical, mental

Plant Family

Umbelliferae

Part of Plant Used

leaves

Application

Cilantro should be diluted and applied as needed. It may also be diffused.

Aromatic Considerations

Although they are made from very different parts of the plant, cilantro and coriander have similar aromas.

Emotional/Spiritual Aspects

Cilantro is distilled from the leaves of the Coriandrum sativum plant; the seeds of this plant are distilled to obtain coriander essential oil. There are many similarities in these two oils, but the plant part used changes the focus of the therapeutic properties. This is particularly true in the emotional aspects. Essential oils derived from the leaf tend to be needed by people who focus outside themselves on the needs of others, often in such excess that it is to their own detriment. These oils can aid us in developing compassion and sympathy for others. Essential oils derived from seeds focus more on potential for personal growth. They can bring feelings of joy and satisfaction with ourselves and the circumstances of our lives.

Physical Aspects

Like coriander, which is distilled from the same plant, cilantro is both a gentle stimulant and a mild sedative. It can be used to raise energy levels and calm nerves, when stress or over-work has brought on a state of nervousness with fatigue. Cilantro's therapeutic properties make it a good addition to blends for the digestive system.

General Information

Recent research indicates that cilantro essential oil is highly effective at inhibiting the growth of some bacteria that are responsible for food borne illnesses. I find this study interesting, especially when I consider that cilantro has been used in cooking in warm climates for a very long time.

Cautions

Cilantro is generally considered to be non-toxic and non-irritating, although it can be very potent in large doses. Like most essential oils, it is best used with judgement and moderation.

Cinnamon Bark

(Cinnamomum verum var. zeylanicum)

Ingredient In

LeBountiful, LeDeliverance, LeEnergy, LeFocus, LeHoliday Spirit, LeInner Peace, LeJourney, LeMoonlight, LeSpice C

Therapeutic Properties

stimulant, antiseptic, antibiotic, antiviral, anti-putrescent, analgesic, antispasmodic, emmenagogue

Affinity For

enhances the properties of other essential oils
circulatory system
cell structure and activity
sacral chakra
root chakra
astral body

Resonance

physcal, emotional, spiritual

Plant Family

Lauraceae

Part of Plant Used

bark

Application

Cinnamon bark is a very strong oil. It ***must*** be diluted well before being applied to the body or the feet.

Aromatic Considerations

Cinnamon is very strong, perhaps too strong to be diffused by itself. As part of a blend such as LeDeliverance, it diffuses very well, and would certainly be effective against a wide range of microbes.

Emotional/Spiritual Aspects

The aroma of cinnamon seems to reach deeply into our souls, asking hard questions and bringing deep issues to the surface. Situations and questions we have left unresolved are brought back to our attention. If we choose to deal with them we will be able to move forward toward healing and peace. Cinnamon can provide courage to look into the darker places in ourselves, as well as sufficient courage to look squarely at each situation in our lives. If you feel that your heart and emotions have gone cold and are buried deep inside, cinnamon will warm them up and help you bring them into the light.

Physical Aspects

Cinnamon bark essential oil has very specific purposes and applications. 1) It is a very powerful antimicrobial. Virus spores, bacteria, and fungus cannot live in the presence of this oil. Cinnamon is effective for all types of infections. 2) Cinnamon oil enhances the action and activity of other oils with which it is combined, creating synergistically amazing combinations. 3) Cinnamon carries oxygen into the cells. It is stimulating and toning to the entire body. Cinnamon is of particular benefit to the circulatory system. Cinnamon, preferably in a blend, should be used for arthritis, muscular aches and pains, coughs, and colds. 4) Cinnamon aids the body in the regulation and utilization of insulin.

General Information

Cinnamon is part of the formula the Lord gave Moses (recorded in Exodus 30:22-27).

Cautions

Cinnamon oil is best used in low doses or as part of a blend of essential oils. Cinnamon is too strong for use in the tub or shower. It should be used cautiously with children and people with sensitive skin.

Cinnamon Berry

(Cinnamomum polyandrum)

Ingredient In

LeFocus, LeStefanie, LeAway

Therapeutic Properties

analgesic, antibiotic, antiseptic, astringent, carminative, digestive, emmenagogue, relaxant, stomachic, nerve tonic, stimulant

Affinity For

circulation	joints	sacral chakra
nerves	digestion	muscles

Resonance	**Plant Family**	**Part of Plant Used**
physical, emotional	Lauraceae	fruit

Application

Cinnamon berry should be diluted well when applied to the body. Application can be on the feet or directly on areas of pain or poor circulation.

Aromatic Considerations

The essential oil made from the berries of this *cinnamomum* species is a little bit milder than oil made from the bark of *cinnamonum verum*. Care should still be taken with inhalation and diffusion. Cinnamon can be irritating to tender mucous membranes.

Emotional/Spiritual Aspects

Cinnamon berry is useful in treating stress related conditions such as headache, insomnia, indigestion, and nervous tension.

Physical Aspects

Cinnamon berry acts as a stimulant to circulation. Increased circulation can be beneficial for arthritis, muscle and joint stiffness, inflamed or painful joints and muscles, and sprains. Cinnamon berry is said to improve appetite. Cinnamon berry, like cinnamon bark, is antimicrobial, but is less caustic and irritating.

Cautions

Use cautiously if pregnant, when working with infants and children, or if your skin is particularly sensitive.

Cistus - Rockrose

(Cistus landaniferus)

Ingredient In

LeAngel, LeDiscernment, melissa blend

Therapeutic Properties

antimicrobial, antiseptic, astringent, diuretic, expectorant, emmenagogue, anti-inflammatory, tonic

Affinity For

skin
nerves
lymphatic system
urinary tract
immune system
respiratory system
kidney meridian
solar plexus chakra

Resonance

physical, emotional, mental

Plant Family

Cistaceae

Part of Plant Used

leaves and twigs

Application

Cistus is particularly nice applied, diluted, on the chest.

Aromatic Considerations

Cistus has a beautiful aroma. The aroma is floral with a hint of honey, but it is not heady, cloying, or overwhelming. Cistus would make a unique and beautiful perfume, in my opinion. The aroma of cistus is something you will either just love or really dislike. Cistus is stimulating to the upper quadrant of the brain and to the senses, amplifying our sense of touch, hearing, and sight. Cistus is useful diffused during meditation or when pondering deeply.

Emotional/Spiritual Aspects

The aftermath of traumatic events, quarrels, or painful losses can leave us feeling empty inside with nothing to left to give and a diminished capacity to feel and show emotion. Emotionally warming, cistus can start the process of thaw throughout the wastelands of such frozen emotions.

Physical Aspects

Cistus is used in skin care regimens, for the prevention and minimization of wrinkles, and in the treatment of skin disorders such as psoriasis and eczema. Because of its regenerative properties, cistus has also been used for many years in the treatment of wounds, abrasions, and boils. The phenols in cistus make it stimulating to the immune system and to the lungs. Cistus can be useful in the treatment of coughs and bronchitis.

General Information

Cistus is one of the earliest aromatic substances. References are made to it is some ancient texts. The rose of Sharon referred to in the Bible is believed to be cistus.

Cautions

Considered a safe, mild, and effective essential oil.

Citronella Java and Citronella Ceylon

(Cymbopogon winterianus) — *(Cymbopogon nardus)*

Affinity For

cardiovascular system, circulation, digestion, skin, muscles, bones

Ingredient In

LeAway, LePurify, LeSunburst

Therapeutic Properties

antibacterial, anti-fungal, anti-inflammatory, antiseptic, antispasmodic, deodorant, insecticidal, parasitic, stimulant

Resonance

physical, spiritual, emotional

Plant Family

Graminae

Part of Plant Used

leaf (grass)

Application

Citronella should always be diluted well before applying to skin.

Aromatic Considerations

Citronella's bright, fresh aroma is nourishing to the spirit. It is also stimulating to the cardiovascular system. Citronella increases the heart rate when it is abnormally low. The aroma of citronella is recognized around the world as an insect repellent.

Emotional/Spiritual Aspects

Citronella is said to clear the soul of the negative influences others may be having on us. It helps us look at our relationships, being able to evaluate whether they are a positive or a negative influence in our lives.

Physical Aspects

Citronella can be used safely as an antiseptic to sanitize and deodorize surfaces being used in food preparation. Citronella, diluted with a carrier oil, makes a refreshing massage therapy oil. The citronella oils are used for colds, flu, fatigue, headaches, migraines, and neuralgia. They are also good for balancing excessive perspiration and excessive oiliness of skin and hair.

General Information

These two oils belong to the same family as lemongrass and palmarosa, and are similar in their therapeutic uses. Most literature does not distinguish between the citronella ceylon and citronella java. MS (mass spectrograph) readouts reveal some interesting differences, however. Java has a much higher percentage of *citronellal.* This is the component most responsible for the lemony aroma and is also responsible for the insect repellent properties of citronella oils. Java has a lower percentage of *geraniol* than the ceylon variety. Geraniol is an ingredient which is suspected of attracting certain kinds of bees—not a good attribute for an insect repellent! Obviously, java makes the best insect repellent, but both varieties are often combined with cedarwood to make insecticides and insect repellents. Ceylon is probably used, not because it is the best choice, but because it is less expensive that java.

Cautions

Too frequent use of citronella on the skin can cause contact sensitization and irritation. Citronella should be used with caution during pregnancy.

Clary Sage

(Salvia sclarea)

Ingredient In

LeBalance, LeExhilaration, LeMoonlight, LeTomorrow, LeWoman Wise

Therapeutic Properties

regulates cells and balances hormones, antiseptic, calming, emmenagogue, anti-infectious, antispasmodic, anti-sudorific, aphrodisiac, nerve tonic, estrogen-like properties

Affinity For

digestive system | supports yang energy and moderates yin energy
respiratory system | spleen meridian | governing vessel meridian
hormone balance

Resonance	Plant Family	Part of Plant Used
physical, emotional	Labiatae	whole plant when flowering

Application

Dilute well and apply to the feet or on the body.

Aromatic Considerations

The aroma of clary sage promotes confidence and clarity about what you want your life to be.

Emotional/Spiritual Aspects

The emotional actions of clary sage are explained by the balance it establishes between stimulation and relaxation (yang and yin). Clary sage calms tension, nervousness, and hypersensitivity, yet revives and revitalizes us when we are fatigued.

Clary sage is a good oil for those who, when overtired, become hypersensitive and either weep or find fault with everyone around them. It is also a good choice for people whose lives show a pattern of continually choosing the wrong kind of friends. The aroma of clary sage calms the nerves and enhances the dream state of sleep. It brings about feelings of contentment.

Physical Aspects

Clary sage moderates excessive estrogen and yin energy. It is very effective for PMS, menstrual problems and cramping, infertility, frigidity and impotence, and some of the difficulties experienced during menopause. An excess of estrogen is linked to several women's cancers. Clary sage is useful in kidney infections, sore throat, and bronchial infections. It strengthens cellular structure and regulates cellular activity. It is an excellent oil, especially as part of a blend, for muscular fatigue and excessive perspiration.

Cautions

Clary sage has a lower percentage of thujone than does common sage *(Salvia officinalis),* which must be used in smaller quantities and with greater care. Clary sage is completely safe for most people in most applications when used in normal dosages. However, clary sage has a strong action on hormones and should be avoided, or used with ***extreme caution***, during pregnancy. Clary sage is not to be used with children because of these hormonal properties. It should be avoided if alcohol is going to be consumed. It is best not to use clary sage in the bath and small amounts at a time are sufficient when difussing.

Clementine

(Citrus nobilis)

Ingredient In

[Le]Insight

Therapeutic Properties

tonic, stomachic, digestive, calming, antispasmodic, antiseptic

Affinity For

nerves | emotions

Resonance	Plant Family	Part of Plant Used
emotional, spiritual	Rutaceae	fruit

Application

Clementine may be applied on the feet or on the body. It is excellent in a bath or diffused. Clementine is a citrus oil that is ***not*** considered photo-toxic!!

Aromatic Considerations

The aroma of clementine is delightful. It can only be described as absolutely 'yummy.'

Emotional/Spiritual Aspects

Clementine is gentler, softer, and sweeter than its parent plant, red mandarin. It is uplifting and gently revitalizing. Clementine is often used for insomnia.

Clove

(Syzgium aromaticum)

Ingredient In

LeAway, LeBountiful, LeDeliverance, LeEnergy, LeEternity, LeHoliday Spirit, LeLife Force, LeMela Plus, LePaine, LeRefresh-Mint, LeSpice C

Therapeutic Properties

antiseptic, antibiotic, ***strongly antiviral***, anti-fungal, analgesic, anti-neuralgic, antispasmodic, stimulant, carminative, aphrodisiac, stomachic, tonic, anti-parasitic, anti-tumoral

Affinity For

muscles
brain
urinary tract
digestive system
immune system
lymphatic system
circulatory system
solar plexus chakra
root chakra
all of the meridians

Resonance

physical, emotional

Plant Family

Myrtaceae

Part of Plant Used

fruit

Application

Careful attention should be paid to the dilution of clove essential oil before putting it on the skin. Clove essential oil can be applied to the feet or to any area of the body where its properties are needed.

Aromatic Considerations

The aroma of clove improves memory, alleviates mental and physical exhaustion, protects from negative energy, and creates feelings of cooperation and courage. Clove helps us to move forward, exploring new possibilities and experiences, with enthusiasm.

Emotional/Spiritual Aspects

The aroma of clove is, literally, heart-warming. It helps us to look away from ourselves and our own needs, so we can see the needs of family members and friends. Clove helps us translate this 'seeing' into practical, every day living and giving. Clove bud oil lifts depression, leaving behind a feeling of optimism and lightness. Clove bud oil can create and sustain a positive outlook and attitude.

Physical Aspects

Spices are among the most nutritional herbal remedies, and clove is one of the best. When clove bud essential oil is absorbed into the body, it provides missing nutrients. Because clove oil improves the overall nutrition in the body, it can be of benefit in many physical conditions. Clove bud is excellent in the early stages of illness to kill viruses and bacteria. Clove's stimulative and nutritive properties are helpful later on, during the recovery phase, to rebuild energy and stamina.

Clove bud is a strong topical anesthetic and pain reliever. It is often used to lessen the pain of a toothache until the problem can be remedied by a dentist. Clove acts on the digestive system for flatulence, nausea, and diarrhea. Clove bud essential oil is strong enough to dissolve warts. It should be used undiluted several times a day directly on the wart. Putting a drop or two on a little round band aid keeps the clove oil directly against the wart. This method is very effective.

Clove can be used for skin afflictions such as ringworm, scabies, and skin parasites. Clove is effective against bacteria, viruses, and funguses, so a diagnosis of exactly what is causing the problem is unnecessary.

General Information

Clove bud essential oil has been used in the treatment of Hodgkin's Disease.

Cautions

Clove, except as part of a blended oil, should be avoided by pregnant women. It should be used with caution and diluted well for use with children and anyone with sensitive skin. Clove is too strong to be used in the bath. Repeated use of clove as a single can cause contact sensitization and allergic reactions.

Copaiba Balsam

(Copaifera langsdorfii)

Ingredient In

LeAngel, LeInner Peace, LeIQ, LeMy-Graine, LePaine, LeSego Lily, LeVitality, LeBelieve

Therapeutic Properties

antiseptic, astringent, diuretic, expectorant, sedative to the nerves, tonic

Affinity For

skin, respiratory system, liver meridian, circulation, vascular system

Resonance	Plant Family	Part of Plant Used
physical, emotional	Fabaceae	resin

Application

Copaiba balsam can be applied anywhere on the body. The aroma of balsam, applied lightly, makes a wonderful perfume.

Aromatic Considerations

Copaiba balsam is referred to as 'nature's air freshener.' This is because of balsam's remarkable ability to absorb odors.

Emotional/Spiritual Aspects

The aroma of balsam seems to fill the room with feelings of friendship and neighborliness. This oil is very supportive of relationships.

Physical Aspects

Balsam oils are traditionally used for skin problems such as chapped skin, rashes, sensitive skin, poor circulation, and eczema. Balsam adds a woodsy, vanilla-like scent to blends. These blends make pleasant hand lotions and skin care products. Copaiba balsam has been used for years as an expectorant for bronchitis, coughs, and colds. This oil increases circulation without being a general stimulant. Copaiba balsam is effective for venous congestion, hemorrhoids, and varicose veins.

Cautions

Copaiba balsam makes the skin mildly photo-toxic where it has been applied. It is best to avoid sunlight on the treated areas of skin if you are applying this oil regularly.

Coriander

(Coriandrum sativum)

Ingredient In

LeEndo Relief, LeGrateful Heart, LeWithin, LeIQ

Therapeutic Properties

sedative, antibacterial, antispasmodic, carminative, antiseptic, deodorant, diuretic, lymphatic decongestant, prostate decongestant, vasoconstrictor, stimulant, tonic, regenerative

Affinity For

digestive system, endocrine system, meridians: earth, fire, air, water, nerves, circulation

Resonance	Plant Family	Part of Plant Used
physical, mental	Umbelliferae	seeds

Application

Coriander should be diluted well and applied as needed.

Aromatic Considerations

The aroma of coriander is like taking a deep breath—breathing out the old ideas, breathing in a new perspective.

Emotional/Spiritual Aspects

Coriander combines a warm, woodsy serenity with the peppery stimulation of a fire meridian remedy. This essential oil is especially appropriate for creative individuals who struggle when locked into situations of predictability and routine. While they need stability and emotional security, they seek these things through passionate involvement with people and causes and not through fear or self-protection. Coriander refreshes and revives our spirits. It can be helpful in overcoming fear of failure or fear of making decisions.

Physical Aspects

Coriander is both a gentle stimulant when energy levels are at a low ebb and a sedative in times of stress. Coriander is particularly valuable during convalescence from illness, when energy levels are low and stress is often high. This oil is of benefit for physical, mental, and nervous exhaustion. In an odd combination of sensations, coriander raises our energy levels and makes us feel less irritable and nervous. Coriander relieves muscle aches due to fatigue.

Coriander has a marked effect on various aspects of the endocrine system. One of the most important uses for this oil is in balancing glucose levels and supporting pancreatic function. Coriander is estrogenic. It is often beneficial in regulating menstrual cycles and relieving cramping.

Coriander is used for digestive problems such as flatulence, nausea, and stomach cramps. It has been used in treatment programs for anorexia.

General Information

Coriander seeds have been used for centuries. Some coriander seeds were found in King Tutankhamen's tomb. Coriander comes from the seeds of the plant we know as cilantro.

Cautions

Coriander should be used in small quantities and for short periods of time. Over use of this oil can result in a cloudy or stupefied feeling.

Cumin

(Cuminum cyminum)

Ingredient In

LeEndo Relief, LeStefanie

Therapeutic Properties

antibacterial, antiseptic, antiviral, antioxidant, antiparasitic, aphrodisiac, digestive, diuretic, emmenagogue, antispasmodic, anti-inflammatory

Affinity For

digestive system, respiratory system, endocrine system, nervous system, lymphatic system, muscles

Resonance

physical, emotional

Plant Family

Umbelliferae

Part of Plant Used

seeds

Application

Cumin oil should be diluted well or used as part of a blend.

Aromatic Considerations

Cumin essential oil has a very strong aroma. It can be quite appealing if it is diffused for a short period of time. The aroma lingers in the air for a long time after the diffuser has been turned off.

Emotional/Spiritual Aspects

People who would benefit from cumin oil are usually very determined individuals. They are proud of their strength and determination. They do not tolerate people they consider to be fools or lazy. Unfortunately, they put most everyone but themselves into these categories. It is possible for these people to become wise and beloved as they mature.

Physical Aspects

Cumin is anti-inflammatory and warming to strained or damaged muscles. It relieves muscular pains and the pains of arthritis. Cumin is a stimulant to the digestive system. It should be considered for colic, flatulence, bloating, and indigestion. Cumin is an excellent nervous system tonic. It is often employed to relieve headaches, migraines, and to boost energy levels with nervous exhaustion. Diluted and applied to the chest, cumin can be useful for asthma, bronchial spasms, and spasmodic coughs. One of the outstanding characteristics of cumin oil is its action in clearing the lymphatic system and ridding the body of excess fluids and toxins. Cumin also increases circulation. Recent studies show strong indications that cumin oil acts as a thyroid stimulant.

General Information

Cumin has an over-powering aroma. This is a very strong, almost caustic essential oil.

Cautions

Cumin is an oil that I appreciate in a blend, but use very rarely by itself. You should avoid cumin if you have sensitive skin or if you are pregnant. ***This essential oil is best as part of a blend of essential oils.***

Cypress

(Cupressus sempervirens)

Ingredient In

LeAspire, LeBalance, LeCandila, LeCypernium, LeDandy, LeDelicate, LeEndo Relief, LeIQ, LeRefresh-Mint, LeTomorrow, LeVisibility, LeVitality, LeWarm Down

Therapeutic Properties

mucolytic, hepatic, astringent, antispasmodic, anti-sudorific, diuretic, restorative, vasoconstrictor, respiratory tonic, calmative, astringent

Affinity For

circulation	muscles, joints	throat chakra
pancreas	lymphatic drainage	solar plexus chakra
respiratory system	liver	central vessel meridian
reproductive system	yin energy	large intestine meridian
		spleen meridian

Resonance	Plant Family	Part of Plant Used
physical, emotional, spiritual	Coniferae/Cupressacea (sub)	wood, leaves

Application

Cypress can be diluted and applied anywhere on the body. It is also excellent applied to the bottoms of the feet.

Aromatic Considerations

Cypress is a wonderful healer for the spirit. It brings the feeling that each new day is a fresh start on our road to glowing life and health. Change is a part of life. Times of transition can be positive if we allow them to be. If we struggle against the changes, trying to hang on to what was, our life can feel like an unending struggle. Interestingly, cypress—while not a sedative—is useful for insomnia. Perhaps the optimism it brings quiets the usual worry that is keeping one awake.

Emotional/Spiritual Aspects

Cypress is considered in many cultures to be symbolic of life after death. It may be useful when facing death or other separations. The aroma of cypress opens us to direction from heaven. Cypress can help soften unbending and inflexible attitudes. Cypress seems to bring balance to our attitudes about money. It has the effect of loosening purse strings that are being held too tightly. Cypress can help us learn to enjoy the bounty that we have. Perhaps those who need to can even learn to spend a little on something that is not an absolute necessity.

Physical Aspects

Cypress strengthens capillary walls, reducing varicose veins and hemorrhoids. Cypress is a respiratory, lymphatic, liver, pancreas, and prostate decongestant. This makes cypress useful for a wide variety of ailments. Cypress is a mild, but effective, diuretic. It should be tried for water retention, cellulite, menstrual bloating, and menopausal problems. Cypress is one of the best oils for muscle cramps and healing wounds. In fact, cypress is one of the best single oils to reach for in many circumstances. I love and use mostly blends, but cypress is so complex and far reaching that it is almost like a blend all by itself.

Cautions

Cypress is mildly estrogenic and should be avoided by most pregnant women. It is, however, used for toxemia when at least part of the cause ***is*** an estrogen imbalance.

Davana

(Artemisia pallens)

Ingredient In

LeRevitalize, LeTurmoil

Therapeutic Properties

anti-infectious, aphrodisiac, stimulant, endocrine system stimulant, expectorant, antidepressant

Affinity For

endocrine system	respiratory system	hormones

Resonance	**Plant Family**	**Part of Plant Used**
physical, emotional	Compositae	stems, leaves

Application

Davanna is best worn somewhere on the body.

Aromatic Considerations

Davana is popular in the perfume industry where it has the reputation of making a scent unique to the individual wearing it. This property is obvious in the pure essential oil as well. The aroma of davana is difficult to describe because it usually smells quite different from person to person. The aroma of davana is very different on the skin than whiffed from a container or when it is diffused.

Emotional/Spiritual Aspects

Davana eases anxious feelings and nervousness. It is helpful in recovering from shock, trauma, disappointment, and perceived failure. (Notice the properties and uses of the blends in which it is found.) Davana is considered a potent aphrodisiac.

Physical Aspects

Davana is used to relieve spasmodic coughing and loosen thick mucous in the lungs. Davana fights infections, particularly tetanus. It should be applied without delay to cuts and wounds, especially if the cut was made by iron objects and tetanus is a real possibility. Davana has been shown to rupture the protective outer layer of viruses, thus killing them quickly. Davana is regarded as a stimulant to the endocrine system, and has some hormonal balancing properties.

Cautions

There are no known contra-indications, but care should always be taken with pregnancy.

Dill

(Anethum graveolens)

Ingredient In

LeEndo Relief, LeLife Force

Therapeutic Properties

antispasmodic, antibacterial, antiseptic, expectorant, stimulant, digestive, sedative, stomachic, sudorific, galactogogue

Affinity For

digestive system	endocrine system: particularly the pancreas	stomach meridian
autonomic nervous system	bloodstream	
respiratory system		

Resonance	Plant Family	Part of Plant Used
physical, emotional	Umbelliferae	seeds

Application

Dill can be applied anywhere on the body—if you don't mind smelling like a dill pickle!

Aromatic Considerations

The autonomic nervous system controls such things as heartbeat, the function of our kidneys, the flow of hormones, and blood pressure. We have been taught that we have no *conscious* control of these functions. Studies and common sense both indicate that this is not entirely true. For example, army snipers are taught to mentally slow their pulse and heartbeat and sharpen the acuity of their vision as they prepare to make their shots. In the nerves and impulses of this area of the nervous system, dill brings sustenance, strength, and calmness.

Emotional/Spiritual Aspects

A sluggish colon often manifests itself in the emotions as depression or repression of emotions. Dill's action on the digestive system can help lift depression and bring buried emotions to the surface where they can be processed.

Physical Aspects

Dill supports pancreatic functions, helping to normalize glucose and insulin levels. As glucose and insulin stabilize, energy levels remain steady—there are no glucose spikes followed by periods of abnormally low glucose levels. This effect of the aroma of dill is almost instantaneous. A more complex blend containing dill, such as LeEndo Relief, should be used for long-term treatment. Dill is used to stimulate digestion. In pioneer times and in much of Europe even today, meals began with something sour such as dill pickles. It might be a good thing to emulate this practice in our own eating habits. Dill is also a mild way to cleanse the liver and blood. It promotes milk flow in nursing mothers. Perhaps there is a connection to the cravings for pickles that are associated with pregnancy, and either the mild cleansing or milk producing properties of dill.

Cautions

Occasionally safety literature will mention that dill should be used cautiously by people with seizure disorders.

Elemi

(Canarium luzonicum)

Ingredient In

LeMillenia, LeNo-More

Therapeutic Properties

anti- catarrhal, antidepressant, antiseptic, expectorant, calming

Affinity For

respiratory system	skin and wound care	yang energy large intestine meridian

Resonance	Plant Family	Part of Plant Used
physical, emotional, mental, spiritual	Burseraceae	resin

Aromatic Considerations

Elemi has more of a citrus aroma than does frankincense, but elemi has the distinctive spicy/peppery tone of frankincense. Elemi is often diffused during meditation or energy work sessions to aid in visualizations. Elemi should be diffused in times of stress or mental exhaustion.

Application

Elemi can be applied to the feet or any part of the body. It makes an excellent addition to massage oils and compresses. Elemi is a good oil to add to the bath.

General Information

Elemi is known throughout the world as 'poor man's frankincense.' It has somewhat similar properties and uses as frankincense. See the section on frankincense for additional uses.

Emotional/Spiritual Aspects

Elemi lifts the spirits and provides the energy and desire to seek out better things and more uplifting experiences. The aroma of elemi encourages compassion and a desire for going beyond the ordinary in serving others.

Physical Aspects

Elemi makes a wonderful addition to blends intended for skin care and rejuvenation. Elemi can be used to treat allergic rashes, chapped skin, skin ulcers, and wounds. It is particularly recommended for cuts that have become infected. Elemi has a reputation for being effective in the treatment of gangrene and breast and uterine infections. Elemi has a rebuilding and strengthening effect on respiratory weakness. Elemi may be of use to people who suffer from chronic bronchitis. This essential oil, like frankincense, is recommended for bronchial or sinus infections.

Eucalyptus

(Eucalyptus globulus)

Ingredient In

LeAspire, LeBreezey, LeDeeper, LeDeliverance, LePaine, LeRefresh-Mint, LeTenda Care

Therapeutic Properties

anti-inflammatory, antiseptic, balsamic, expectorant, antibiotic, anti-fungal, febrifuge, anti-infectious, anti-parasitic, anti-neuralgic, pectoral

General Information

I do not recommend taking essential oils internally, but I want to issue a particular warning about all varieties of eucalyptus and internal use. The literature around the world and in most schools of thought about essential oils agree that eucalyptus is toxic when taken internally. Nevertheless, the FDA (what do they know about this kind of thing?) have approved it for use as a dietary supplement. You can do most anything with the topical application of an essential oil that you would hope to do with internal consumption. Please be sensible and cautious about the internal use of any essential oil, especially with children, and do not take or administer eucalyptus oils internally at all.

Affinity For

endocrine system
respiratory system
muscles
bones
yin energy
brow chakra

Resonance	**Plant Family**	**Part of Plant Used**
physical, emotional	Myrtaceae	leaves

Aromatic Considerations

Eucalyptus is energizing and promotes feelings of steadfastness and confidence in oneself. The aroma of eucalyptus can help us release resentment calmly, without the usual explosions of temper and hostility. Eucalyptus, diffused, purifies the air.

Application

Eucalyptus should be applied to the feet, and on areas when anti-inflammatory properties are needed. Eucalyptus, or a blend containing it, can be diluted and applied to the chest for respiratory congestion and infections. If used in small amounts, eucalyptus makes a good addition to massage oils. Eucalyptus applied under and on each side of the nose brings quick relief for clogged sinus cavities.

Emotional/Spiritual Aspects

Eucalyptus helps us find our survivor spirit. Eucalyptus taps into the inner strength in each of us. It can help us develop unfaltering faith in ourselves and in divine assistance. Eucalyptus strips away doubt about our abilities, removes negativity and hesitation, and pushes us forward. Eucalyptus calms our spirits and opens our minds to see the way ahead clearly.

Physical Aspects

Eucalyptus is a very versatile and useful essential oil. It can be used to cool the body in summer and protect us from bacteria and viruses in the winter. Eucalyptus is useful for bronchitis, colds, flu, asthma, and any problem in the respiratory system. Eucalyptus is one of the best oils for bringing down a fever. It is a strong analgesic. It can be applied alone or as part of a blend for muscle aches and headaches. Eucalyptus alleviates mental exhaustion and stabilizes blood sugar levels in both hypoglycemia and diabetes. Well diluted, eucalyptus is good for skin rashes and makes a very good energizing massage oil.

General Information

Eucalyptus becomes more antiseptic with age, if it has been stored and handled properly.

Cautions

Eucalyptus can be caustic to the skin if used undiluted. ***Not to be taken internally—see General Information***

Eucalyptus (Blue Mallee)

(Eucalyptus polybractea)

Therapeutic Properties

Eucalyptus blue mallee is similar in properties and uses to eucalyptus globulus discussed above.

Affinity For

especially suited to the respiratory system
any where eucalyptus globulus would be used
yin energy
triple warmer meridian
spleen meridian
lung meridian

Resonance	**Plant Family**	**Part of Plant Used**
physical, emotional	Myrtaceae	leaves

Aromatic Considerations

Blue mallee eucalyptus has a milder aroma than the more commonly used eucalyptus globulus. The milder aroma makes it more pleasant for children. This eucalyptus is very good when used in emotional release and energy work.

Application

Use eucalyptus blue mallee exactly as you would use any other variety of eucalyptus.

Emotional/Spiritual/ Aspects

See eucalyptus globulus above

Physical Aspects

This variety of eucalyptus, though milder in aroma than globulus, seems to penetrate more deeply into the lungs and bronchial tubes. The aroma makes one feel like trying to take a deep cleansing breath.

General Information

Like other eucalyptus varieties, blue mallee gets more antiseptic and effective as it ages.

Cautions

All eucalyptus varieties can be caustic to the skin if used undiluted. ***Internal use: see General Information in eucalyptus notes on the previous page.***

Eucalyptus, peppermint

(Eucalyptus dives)

Ingredient In

[Le]Away

Therapeutic Properties

anti-catarrhal, antiseptic, antiviral, astringent, expectorant, mucolytic, analgesic, anti-inflammatory, anti-neuralgic, decongestant, diuretic, febrifuge, calming

Affinity For

respiratory system
circulation
muscular system
yin energy
triple warmer meridian
spleen meridian
lung meridian

Resonance	Plant Family	Part of Plant Used
physical and emotional	Myrtaceae	leaves

Aromatic Considerations

This essential oil combines the aromas of eucalyptus and peppermint, just as the name implies. As it dries or hangs in the air, it develops a balsamic, woody undertone that is centering and calming. If I am going to diffuse a eucalyptus, this is my first choice.

Application

Use this oil exactly as you would other varieties of eucalyptus.

Emotional/Spiritual Aspects

The emotional qualities of all eucalyptus varieties are similar. This variety, with its slight peppermint aroma, seems to be more calming than the others.

Physical Aspects

Eucalyptus peppermint encourages deep, slow breaths that aid bronchial dilation when inflammation or fluids are present. This essential oil encourages circulation and eases muscular pain and tightness. This is an appropriate eucalyptus to use in athletic massage oils. Eucalyptus peppermint has a very strong and specific antiseptic action. It really targets and eliminates bacteria, viruses, and fungi. Many people find it useful and quite pleasant as an insect repellent.

General Information

Eucalyptus peppermint is lower in ecualyptol content but higher in menthols. These differences in constituents make this eucalyptus slightly less caustic for skin applications but still excellent for the treatment of respiratory ailments. This eucalyptus is sometimes referred to as peppermint eucalyptus or broad-leafed pepperming.

Cautions

All eucalyptus varieties can be caustic to the skin if used undiluted.

Internal use: see General Information in eucalyptus notes on the previous page.

Eucalyptus, radiata

(Eucalyptus radiata)

Ingredient In

[Le] Spice C

Therapeutic Properties

anti-catarrhal, antidepressant, antiseptic, expectorant, calming

Affinity For

respiratory system
circulation
muscular system
yin energy
triple warmer meridian
spleen meridian
lung meridian

Resonance	Plant Family	Part of Plant Used
physical, emotional	Myrtaceae	leaves

Aromatic Considerations

Eucalyptus radiata, like the blue mallee variety, is gentler and softer than globulus.

Application

Use exactly as you would other varieties of eucalyptus.

Emotional/Spiritual Aspects

The emotional qualities of all eucalyptus varieties are similar, but this one is preferred by many for use in meditation and energy work.

Physical Aspects

This eucalyptus is used much the same as the globulus variety but it is reputed to be less likely to irritate the skin when used repeatedly for sore muscles. Radiata has a high percentage of cineol, also known as eucalyptol. This is the component believed to relieve colds and congestion.

General Information

Eucalyptus radiata was actually the first eucalyptus distilled commercially as an essential oil. It is commonly known as 'narrow-leafed peppermint,' although it is a member of the eucalyptus family.

Cautions

The cautions for this variety are the same as for other varieties of eucalyptus. ***Internal use: see General Information in eucalyptus notes on the previous pages.***

Fennel

(Foeniculum vulgare)

Ingredient In

[Le]Inside-Out, [Le]Revitalize, [Le]Woman Wise

Therapeutic Properties

hepatic, carminative, emmenagogue, hormonal, galactagogue, depurative, diuretic, stimulant, regenerative, antispasmodic, antiseptic, antibiotic, vermifuge, expectorant

Affinity For

digestive system	sacral chakra	stomach meridian
urinary tract	large intestine/lung meridian	gallbladder meridian
liver	hormones	

Resonance	**Plant Family**	**Part of Plant Used**
physical, emotional	Umbelliferae	seeds

Aromatic Considerations

The aroma of fennel can help us establish a balance between appropriate service and total burnout. It can help us stand by decisions and stabilize our mood swings.

Application

Dilute and apply to appropriate areas of the feet, on the abdomen, and on the lower back.

Emotional/Spiritual Aspects

Fennel, because of its affinity for the liver, can have a positive impact on a whole range of emotions. Fennel can help when we are feeling overwhelmed by our responsibilities and workload. It can also stimulate our minds with creative ideas when we are bored or out of sorts. Fear of failure is often the root cause of procrastination. Fennel, with its impact on creativity and confidence, can help us get started on a project we have been putting off.

Fennel essential oil is well suited to individuals who are out of balance in the metal (meridian #3) aspect of their energy. They tend to over think and over analyze until indecision freezes them in place.

Physical Aspects

Fennel supports the liver in producing the enzymes necessary for good digestion. It is often used for indigestion and to relieve gas pains. Fennel also helps balance the hormones. It is often found in blends for PMS. Because fennel is mildly diuretic, it is helpful with the fluid retention of PMS.

Cautions

Fennel should be avoided if you are pregnant or epileptic. Fennel should not be used on babies or very small children. Fennel should be avoided by women with high estrogen levels and/or breast cancer. Experts disagree about the use of fennel with kidney problems and kidney stones. Some texts list fennel as strongly contra-indicated for these conditions, while others say that fennel is specific for these ailments. I prefer to use something else for these ailments.

Fenugreek
(Trigonella foenum)

General Information

Fenugreek seeds have been used for many years as an herbal remedy, but it is fairly new in the essential oil market.

Therapeutic Properties

emollient, expectorant, anti-inflammatory, antiseptic, sudorific

Affinity For

digestion	respiratory system	endocrine system
Resonance	**Plant Family**	**Part of Plant Used**
physical	Fabaceae	seeds

Aromatic Considerations

The aroma of fenugreek is reminiscent of Indian curry, of which it is a key ingredient. There is just a hint of balsam and the earthy aroma of angelica.

Application

Fenugreek should be diluted well for topical application.

Emotional/Spiritual Aspects

There is not enough known yet about fenugreek essential oil to comment on its emotional aspects.

Physical Aspects

Fenugreek is used as an aid to digestion and as an expectorant for the lungs and bronchials. The herb is often used as a poultice for boils, cysts, and inflamed tissues. The oil should be even more powerful in those applications. Fenugreek stimulates perspiration, lowering fever while helping the body to rid itself of bacteria and toxins.

Fenugreek is an excellent source of natural iron, silicon, sodium, and thiamine. You do not need to ingest the oil to reap the nutritional benefits. Fenugreek seeds have an excellent reputation for use with diabetes. In the studies conducted, fenugreek was used in conjunction with insulin administered either by mouth or by injection.

Cautions

There are no known cautions for fenugreek oil, but I have seen overdoses of the herb with infants. Please use reasonable caution, as always, with babies and small children

Fir, Balsam
(Abies balsamea)

Ingredient In

LeConnection, LeDeeper, LeMillenia, LeSanctuary, LeWarm Down

Therapeutic Properties

antiseptic, antibacterial, deodorant, antitussive, expectorant, astringent, laxative, antispasmodic, analgesic, diuretic, immune stimulant, nervine

Affinity For

central nervous system	heart chakra	solar plexus chakra
endocrine system	immune system	urinary tract
lymphatic system	respiratory system	muscles, tendons, joints
Resonance	**Plant Family**	**Part of Plant Used**
physical, emotional	Coniferae	needles (leaves)

Aromatic Considerations

The various varieties of fir oil are quite similar to one another in therapeutic properties, but the *balsamea* is more mellow, with an increased ability to center and ground the emotions. This fir has a wonderful aroma when diffused.

Application

Fir, balsam should be diluted and applied to areas of concern or to the feet.

Emotional/Spiritual Aspects

Fir essential oil is excellent during the recovery stage of serious illness, whether the illness is of the body, the mind, or the spirit.

Physical Aspects

The essential oil of fir, balsam, like all conifer oils, is an immune and endocrine stimulant. It is often used to treat urinary infections and remove deposits from the lymphatic system. Fir, in any form, has been well regarded for many years and in many cultures for treatment of respiratory complaints and fevers. Fir essential oil is excellent for muscle pain relief and to loosen muscles before strenuous exercise. It is also soothing for overworked or tired muscles, tendons, ligaments, and joints. Fir oils are useful for back pain.

Cautions

Fir essential oil is a possible skin irritant if used for long periods of time, or when used undiluted.

Fir, Siberica

(Abies siberica)

Ingredient In

[Le] Holiday Spirit

Therapeutic Properties

antiseptic, antibacterial, deodorant, anti-tussive, expectorant, astringent, laxative, antispasmodic, analgesic, diuretic, immune stimulant, nervine

Affinity For

central nervous system

all of the chakras

Resonance

physical, emotional

Plant Family

Coniferae

Part of Plant Used

needles (leaves)

General Information

Fir, siberica can be used almost interchangeably with fir balsamea.

Aromatic Considerations

Fir, siberica is sightly more pungent than the *balsamea* variety that is described above, but still wonderfully resinous and woodsy. The aroma of fir, siberica is pleasing to both men and women. Men like the conifer oils because they lack any hint of feminine flower aromas. All conifer oils, while very nice applied to the body, are absolutely wonderful when diffused.

Application

Fir, siberica should be diluted and applied to areas of concern or to the feet.

Emotional/Spiritual Aspects

Conifer trees stand straight and tall with their heads in the clouds of heaven and their feet firmly planted in the earth. They have a tremendous resilience, maintaining their foliage in both summer and winter. In an evergreen tree, the foliage is centered around a central strong and solid center. Conifer trees provide protection for the other residents of the forest. These features tell us much about the use of the essential oils that are distilled from them. They are protecting and grounding and they help us structure our lives around a firm and solid center.

Physical Aspects

Fir siberica has a very pleasing aroma. Nevertheless, it is an intense antiseptic and antibacterial. It is a pleasant alternative to tea tree oil in many instances and certainly has a more pleasant aroma.

Cautions

Fir, siberica oil could be a possible skin irritant if used for long periods of time, or when used undiluted.

Frankincense

(Boswellia carterii)

Ingredient In

LeAcknowledge, LeAssurance, LeBelieve, LeBountiful, LeEternity, LeEverlasting, LeExpressions, LeEZ-Traveler, LeFaith, LeGrateful Heart, LeInner Peace, LeIQ, LeJourney, LeLife Force, LeMagi, LeMeditation, LeMillenia, LePatches, LeTomorrow, LeRefresh-Mint, LeTrust, LeTurmoil, LeUnity

Therapeutic Properties

tonic, stimulant, expectorant, antidepressant, antiseptic, revitalizer, anti-catarrhal, anti-tumoral

Affinity For

cellular structure and strength
digestive system
immune system
respiratory system

skin
circulation
urinary tract

meridians
particular affinity for earth
chakras
particularly the crown

Resonance	Plant Family	Part of Plant Used
mental, emotional, physical	Burseraceae	resin

Aromatic Considerations

Frankincense should be used to reduce anxiety and nervous tension, and in times of stress or fear.

Application

Frankincense can be applied to any area of the body. It is of great benefit diffused.

Emotional/Spiritual Aspects

Frankincense is an excellent choice for those who are afraid of death, fear coming changes in their lives, or have suffered the loss of a loved one. Frankincense helps us link the past with the future, allowing us to connect cause and effect, actions and consequences, to one another. As we make these connections, we can choose our course more wisely in the future.

Physical Aspects

Frankincense has a reputation world-wide for crossing the blood/brain barrier, carrying oxygen and nutrients to the pineal and pituitary glands within the brain. It is the sesquiterpenes contained in frankincense that give it this ability. (There are many essential oils besides frankincense which contain sesquiterpenes. Some of them even contain more sesquiterpenes than frankincense.)

Frankincense is useful for skin disorders and circulation problems. It has a very beneficial effect on respiratory conditions such as cough, bronchitis, and pneumonia. Frankincense is of benefit in any condition that is caused or worsened by nervous tension and emotional trauma.

General Information

Frankincense is considered a holy oil in the Middle East. It has been used since ancient times in meditations. It is said that frankincense improves communication between us and our Creator.

Frankincense, frereana

(Boswellia frereana)

General Information

The frereana variety of frankincense grows in the high mountain regions of Somalia. In Somalia and Arabia, frereana is considered the 'King' of all the Boswellia species.

Resonance	Plant Family	Part of Plant Used
mental, emotional, physical	Burseraceae	resin

Therapeutic Properties

There is very little information in the literature to distinguish frereana from its cousin, carterii. The general opinion is that the two species are very similar in therapeutic properties, although their aromas differ quite a bit. It is recognized that the gentler frereana is very good for skin care.

Aromatic Considerations

Frankincence frereana's aroma is similar to frankincense carterii, but it has a delightful balsam undertone with just a hint of lemon. Frankincense frereana is lower in thujene. The missing thujene leaves frereana with a softer, sweeter aroma that is quite appealing.

Application

Frankincense frereana can be applied to any area of the body. This variety is particularly nice diffused.

Emotional/Spiritual Aspects

The keynote of frankincense frereana is the calming and centering effect it has on the energy grid of the body. Frankincense frereana is said to enhance and balance the spiritual aspects of an individual more so than the carterii or serrata varieties. It is the frankincense of choice for religious ceremonies in many Arabic countries. Frankincense frereana is useful in treating stress, tension, depression, and other nervous disorders.

Physical Aspects

Frankincense frereana improves immune system function, partially because of its antibiotic properties and partially because it raises the overall frequency of the body. Frereana's other therapeutic properties seem to be similar to carterii.

A science journal published by the U.S. National Library of Medicine, National Institute of Health reports, "We have demonstrated that Boswellia frereana prevents collagen degradation, and inhibits the production of pro-inflammatory mediators. Due to its efficacy, we propose that Boswellia frereana should be examined further as a potential therapeutic agent for treating inflammatory symptoms of arthritis."

Frankincense, Indian

(Boswellia serrata)

Ingredient In

LeFaith

Therapeutic Properties

tonic, expectorant, antiseptic, analgesic, anti-arthritic, revitalizer, anti-tumoral

General Information

Boswellia serrata is quite similar to *Boswellia carterii.* This is a fairly new oil in the essential oil market and few comparison studies have been conducted.

Affinity For

cellular structure and strength	all chakras	all meridians
digestive system	respiratory system	skin
immune system	urinary tract	circulation
Resonance	**Plant Family**	**Part of Plant Used**
mental, emotional, physical	Burseraceae	resin

Aromatic Considerations

Frankincense serrata is slightly less mellow and balsamic than frankincense carterii. Many people prefer serrata because, they say, it has a freshness about it that is lacking in carterii. Frankincense, diffused, can help us develop a better attitude. When we have a better attitude, we have a stronger immune system.

Application

Frankincese has been applied to the body for centuries. It has stood the test of time as a healing oil.

Emotional/Spiritual Aspects

This frankincense relieves feelings of bitterness, skepticism, and cynicism. It promotes forcefulness of spirit, gives energy, and strengthens the will to live. This oil can help us to be more warm-hearted and generous.

Physical Aspects

There is a lot of scientific data around the world indicating that the anti-inflammatory properties of resin oils (frankincense is a resin oil) are useful to inflammatory diseases such as Crohn's disease.

Preliminary studies conducted by medical research teams are also promising for shrinking tumors, particularly those in the brain. The studies are being conducted using the isolated single components of the frankincense oils. These studies apply equally to the carterii and serrata varieties. Experience and understanding would indicate that frankincense, whole and undamaged by laboratory procedures, would be even more effective. This is certainly the reputation that frankincense has enjoyed for generations.

Galbanum

(Ferula galbaniflua syn Ferula fummosa)

Ingredient In

[Le]Life Force

Therapeutic Properties

anti-infectious, analgesic, lightly antispasmodic, anti-inflammatory, stimulant, diuretic and kidney support, expectorant in chronic bronchitis and asthma

General Information

Galbanum adapts itself to the body chemistry of the user more than most essential oils do, even as part of a blend. Galbanum is a low frequency essential oil, but when combined with frankincense or sandalwood, the frequency of the blend is much higher than the components lead one to expect. In spite of having a low frequency, it acts as a top note (one of the last added) in most blend recipes.

Affinity For

nerves | circulation | cellular strength and structure

Resonance	Plant Family	Part of Plant Used
emotional, physical	Umbelliferae	wood, leaves

Aromatic Considerations

Galbanum is especially nice when combined with frankincense or sandalwood. It is so calming that it is useful for any type of anxiety or hysteria.

Application

Galbanum is often combined with myrrh for use in the tub and as a massage oil to tone skin and remove wrinkles.

Emotional/Spiritual Aspects

Galbanum essential oil was used by most ancient civilizations as an incense and is recognized as an oil for nervous tension. Galbanum soothes the soul, bringing calmness and a sense of peace with the way things are.

Physical Aspects

Galbanum is an oil that strengthens and supports the entire system. It is useful for treating skin disorders, muscle aches, and inflamed wounds. It is also useful for circulation problems and arthritis.

Cautions

There are no known contra-indications for this essential oil.

Garlic

(Allium sativum)

General Information

This oil is mentioned here mainly so that I can list the cautions that should be used. Essential oil of garlic is not the same as the extracted and very diluted garlic oil that is found in capsules for sale in health food stores. Essential oil of garlic is strong and potent—actually very caustic!!! Two drops of garlic essential oil, undiluted, in the ear would burn sufficiently to possibly require medical assistance.

Therapeutic Properties

antibiotic, antibacterial, anti-fungal

Resonance	Plant Family	Part of Plant Used
physical	Lilliceae	bulb

Aromatic Considerations

Garlic oil is not recommended for diffusion. You will have more 'aroma' than you need on your fingers any time that you touch a bottle of garlic essential oil.

Application

Garlic oil ***must*** be diluted extremely well each time it is used.

Physical Aspects

Garlic, in the world of herbal medicine, is considered to be nature's most perfect antibiotic. It is used for particularly nasty viruses or bacteria because its antimicrobial action is so strong. ***2 drops of garlic essential oils in 1 ounce of carrier oil (shake very well!) is an excellent treatment for earaches or bacterial skin rashes.*** Garlic essential oil has been added, sparingly, to animal feed with good results and has been used for centuries to combat every known virus or bacteria. Never forget how concentrated the essential oil is, but don't be so afraid that you miss the amazing benefits of garlic essential oil.

Cautions

Garlic oil should be used with extreme caution and always diluted well!

Geranium

(Pelargonium graveolens)

Ingredient In

LeAcknowledge, LeAngel, LeBeloved, LeBenediction, LeVisibility, LeCypernium, LeDiscernment, LeEndo Relief, LeEverlasting, LeGrateful Heart, LeHeart Song, LeLetting Go, LeLife Force, LeMillenia, LeMoonlight, LeRevitalize, LeTomorrow, LeTranquility , LeUnity, LeVitality

Therapeutic Properties

astringent, diuretic, antiseptic, antidepressant, regenerative, tonic, anti-biotic, antispasmodic, anti-infection

Affinity For

cellular structure	nerves	skin	spleen meridian
urinary tract	gallbladder	liver	solar plexus and heart chakras
			yin energy

Resonance	Plant Family	Part of Plant Used
physical, emotional	Geraniaceae	leaves

Aromatic Considerations

Geranium fosters positive thought patterns. It helps us to feel hope for the future and peace with today.

Application

Dilute and apply anywhere on the body

Emotional/Spiritual Aspects

Geranium is a very potent and aromatic oil. It is a good oil for people whose negative patterns need to be swept away in spite of their desire to hang on to them. Geranium helps one to release negative memories. It is a good oil for nervous fatigue where the body is exhausted but the mind just won't let the body sit and rest. Geranium is a potent oil for those whose moods are 'up' one minute and 'down' the next. Geranium is a good choice for people whose drive and ambition interferes with sensitivity and spontaneous joy.

Physical Aspects

Geranium regenerates tissues and nerves. It is excellent for skin disorders and skin care, and is especially nice for the skin of expectant mothers. Along with the essential oil blend LeDeeper, geranium heals the sores of shingles. Geranium discharges toxins from the liver and dilates the bilary ducts, aiding liver, gallbladder, and kidney function. This oil can bring relief from gastric ulcers, diarrhea, jaundice, and kidney stones. Geranium is one of the best oils for circulation problems such as hemorrhoids, and is helpful in slowing down bleeding.

General Information

Geranium is a very versatile and important essential oil. It is among a handful of essential oils considered to be *cool* and *moist* energetically.

Ginger

(Zingiber officinale)

Ingredient In

[Lee]Exhilaration, [Le]Focus, [Le]Within

Therapeutic Properties

antiseptic, stimulant, stomachic, aphrodisiac, febrifuge, expectorant

Affinity For

circulation	memory	stomach meridian
digestive system	base chakra	small intestine

Resonance	**Plant Family**	**Part of Plant Used**
physical, emotional, mental	Zingiberaceae	root

Aromatic Considerations

Ginger essential oil increases physical energy and stamina. It influences how we relate to money and how we feel about our material possessions. Ginger essential oil has long been considered to be an aphrodisiac.

Application

Ginger is extremely strong. It must always be diluted very well.

Emotional/Spiritual Aspects

Ginger is for the usually dynamic individual who has lost their drive and ambition and has become apathetic and confused. The emotional impact of ginger is absolutely uncompromising. It insists on burning away illusions and mis-perceptions and replacing them with clarity and vision. Ginger insists that we take the initiative and be willing to tackle and complete the hard tasks facing us in our life. The aroma of ginger strengthens our will power, activates initiative, and restores our determination. It can boost our confidence in ourselves and give us additional vitality and ambition.

Physical Aspects

Ginger warms the body and the soul, helping one to tap into hidden reserves of energy. Ginger has been widely recognized since ancient times as being toning and stimulating to the digestive tract and for circulation. Because it increases capillary strength and circulation, it is of benefit to a long list of physical and mental complaints. A few unusual ones are: alcoholism, loss of appetite, impotence, memory loss, and motion sickness.

General Information

Ginger mixed with lime is one of my favorite combinations in aromatherapy. I enjoy it for the emotional and physical lift it provides. This combination disinfects and purifies while leaving a uniquely pleasant aroma behind.

Cautions

Ginger is extremely potent, almost caustic. Undiluted or used too often, it may irritate sensitive skin. Ginger is photo-toxic; you must avoid direct sunlight on skin to which it has been applied for at least 12 hours. ***Never use more than 1 drop in the bath.*** Ginger opens the capillaries so quickly that a severe headache can result if more than a single drop is used.

Gingergrass

(Cympopogan martini variation sofia)

Ingredient In

[Le]Patches, [Le]Tenda Care

Therapeutic Properties

antiseptic, stimulant, stomachic, aphrodisiac, febrifuge, expectorant

Affinity For

circulation	muscles and joints	congestion

Resonance	**Plant Family**	**Part of Plant Used**
physical, emotional	Gramineae	leaves, grass

Aromatic Considerations

Gingergrass is a close relative of lemongrass and a distant cousin of palmarosa. These family connections give a glimpse of its aroma. Gingergrass has a gentle, spicy aroma with marvelous earthtones. Just when you think you have experienced all the layers of the aroma, a hint of rose surfaces, calming the nerves and raising the spirits.

Application

Dilute gingergrass and apply to appropriate areas of the feet and anywhere on the body where it is needed. Gingergrass is wonderful added to the tub. You should use only one or two drops at a time.

Emotional/Spiritual Aspects

The aroma of gingergrass makes me want to smile and forget about petty annoyances. Gingergrass is said to be an aphrodisiac.

Physical Aspects

The main action of gingergrass is on the circulation. It encourages blood flow to any area of the body to which it is applied. This action, and the anti-inflammatory properties of this essential oil, make it an excellent choice for massaging sore muscles and relieving stiffness in joints. Gingergrass is useful for headaches that originate in tense muscles in the neck or upper back.

Cautions

Gingergrass may cause irritation to sensitive skin if used undiluted.

Grapefruit

(Citrus paradisi)

Ingredient In

LeEverlasting, LeHeart Song, LeMy-Graine, LeSego Lily, LeSunburst, LeWake-Up LeWeightless, LePurify

Therapeutic Properties

tonic, digestive, antiseptic, anti-infectious, restorative

Affinity For

urinary tract	triple warmer meridian	heart chakra
lymphatic system	spleen meridian	

Resonance	**Plant Family**	**Part of Plant Used**
physical, emotional, mental	Rutaceae	fruit

Aromatic Considerations

Grapefruit is uplifting to the mind and spirit. It is hard to be negative or anxious in the presence of this oil, because it promotes feelings of joy, confidence, and spontaneity. Grapefruit should be diffused or inhaled for performance stress or to cope with jet lag.

Application

Grapefruit should be diluted and applied to the feet or to areas of the body needing to release emotions, cellulite, or both.

Emotional/Spiritual Aspects

Grapefruit is a very joyous and positive essential oil. It can be a ray of bright light guiding us out of darkness and depression. Grapefruit is equally good for mental exhaustion and mental tension. Grapefruit seems to address the emotional issues of self-worth and discontent with one's body that are so often a part of anorexia and other eating disorders.

The aroma of grapefruit is particularly suited to people who, when tense or under pressure, eat as a means of relieving stress or finding comfort. Often, the driving emotion is frustration because their too high expectations have not been met in some way. If they reacted to their frustration with anger or blame of themselves or others, a layer of guilt is added to the frustration. Grapefruit is used in treatment programs for drug withdrawal and to cope with the after-effects of drinking too many alcoholic beverages.

Physical Aspects

Grapefruit detoxifies the lymphatic system. This makes it a useful tonic for many body systems. It is specific for water retention and the dissolving of cellulite. Grapefruit aids with gallstones, water retention, kidney and liver disorders. Grapefruit, diluted in water, can be used as an astringent face wash for acne. Grapefruit can relieve a migraine headache and return the energy system to normal after long jet flights. Grapefruit is one of the best oils for premenstrual water retention and headache.

Cautions

Grapefruit is photo-toxic. You should avoid exposing areas of skin to which grapefruit has been applied to sunlight or UV rays for at least 12 hours.

Green Pepper

(Piper nigrum)

Ingredient In

LeWeightless

Therapeutic Properties

anti-inflammatory, muscle relaxant, carminative, circulatory stimulant, detoxifying, diuretic, expectorant, laxative, aphrodisiac

Affinity For

respiratory system
muscles

Resonance	**Plant Family**	**Part of Plant Used**
physical, mental	Piperaceae	fruit

Aromatic Considerations

Green pepper is slightly milder when diffused than black pepper. It is uplifting to the mind and soothing to the senses.

Application

Green pepper should be diluted well. It can then be applied to the feet or to any area of the body.

Emotional/Spiritual Aspects

When the mind becomes tired or dull before an important project is completed, green pepper essential oil can revive the mind and the spirits, helping one to stay awake and focused for a bit longer. Green pepper is considered an aphrodisiac.

Physical Aspects

Like black pepper, green pepper can be used as an expectorant. It can also be used to improve muscle tone.

General Information

Green pepper essential oil is derived from the *green* berries of the Piper nigrum plant, while black pepper essential oil is derived from the *ripened and dried* berries.

Cautions

Green pepper should be used well-diluted, but is less likely to cause skin irritation than black pepper.

Helichrysum

(Helichrysum italicum and Helichrysum and agustifolia)
(also know as Immortelle)

Ingredient In

LeDeeper, LeEverlasting, LeExhilaration, LeIQ, LeMariah LeMy-Graine, LePaine, LeRevitalize, LeStefanie, LeTrust, LeTurmoil, LeVallee, LeVitality

Therapeutic Properties

antispasmodic, analgesic, expectorant, anti-coagulant, hepatic, anti-inflammatory, stimulant, antibacterial, antiviral, anti-fungal

Affinity For

cardiovascular system
respiratory system
endocrine system
liver
bones
joints
muscles
skin
right side of the brain
throat chakra
gallbladder meridian

Resonance

physical, emotional

Plant Family

Compositae

Part of Plant Used

flowers

Aromatic Considerations

When there are emotional blockages or repetitive behavior patterns as the result of abuse or trauma, helichrysum can help us discover and remove them. Once these blockages have been removed, we can move on with our lives.

Application

Dilute and apply to appropriate areas such as the feet, the chest, or behind the ears.

Emotional/Spiritual Aspects

Helichrysum has an affinity for the creative right side of the brain, which our culture and schooling often pushes into the background. Because helichrysum stimulates this side of the brain, we are able to view our world and make our choices from a more balanced perspective.

Helichrysum is often used in emotional healing. It helps us get in touch with unresolved emotions and gently restores memories that have been deeply buried in the subconscious mind. Helichrysum helps release defense mechanisms and offers comfort while we are processing difficult emotions. Helichrysum promotes a calm acceptance of the changes within ourselves that may result from the processing of emotions and memories. It also helps supply the needed self-confidence to make hard decisions.

Physical Aspects

Helichrysum is renowned for its use in rejuvenation of skin and muscle. It drains congestion and re-establishes blood flow to traumatized areas, helping bruises and hematomas to disperse more quickly. Helichrysum regenerates damaged tissue and can help prevent scarring at the site of an injury. Helichrysum is recommended for lowering cholesterol. Helichrysum is anti-inflammatory and analgesic, making it excellent for sciatica and arthritis.

Helichrysum is an excellent oil for respiratory conditions and for lymph drainage. It is stimulating to the liver, pancreas, gallbladder, and vascular system.

Helichrysum, diluted with a carrier oil, has been used in many cultures as a sunscreen.

General Information

Helichrysum (immortelle) is a very delicate, yet hardy in its own way, plant. There is often a great deal of difference in aroma and therapeutic properties from one year to the next. Difference can occur from one distillation to the next even in the same season. Growing conditions, such as the amount of rain, can have a tremendous impact. The higher the quality of a helichrysum oil, the more mellow and pleasant the aroma will be. The price will certainly reflect this quality. The lower priced (more pungent) helichrysum essential oils are often very therapeutic and more practical for use in some applications. For this reason, many essential oil companies provide more than one helichrysum oil at widely divergent prices.

There is a lot of confusion about the helichrysum species. Many distributors claim that helichrysum augustafolia and helichrysum italicum are the same plant. They are certainly quite similar. As stated previously, the difference in quality of these two species of helichrysum seems to be in the growing conditions of each year's crop. There are many other species of helichrysum besides italicum and augustifolia. Each one has unique advantages, however, none of them are as therapeutic as these two.

Cautions

Helichrysum should be used with caution if pregnant. It should also be used cautiously with small children.

Hinoki Wood

(Chamaecyparis obtusa)

Ingredient In

LeDiscernment, LeLetting Go, LeWisdom

Therapeutic Properties

antiviral, anti-fungal, antibacterial, decongestant, relaxant

Affinity For

nerves	respiratory system	lymphatic system
skin	sinus cavities	

Resonance	**Plant Family**	**Part of Plant Used**
physical, emotional	Coniferae/Cupressaceae (sub of conifer)	needles, twigs

Aromatic Considerations

The aroma of hinoki wood is reminiscent of cedar, but is milder and much less woodsy, with a delightful hint of lemon. Hinoki is excellent in lighter, more floral blends because it does not add an overpowering cedar tone. Hinoki is a wonderful way to relax and unwind at the end of the day. Taking a relaxing bath in hinoki wood essential oil provides a quiet, serene form of energy that carries through the rest of the evening. Hinoki oil can be used to carve out a soothing and relaxing moment anywhere in your busy life.

Application

In Japan, where this tree grows, there is nothing more important than the relaxing bath upon returning home in the evening. It is considered a time of emotional growth and purification. Hinoki is the prized wood used for building temples, shrines, and structures that will be used in daily bathing rituals.

Physical/Emotional/Spiritual Aspects

The hinoki tree, while resistant to rot and bacteria, has never adapted very well to polluted urban environments. Hinoki is a 'pure' wood. It absorbs, isolates, and then removes poisons from its system. Hinoki is a product of fresh mountain water and air. These growing conditions are reflected in the aroma and energy of the essential oil. Hinoki oil effectively creates a wonderful sensation of peace and relaxation when applied or diffused.

Physical Aspects

Hinoki essential oil contains an abundance of phytoncidere. This constituent, when found in plants, enables them to eliminate harmful living things, such as bacteria, toxins, and pollutants, from within themselves and from their surroundings. Hinoki has grown in Asia for centuries and is naturally resistant to insect infestation and decay. The essence distilled from this wood is well known for its ability to kill bacteria, viruses, and fungus. Hinoki essential oil is used to increase immune function and, automatically, to improve the quality of the environment around us.

Hinoki essential oil has a decongestant effect on the respiratory and lymphatic systems. It is particularly effective for relieving congestion in sinus cavities.

Essential oils from evergreen trees have a tendency to cause skin irritation. Hinoki essential oil is an exception. It is gentle on the skin, making it very useful in the healing of rashes, cuts, abrasions, and minor injuries.

General Information

Hinoki wood is so valued in Japan that, by law, the essential oil can only be extracted from trees that have fallen or already died.

Howood

(Cinnamomum camphora)

Ingredient In

[Le]Grateful Heart

Therapeutic Properties

antibacterial, anti-fungal, anti-infectious, emollient, analgesic, antispasmodic, immune tonic, sedative, tonic, antidepressant, aphrodisiac

Affinity For

immune system | bones, muscles, and joints | skin

Resonance	**Plant Family**	**Part of Plant Used**
physical, emotional, spiritual	Lauraceae	twigs, bark

Aromatic Considerations

Howood is similar in composition and nature to rosewood. It can be used for most applications in which you would use rosewood, yet howood is a beautiful oil in its own right. Howood is emotionally uplifting to the mind. It promotes alertness and clarity, but is relaxing and refreshing at the same time.

Application

Howood is especially nice when added to a bath. It can be diluted and applied to the appropriate areas of the feet and body. It makes an excellent addition to massage oil. Some people like to add a few drops to their shampoo.

Emotional/Spiritual Aspects

Howood can prepare our minds and spirits for emotional, spiritual, and energy healing work. Howood calms the nerves and is an antidepressant.

Physical Aspects

Howood is a cellular stimulant and regenerator (cytophylactic), much like helichrysum. This makes it a very valuable oil, especially for the price. Because howood has an exceptionally high linalol content, it is thought to be very nourishing and supportive to the immune system. It should be used routinely as part of a preventative health care regimen.

Howood is an excellent oil for reducing inflammation, spasms, and pain in muscles and joints. It can be used effectively for injuries or arthritis.

General Information

The aroma of howood contains NO camphor-like notes, in spite of its latin name. This is a very mild and pleasant essential oil.

Howood is being promoted around the world as a viable substitute for rosewood, which is becoming an endangered species. It seems to be quite a good substitute, actually, but I hope we can always purchase and use both.

Hyssop

(Hyssopus officinalis)

Ingredient In

LeBenediction, LeVisibility, LeEverlasting, LeJourney, LeLife Force, LeUnity, LeVision

Therapeutic Properties

anti-inflammatory, antiviral, digestive, diuretic, expectorant, febrifuge, hypertensive, nervine, sudorific

Affinity For

digestive system
respiratory system
circulatory system
yang energy
nervous system
heart meridian
stomach meridian

Resonance	**Plant Family**	**Part of Plant Used**
physical, emotional	Labiatae	stems, leaves

Aromatic Considerations

Hyssop is often diffused at the beginning of energy work or emotional healing sessions to clear and protect the enviornment. Hyssop is said to protect the auric field and strengthen personal boundaries. In an energy work situation, hyssop puts the customer in charge and in control of the direction and the depth to which the work will go. In many traumas and nearly all cases of abuse, the situation was out of the person's control. A sense of being in charge, being able to control the pace, and being able to choose the direction of the work is absolutely essential to healing.

Application

Hyssop should be diluted and applied to the feet, the chest, or the back of the neck.

Emotional/Spiritual Aspects

The herbaceous aroma of hyssop is about freedom—freedom of movement in the body, freedom of expression, and freedom from sin. Hyssop is a symbol of spiritual cleansing and is used in purification rituals in many cultures and religions. The feeling it creates of freedom to express one's opinions makes hyssop oil beneficial for family or group planning sessions. It is a good oil to diffuse or wear when you sit down to journal and set goals. From a strong sense of our personal space and boundaries, we are better able to be tolerant, understanding, and accepting of others as they learn and grow. With the help of hyssop, we can better live the commandment to love one another.

Physical Aspects

Hyssop is used to strengthen the lungs and prevent the recurrence of colds and flu. It is particularly helpful in drying up the secretions and mucous of pneumonia, bronchitis, and asthma.

In the digestive system, hyssop is used to improve appetite, digestion, abdominal bloating, and the absorption of nutrients. It is considered helpful in expelling parasites.

Hyssop's effect on circulation and lymph drainage make it useful for discharging toxins and mucous, treating dermatitis and gout, raising low blood pressure, preventing or minimizing scar tissue, and the healing of infections and wounds. Hyssop increases perspiration. Sweating is one of the body's ways of removing toxins and impurities. It also lowers body temperature. When the circulation is poor and the lymph glands are clogged, perspiration is unable to occur. This is a serious and health threatening situation.

General Information

Hyssop is mentioned several times in the Bible (Exodous, Leviticus, Numbers, 1 Kings, and Psalms).

Cautions

Hyssop is not recommended for use as a single oil; it is better used in a blend. Hyssop, as a single oil, should be avoided if pregnant, epileptic, or if you have high blood pressure. Always use caution and be sure to dilute well.

Idaho Tansy

(Tanacetum vulgare)

General Information

Because Idaho tansy has a high percentage of thujone, it is considered by conservative aromatherapists to be an oral toxin. Some of them severely caution against its use in aromatherapy at all. As is so often the case, the test data being quoted to support this position was done by isolating individual components and then testing each component on rats or mice. Thujone, tested without the presence of the 'balancing' components found in the natural oil (see Chapter 14 page 7 for a comparable testing situation) and in extremely high concentrations, produced convulsions in mice. Does this mean that Idaho tansy (or any other oil containing thujone) is contra-indicated for human use? It is doubtful, but the data gives us a reason to be extra cautious and dilute extra well with this oil until further information has been gathered.

Ingredient In

[Le]Mariah

Therapeutic Properties

anti-inflammatory, antiviral, antibacterial, anti-fungal, anti-histiminic, vermifuge, sedative and/or stimulant, antispasmodic, nervine, insecticide

Affinity For

Idaho tansy seems to have an effect across the various systems of the body. It appears to awaken our inner strengths and resources on both the physical/immune system levels and on the emotional/spiritual planes as well. When using this oil it is difficult to think thoughts of failure and disease.

Resonance	**Plant Family**	**Part of Plant Used**
physical, emotional, spiritual	Compositae	leaves, flowers

Aromatic Considerations

Idaho tansy encourages a positive attitude and general feeling of well-being.

Application

Idaho tansy should be diluted and applied to the feet or specific areas of the body at reasonable intervals. Continuous use is not recommended.

Emotional/Spiritual Aspects

Idaho tansy acts as a sedative for nerve disorders and emotional impulses. It is useful for the emotional aspects of anxiety, depression, anger, irritability, convulsions, and hysteria. This oil is specific for people who need deep emotional healing in order to heal physically. Often, physical healing is impossible if our hearts are heavy, weary, or broken.

Physical Aspects

Idaho tansy, because of the high concentration of certain components not usually found in essential oils, is ***very*** antiviral and antibacterial. It could be used, with caution, to expel parasites. Beneficial effects from using this oil have been recorded for heart, lungs, liver, bowels, kidneys, circulation and vascular health, respiratory infections, inflamed joints and muscle sprains, to name just a few. This oil is also considered to be a potent anti-histamine and hormone stimulant.

Cautions

This essential oil is best used as part of a blend, rather than by itself. It should be avoided completely by pregnant women.

Idaho tansy is generally considered strongly contra-indicated for any one with epilepsy or a tendency to seizures or convulsions. Mild doses, under the supervision of an experienced aromatherapist however, have proven helpful for epileptic-type attacks.

Idaho tansy is very high in thujone and camphor. Used as a single oil (rather than as a small percentage of a blend), it may contain enough camphor to negate a homeopathic remedy.

Jasmine, grandiflorum *and* Jasmine, sambac

(Jasminum grandiflorum) *(Jasminum sambac)*

General Information

Jasmine grandiflorum and jasmine sambac are very similar in aroma and therapeutic use. Grandiflorum blooms in the early morning and the sambac variety blossoms late in the evening. This strength at the end of the day subtly affects the properties of the sambac oil. It is particularly appealing to those who tend to work late into the evening—or would do so if they only had the energy left to match their desire.

Ingredient In

LeExhilaration, LeWoman Wise, LeExpressions, LeMoonlight

Therapeutic Properties

antidepressant, stimulant, aphrodisiac, antispasmodic, sedative

Affinity For

respiratory system	yang energy	triple warmer
skin	heart chakra	crown chakra
hormones		

Resonance	**Plant Family**	**Part of Plant Used**
physical, emotional, spiritual	Oleaceae	flowers

Aromatic Considerations

Both jasmines have beautiful fragrances. They are heavy, exotic, sensual, and soothing essential oils. The aroma of either jasmine is multi-faceted; much more so than most essential oils. They speak to the soul of both femininity and core strength.

Jasmine, both grandiflorum and sambac, are absolutes rather than distilled essential oils. All absolutes, because of their concentration and intensity, should be evaluated in extremely small quantities. Large amounts of these oils can overcome the receptor sites in the nose. The complexity of the fragrance, especially the rare and exotic notes, become entirely lost to our sense of smell.

Application

Jasmine should be diluted (a drop or two is sufficient for any application) and massaged onto any area of the body.

Emotional/Spiritual Aspects

Jasmine is good for women who want to find and utilize their strength of character and purpose without losing their feminine side. It is appropriate for men who want to find and utilize their strength of character and purpose while developing their sensitivity and caring. Historically and in many religious traditions, jasmine flowers symbolize hope, happiness, and love.

Physical Aspects

Because of its powerful effect on the emotions and hormones, jasmine is often effective for a very long list of physical, mental, and emotional disorders. Jasmine, either as a single or as an ingredient in a blend, is often used for hormone balancing, menstrual cramps, and PMS. Jasmine is used during childbirth to strengthen the contractions and, at the same time, ease the intensity of the pain.

Jasmine is excellent in skin care products because it increases elasticity. It is often used to prevent or minimize stretch marks. Consistent use of jasmine essential oil can reduce scarring.

Jasmine soothes irritating coughs and relieves hoarseness and laryngitis. It is also beneficial for muscle strains, sprains, and stiffness.

Juniper Berry

(Juniperus communis)

Ingredient In

LeDreams, LeEnergy, LeEverlasting, LeInside-Out, LeMagi, LeRefresh-Mint, LeTenda Care, LeWhispering Hope

Therapeutic Properties

antiseptic, diuretic, expectorant, emmenagogue, anti-parasitic, tonic, depurative

Affinity For

- digestive system
- endocrine system
- urinary tract
- reproductive system
- hormones
- yang energy
- brow chakra
- kidney meridian

Resonance	Plant Family	Part of Plant Used
physical, emotional	Coniferae	fruit

Aromatic Considerations

Juniper berry is said to improve mental clarity and memory without undue stimulation to the nervous system. In fact, juniper berry essential oil is quite relaxing.

Application

Juniper berry oil should be diluted and applied to the feet, on the abdomen, or on the small of the back (over the kidneys).

Emotional/Spiritual Aspects

Juniper berry essential oil is suited for people who fear growing up or growing older. The use of juniper berry essential oil is about maturing into wisdom; not just ordinary wisdom but wisdom with compassion. It is about cultivating an understanding of the continuity of life, coupled with a sense of humor. Juniper gives us a feeling of gratitude for the privilege to have learned from the experiences and lessons of life. Juniper berry helps to elevate spiritual awareness and reverence for sacred things. It can open the soul to direction by inspiration and religious principle.

Physical Aspects

Juniper berry improves circulation, particularly to the kidneys. It helps the body move fluids and toxins out of the cells and tissues. It is a useful remedy for fluid retention, cellulite, premenstrual bloating, gout, and arthritis. It is said that juniper berry oil helps with nerve function and regeneration. Juniper can be a useful oil for the digestive system. It has a beneficial effect on the emotional and physical aspects of over-indulgence in food. Juniper essential oil is effective for acne, eczema, oily skin, psoriasis, and dandruff.

Cautions

Use of juniper berry essential oil should be avoided during pregnancy. It should be used with caution on children. This oil is contra-indicated for people with kidney disease. This is a great oil to balance and strengthen kidney function and deal with kidney infections, but it is not to be used by people with kidney diseases.

Laurel

(Laurus nobilis)

Ingredient In

LeAspire, LeIQ, LeMariah

Therapeutic Properties

analgesic, antiseptic, antiviral, carminative, decongestant, diuretic, emmenagogue, nervous system tonic

Affinity For

- lymphatic system
- hair
- scalp
- skin

Resonance	Plant Family	Part of Plant Used
physical, emotional	Lauraceae	leaves

Aromatic Considerations

Laurel clears the mind while relaxing the emotions; perfect for test taking and other challenges.

Application

Laurel should be diluted and applied to appropriate areas of the feet. It is very nice diffused.

Emotional/Spiritual Aspects

Historically, the leaves of Lauris nobilis were used to crown the victorious. Laurel can help us realize that we are victorious in our own way with the challenges of our own lives.

Physical Aspects

Laurel's antibacterial properties are specifically recommended as a steam inhalation for tonsillitis. Laurel essential oil is considered a valuable remedy for stimulating hair growth and eliminating dandruff. It is recommended in the treatment of acne and other skin disorders. Laurel is said to bring awareness of our strengths, moral courage, and confidence. Laurel aids in lymphatic drainage and promotes healthy sweating and the discharge of toxins.

General Information

Laurel essential oil can be used sparingly (less than 1 drop in most instances) as a substitute for bay leaf in recipes. The flavor is more vital than when using dried bay leaf and you don't have to fish them back out of the pot!!

Cautions

Laurel should be avoided (except in a blend) during pregnancy. It should never be applied undiluted to the skin. If over-used, laurel can be almost narcotic in its sedative effects. The use of laurel should be avoided if you are taking prescription blood thinners.

There is much confusion around the world surrounding the usage of common names for plants. A plant called pigweed on one continent is rarely the same plant that is called pigweed on another. This confusion of names can be true from one community to another, even in the same country. Laurel is a prime example of this confusion!

Laurel (Laurus nobilis) is often referred to as sweet bay laurel, but it is not the same as bay (Pimenta racemosa) which is sometimes referred to as bay laurel. Nor is Laurus nobilis the same as bayberry (which are two different plants depending on whether you are European or American).

Bay (Pimenta racemosa) is a member of the myrtle (Myrtaceae) family and laurel (Laurus nobilis) is a member of the laurel (Lauraceae) family. Because they are from different families, their properties are very different. There is so much confusion about the names that it is difficult to tell which one is being referred to, especially when 'surfing the web.' Many essential oil companies seem to be confused and are adding to this confusion. When working with plants, always pay attention to the Latin names and, in the case of 'laurel' hope that the buyer you are trusting paid attention, too!

Lavender

(Lavandula officinalis)

General Information

Lavender is a universal oil that has been shown to balance the body and to work wherever there is a need. It is called 'the grandmother' of essential oils because it cares for and nurtures us through such a variety of physical and emotional stresses. If you don't know what essential oil to reach for, try lavender.

Ingredient In

[Le]Angel, [Le]Assurance, [Le]Balance, [Le]Candila, [Le]Cypernium, [Le]Dandy, [Le]Delicate, [Le]Discernment, [Le]Everlasting, [Le]EZ-Traveler, [Le]Inner Peace, [Le]IQ, [Le]Letting Go, [Le]My-Graine, [Le]Millenia, [Le]Purify, [Le]Simplicity, [Le]Solitude, [Le]Tranquility, [Le]Trust, [Le]Turmoil, [Le]Unity, [Le]Vision, [Le]Warm Down, [Le]With-In, [Le]Woman Wise

Therapeutic Properties

antiseptic, diuretic, expectorant, emmenagogue, anti-parasitic

Affinity For

digestive system	nerves	all meridians
cardiovascular system	brain	chakras:
lymphatic system		base
immune system		heart
genito-urinary system		solar plexus
reproductive system		

Resonance	Plant Family	Part of Plant Used
physical, mental, emotional, spiritual	Labiatae	flowering tops

Aromatic Considerations

Lavender can help us return to kindness and generosity if we have been in a place of judgement.

Application

There is probably no wrong way to apply or diffuse lavender.

Emotional/Spiritual Aspects

One of the great emotional gifts of lavender is the feeling of total and unchanging support around us. It leaves us with no room for doubt that we are loved and will be supported in life's challenges and in the process of healing. Lavender promotes faith, even in the hard times. Lavender brings balance between masculine and feminine energy and traits.

Lavender is a gentle, but effective, sedative and nervine. It can bring relief from anxiety, panic, hysteria, emotional and mental fatigue, headaches and migraines, and insomnia.

Physical Aspects

Lavender can be used for nearly all skin conditions. It can be applied to cuts, sunburns, burns, rashes, dermatitis, eczema, and insect bites. Consistent use of lavender with burns and injuries minimizes scarring. Lavender, usually as part of a blend, is often used to prevent or remedy conditions of dandruff and hair loss. Lavender is antiseptic, anti-inflammatory, cytophylactic, and antispasmodic, making it effective for muscle strains and sprains, cramps, and wound healing.

Lavender clears excess waste products from the lymphatic system and is an aid to digestion. Lavender is sometimes all that is needed to prevent or alleviate nausea. Mildly diuretic, lavender can be useful in alleviating edema and premenstrual water retention. Whether the root of the problem is emotional or physical, lavender is often effective in stabilizing both high or low blood pressure and regulating the pulse. Lavender, or blends containing it, is used to lessen pain and promote restful sleep. Lavender is useful for babies with thrush.

Cautions

Lavender is wonderfully calming in small amounts, but can be stimulating if used in too large a quantity or too often. This is especially true with babies and small children.

Ledum - Labrador Tea

(Ledum groenlandicum)

General Information—Fat Storage and the Liver

The liver has a very long list of functions. One of these functions is the manufacture of carnitine which is essential if cells in the body are going to break down fat—rather than just store it away. If the liver becomes compromised, carnitine is not created and fat begins to accumulate in the cells. Fat accumulates first in the cells of the liver itself. The result is a fatty liver because the liver can store more fat cells than ***all*** of the other organs combined. A fatty liver used to be seen only in alcoholics. That is no longer true. Today's lifestyle is a recipe for disaster to the liver.

What is the problem with a fatty liver? There are many; let me summarize just two of them here. 1) Fat cells soak up and hold onto toxins. Since detoxification of the blood is one important function of the liver, the liver gets the first shot at soaking up toxins. The more fat cells your liver has, the more toxins the liver can hold . Fat cells in the liver uptaking toxins almost sounds like a good thing, until you consider that a large percentage of new red blood cells are 'born' in the liver. These new blood cells become contaminated and damaged by the toxins. They then travel throughout the body, trying to carry oxygen and nutrients to cells and organs but carrying contaminants instead. 2) The liver, magnified under a microscope looks like a pinkish/red colored filter. If the liver is filled with toxic fat, it cannot do a good job as a filter for the bloodstream.

How common is fatty liver? In the United States, 15-20% of the general population has too much fat in their liver. Your odds are much higher if you are overweight. Fatty liver can, and does, occur in children.

What are the symptoms of a fatty liver?

- You are probably overweight, especially in the abdominal area and you find it very hard to lose weight.
- You may have elevated cholesterol and triglycerides in your blood.
- You may have diabetes type 2.
- You may have been diagnosed as insulin resistant.
- ***You will be very tired, and tired all the time.***
- ***You will probably have a lowered immune response.***

Why this discussion of liver function?

There is clinical evidence that ledum essential oil digests both the fat cells in the liver and their toxic load.

Ingredient In

LeLiv-N (a new blend, soon to be available for purchase from Butterfly Express, llc)

Therapeutic Properties

hepatic (acts on the liver), cholagogue (encourages the flow of bile and the digestion of fats), anti-inflammatory, anti-tumoral, antibacterial, diuretic, decongestant, cytophylactic, depurative, immunostimulant

Affinity For

liver function	respiratory system	liver
kidney/bladder function	mucous membranes	skin

Resonance	**Plant Family**	**Part of Plant**
physical	Ericaceae	leaves

Aromatic Considerations

Ledum has a strong medicinal aroma, but with an herbaceous twist.

Application

Ledum essential oil should always be diluted well before applying it to the body.

Emotional/Spiritual Aspects

Ledum has a high sesquiterpene count. Essential oils containing sesquiterpenes cross the blood/brain barrier carrying nutrients and oxygen to the brain. These oils are very calming. This effect is felt, not just by the nervous system, but throughout the body.

Physical Aspects

Ledum acts as an enzyme to remedy liver dysfunction and aid in liver detoxification. Ledum's action on the liver sets off a chain reaction of improvement throughout the organs of the body. A stronger liver creates a balanced thyroid, a stronger immune system, better functioning kidneys, and clearer skin. Ledum has been used in programs for weight management, obesity, edema, and water retention. A review of recent literature indicates that ledum may be even more anti-cancerous and anti-tumoral than frankincense.

Cautions

Ledum should not be used if you are pregnant. Its use should be avoided with very young children.

Lemon

(Citrus limonum)

Ingredient In

LeBeloved, LeBenediction, LeBreezey, LeDeliverance, LeEverlasting, LeHeart Song, LeInside-Out, LeIQ, LeLetting Go, LeLife Force, LeRefresh-Mint, LeRevitalize, LeSimplicity, LeSunburst, LeTenda Care, LeTomorrow, LeTrust, LeTurmoil, LeVision, LeWeightless, LeWhispering Hope, LeWisdom

Therapeutic Properties

antibiotic, sedative, carminative, diuretic, hemostatic, astringent, digestive, immunostimulant, antidepressant, stimulant, antiseptic, febrifuge, calmative, antispasmodic, anti-sclerotic, depurative, vermifuge, cicatrisive

Affinity For

respiratory system
lymphatic system
cardiovascular system
digestive system
nervous system
skin, muscles
solar plexus chakra
bladder meridian
wood element

Resonance	Plant Family	Part of Plant Used
physical, emotional	Rutaceae	fruit

Aromatic Considerations

Lemon essential oil fills the air with a light, refreshing scent of lemons while it nourishes the nervous systems of everyone close by.

Application

Lemon oil should be diluted and applied to any area of the body. Since it helps dissolve cellulite, applying lemon to areas where cellulite has accumulated would be a good idea. Be sure to dilute to avoid irritation.

Emotional/Spiritual Aspects

Lemon brings clarity of thought, aids in logical thinking, helps us prioritize, and helps us connect cause and effect in our lives. Lemon is a good oil for study sessions, improving attention span, and problem solving. Lemon oil can bring a dose of reality to our thinking. It can help us analyze our resentments, decide if they are based on reality or not, and then help us let go of them—real or not! Lemon makes it easier to handle the stresses of life with a sense of humor.

Physical Aspects

Lemon essential oil supports the respiratory system and is useful for asthma, bronchitis, sore throat, sinusitis, and most other respiratory complaints. Lemon oil tightens smooth muscles and strengthens connective tissue throughout the body. Lemon oil can be used for a liver or lymphatic cleanse. After cleansing is complete, lemon oil can stimulate the pancreas and the entire endocrine system. Lemon is very helpful in passing gallstones and is said to induce labor when the baby is over due. Lemon oil can be used to purify water and leaves no unpleasant taste behind.

Cautions

Lemon essential oil is photo-toxic. Avoid sunlight or UV radiation on skin to which lemon oil has been applied.

Lemongrass

(Cymbopogon flexuosus)

Ingredient In

LeDeeper, LeEnergy, LeInside-Out, LePurify, LeRefresh-Mint, LeSunburst, LeTenda Care, LeTomorrow, LeWake-Up

Therapeutic Properties

astringent, tonic, calmative, antiseptic, anti-infectious, diuretic, digestive, anti-parasitic, depurative, nervine

Affinity For

kidney, bladder
lymphatic system
vascular system
circulation
parasympathetic nervous system
solar plexus chakra
spleen meridian

Resonance	Plant Family	Part of Plant Used
physical, emotional	Graminae	leaves

Aromatic Considerations

Lemongrass has a woodsy but light fragrance which has an uplifting effect on mind, mood, and attitude.

Application

Dilute and apply to the feet or to any area of the body that is causing concern.

Emotional/Spiritual Aspects

The aroma of lemongrass awakens curiosity. It encourages us to go outside our usual boundaries and comfort zones. Lemongrass should be used to cleanse your energy system when you have been in negative situations or around negative people. Lemongrass can give us energy and reawakens compassion following emotional overload or collapse.

Physical Aspects

Lemongrass improves circulation, regenerates connective tissue, and repairs ligaments. Lemongrass is used for acne and for dissolving cellulite during weight loss programs. Lemongrass repairs the parasympathetic nervous system and improves eyesight. It is useful in bladder and kidney disorders and for healing varicose veins. Two of the greatest benefits of lemongrass is that it improves lymphatic drainage and gets oxygen flowing throughout the body. Lemongrass is one of the best oils for disinfecting and purifying around the house.

Cautions

Overuse of lemongrass can cause extreme skin irritation.

Lime

(Citrus aurantifolia)

Ingredient In

LeTomorrow, LeTurmoil, LeWeightless

Therapeutic Properties

antibacterial, antiseptic, antiviral, restorative, tonic

Affinity For

digestive problems
immune function
liver and gallbladder meridians
respiratory problems
lymphatic system
solar plexus chakra

Resonance	Plant Family	Part of Plant Used
physical, mental, emotional	Rutaceae	fruit

Aromatic Considerations

Lime has a beautiful, fresh, and refreshing fragrance. It is a favorite among essential oils for diffusing.

Application

Lime is a delightful addition to baths, body lotions, and deodorants.

Emotional/Spiritual Aspects

Lime essential oil is a perfect choice for the ***very*** weary—those who are so weary of trials and troubles that they feel far older than their years on earth would indicate. The lively fragrance of lime is stimulating and refreshing. It can help one overcome exhaustion, depression, apathy, and listlessness. Lime is a good oil for improving memory and concentration.

Physical Aspects

Lime essential oil is said to soothe broken capillaries, stimulate the muscles around the eyes, brighten a pale, dull complexion by removing dead skin cells, and is capable of tightening skin and connective tissue. Lime is a good oil for digestive difficulties, particularly gallstones and gallbladder inflammation. This oil is recommended for liver deficiencies and liver cleansing in infants and children. Lime stimulates the immune system to increase production of leukocytes that aid in fighting infections. Lime oil is also used to stabilize blood pressure fluctuations.

General Information

Lime oil works extremely well in removing gum, wood stain, oil, and grease spots from clothing.

Cautions

Lime essential oil is photo-toxic. Avoid sunlight or UV radiation on skin where lime has been applied.

Litsea Cubeba

(Litsea cubeba)

(Commonly known as May Chang)

Ingredient In

LeTherma Care

Therapeutic Properties

hypotensive, astringent, digestive, stomachic, disinfectant, sedative or stimulant—as needed and according to quantity used, much like lavender

Affinity For

digestive system, heart, skin, brow chakra, nervous system

Resonance

physical, emotional

Plant Family

Graminae

Part of Plant Used

fruit

Aromatic Considerations

Litsea cubeba has a lovely crisp, lemony scent. It is valued for its calming and antidepressant properties.

Application

Litsea cubeba can be diffused or diluted and worn on the body.

Emotional/Spiritual Aspects

Litsea cubeba brings joy and lightness of spirit. It makes one feel young at heart and enthusiastic about life. This essential oil is often used in Inner Child work, where it is calming and soothing. Litsea cubeba is an oil that often appeals to children.

Physical Aspects

Litsea cubeba is considered useful for high blood pressure and other disorders that have been brought on by nervousness, fear, or stress. Litsea cubeba is useful for indigestion and to dispel gas pains. It is a good oil for treatment of skin disorders such as acne, dermatitis, and oily or discolored skin. Litsea cubeba is useful for controlling excess perspiration.

General Information

Litsea cubeba is often used in soaps and lotions where it tends to stabilize the higher notes of the other essential oils in the product.

Cautions

Litsea cubeba should be avoided if pregnant. It can be a skin irritant to people with very sensitive skin.

Mandarin

(Citrus reticulata)

Ingredient In

LeAspire, LeBalance, LeMy-Graine, LeSolitude, LeTenda Care, LeVitality , LeWarm Down, LeWoman Wise

Therapeutic Properties

tonic, stomachic, digestive, calming, antispasmodic, antiseptic

Affinity For

emotions
nervous system
digestion
gallbladder meridian
governing vessel meridian

Resonance	**Plant Family**	**Part of Plant Used**
physical, emotional	Rutaceae	fruit

Aromatic Considerations

Mandarin essential oil has sedative and slightly hypnotic properties, making mandarin one of the best essential oils for stress and irritability.

Application

Mandarin may be diffused or diluted and applied to the feet or the body. Mandarin is a very gentle oil and could be massaged safely, with any carrier oil, on the abdomen.

Emotional/Spiritual Aspects

Mandarin promotes feelings of deep happiness. This personal happiness often manifests in our lives as kindness and gentleness with all living things. Mandarin also provides a firmness and a sense of self that allows personal growth and spiritual development. This oil is an especially good choice for those who tend to dwell in the past. It is also good for those who tend to dwell on past emotional traumas. They have survived the trauma, but they have not thrived. Mandarin can help us achieve a state of mind where we are able to build or repair our relationships, especially with the children and the elderly in our lives.

Physical Aspects

Mandarin essential oil is a gentle and supportive healer. It is especially good for the convalescence stage of an illness. It is a good choice for very young children and for the old and frail. This oil should be considered whenever the illness is accompanied by great sadness. Mandarin essential oil is also good for digestion where it aids with such conditions as constipation and diarrhea.

General Information

Mandarin *(Citrus reticulata)* is the variety of mandarin that is often referred to as red mandarin.

Cautions

There are no known contradictions. This is a rare citrus essential oil that is **not photo-toxic**.

Manuka

(Leptospermum scoparium)

Ingredient In

Le Candila, LePurify, LeSimplicity, LeStefanie

Therapeutic Properties

antibacterial, anti-fungal, antiseptic, antiviral, immunostimulant, antibiotic, anti-parasitic

Affinity For

immune system
killing bacteria

Resonance	**Plant Family**	**Part of Plant Used**
physical, emotional	Myrtaceae	leaves, seeds

Aromatic Considerations

Manuka has a woodsy scent that is warmer and less caustic than the aroma of tea tree. It is much more pleasant when diffused than tea tree and very antiseptic.

Application

Dilute and apply to the feet or the body.

Emotional/Spiritual Aspects

Manuka is gently cleansing to the energy body. It makes us feel as though we are 'ready and waiting' for something in our lives. The aroma of manuka can start us on the first step toward a goal or project.

Physical Aspects

Manuka is reported to be many times more effective against both gram negative and gram positive bacteria than its close cousins, the many varieties of tea tree (*Melaleuca).* Manuka is milder and more pleasant in aroma and less caustic to the skin than are the tea tree oils. Manuka is strongly anti-fungal and effective against a wide variety of yeasts and molds. Suggested uses for manuka include eliminating athlete's foot and toenail fungus, relieving dry, cracked, and irritated skin conditions, neutralizing pathogens in the air, and healing cold sores. Manuka can be used effectively on insect bites and stings to avoid infection and dull pain. Used undiluted and consistently, manuka oil is strong enough to eradicate warts. Well diluted, manuka oil relieves the itch and burn of chicken pox sores.

Cautions

Manuka is fairly new to the essential oil market. While there are no safety cautions or contraindications in any literature that I can find, it is always wise to use a little caution with an unfamiliar essential oil.

Marjoram

(Marjorana hortensis or Origanum marjorana)

Ingredient In

LeAspire, LeBalance, LeMy-Graine, LeSolitude, LeTenda Care, LeVitality , LeWarm Down, LeWoman Wise

Therapeutic Properties

antispasmodic, arterial vasodilator, expectorant, digestive, analgesic, calming, sedative, antitussive, antiseptic, antibiotic, anti-infectious, diuretic, emmenagogue

Affinity For

respiratory system	reproductive areas	solar plexus chakra
digestive system	cardiovascular system	governing vessel meridian
	yang energy	stomach and spleen meridians

Resonance	**Plant Family**	**Part of Plant Used**
physical, emotional	Labiatae	leaves

Aromatic Considerations

The aroma of marjoram oil can warm the soul in times of grief, sorrow, or loneliness.

Application

Dilute and apply to the feet or any area of the body.

Emotional/Spiritual Aspects

Marjoram is quieting to obsessive worry where negative thoughts circle repetitively in the brain hour after hour. This type of obsessive worry is an indication of depleted or stressed earth energy. Marjoram essential oil is also helpful for those who seem to ***love*** being in the center of some sort of drama all the time. This need for attention is a manifestation of an energetically depleted earth meridian with its 'lack of something' perception. In this instance, the feeling of deprivation focuses on family or friends. We are sure that 'no one cares' about us as they should. The aroma of marjoram oil can eliminate feelings of loneliness or persecution, replacing them with feelings of security and even some compassion for others.

Physical Aspects

Marjoram eases respiratory distress and infections such as bronchitis. It is often beneficial for spasmodic dry coughs. The analgesic properties of marjoram make it an appropriate choice for muscle aches, sprains, strains, and arthritis. Marjoram essential oil helps bruising to clear and fade more quickly. Marjoram increases the dilation of blood vessels, lowers blood pressure, and eases heart palpitations. It can ease headaches that are caused by muscle tension or lack of circulation.

Marjoram oil increases the tone and effectiveness of parasympathetic nerves. One benefit of healthy parasympathetic nerves is an increase in the peristalsis in the colon. Marjoram regulates the menstrual cycle, relieves pain and cramping.

General Information

Marjoram was known as the 'herb of happiness' to the early Romans and 'joy of the mountain' to the Greeks.

Cautions

Marjoram should be used sparingly during pregnancy.

Melissa

(Melissa officinalis)

Ingredient In

[Le]Simplicity, [Le]Stefanie

Therapeutic Properties

antiseptic, antibiotic, antiviral, sedative, calmative, antidepressant, stimulant

Affinity For

immune system	yang energy	brow chakra
respiratory system	reproductive system	fire element
reproductive areas	cardiovascular system	wood element

Resonance	**Plant Family**	**Part of Plant Used**
physical, emotional	Labiatae	leaves, flowers

Aromatic Considerations

Melissa essential oil has a delicate lemony scent. It is both calming and uplifting to the spirits.

Application

Melissa can be applied, diluted, to the feet or any area of the body.

Emotional/Spiritual Aspects

Melissa essential oil has a youthful, revitalizing effect on the body and spirit. It opens our ability to see and understand truth. The aroma of melissa oil helps us receive insights for living our daily lives. It promotes feelings of compassion and love for life.

Melissa is beneficial to emotionally sensitive individuals who do not respond well to pressure or who are easily upset, almost traumatized, by the slightest confrontation. They spend their strength trying to hold in their feelings to prevent or end an argument rather than risk expressing feelings of anger or hurt. This continual repression of fear or anger eventually leads to depression. Melissa essential oil can be helpful anywhere along this soul destroying path.

Physical Aspects

Melissa essential oil has been proven to have powerful antiviral properties. It is considered to be one of the most powerful antiseptic and medicinal essential oils. Studies conducted in Germany indicate that it is useful against various strains of flu virus, smallpox, and mumps. The University of Munich reports a complete remission of herpes simplex lesions (cold sores and impetigo) from the use of melissa oil.

Melissa oil is used for hypertension, palpitations, shock, and conditions where the heart is overstimulated. Melissa is excellent in the treatment of allergies, asthma, bronchitis, chronic coughs, colds, and cold-sore blisters. Melissa is recommended for sterility in women.

General Information

Because pure melissa is so expensive to produce, growers often redistill the plant material and combine the products of the two distillations. This is a process that is also used for oils other than melissa. The product of this type of distillation is referred to as a rectified oil. The melissa that is currently carried by Butterfly Express, llc, is a rectified oil. I have had very good results using this particular melissa oil; the antiviral properties seem to be strong, complete and effective. It is an excellent oil and the best reasonably priced melissa oil that I have ever seen. Hopefully this grower will continue to produce this excellent product consistently in the coming years.

Melissa Blend

Melissa is extremely expensive. Butterfly Express, llc sells a well-done blend of other essential oils put together to simulate the healing properties of melissa oil. This is a blend of pure essential oils, not a chemically produced substitute. I have been very impressed with this blend, but *it is not pure Melissa oil.* If you can possibly afford it, try to get some of the real thing!

Another solution to the prohibitive expense of melissa oil is to purchase a *rectified* melissa essential oil. (See General Information section, above, for melissa essential oil.)

The ingredients of melissa blend are as follows: lemon, lemongrass, melissa, pine, tangerine, ylang ylang

Ingredient In

LeAcknowledge, LeBenediction, LeEverlasting, LeExhilaration, LeFaith, LeGrateful Heart, LeIQ, LeTrust, LeWhispering Hope

Myrrh

(Commiphora myrrha)

Ingredient In

LeBenediction, LeBountiful, LeDeeper, LeEZ-Traveler, LeGrateful Heart, LeJourney, LeMagi, LeMeditation, LeRefresh-Mint, LeWhispering Hope

Therapeutic Properties

anti-inflammatory, pectoral, antiseptic, antispasmodic, cicatrisive, balsamic, expectorant, anti-fungal, astringent, vulnerary, soporific

Affinity For

digestive sysetm	base chakra	earth and metal elements
respiratory system	yang energy	throat chakra
vascular system		

Resonance	**Plant Family**	**Part of Plant Used**
physical, emotional	Burseraceae	resin

Aromatic Considerations

Myrrh has been used in meditation for centuries. It is a wonderful oil, although it doesn't have the most pleasant aroma.

Application

Myrrh essential oil can be diluted and applied to the feet or anywhere on the body. Myrrh is a resin; even diluted it remains tacky on the skin for a few minutes.

Emotional/Spiritual Aspects

Myrrh essential oil helps us see ways and means for the achievement of our dreams. It opens our minds to inspiration and the direction of the spirit while keeping us firmly grounded in reality and common sense. Myrrh has an affinity for the base chakra, which connects this essential oil to issues of abundance and bounty. When we open ourselves to receive the gifts of the spirit and of the material world, these gifts will be given to us.

Physical Aspects

One of the outstanding properties of myrrh is astringency. Astringency means that myrrh causes tissues and blood vessels to contract. Myrrh can tighten the gums, tone the skin, aid muscle contraction in the intestines and other internal organs, and stop bleeding. Myrrh relieves congestion in the lungs and sinuses. As a stimulant, myrrh has an effect on thoughts, blood circulation, the secretion of needed bile in the digestive process, the pumping action of the heart, and makes you more alert by stimulating the brain and nervous system. Myrrh essential oil increases perspiration during times of illness, ridding the body of toxins and cleansing the pores of the skin. Myrrh's stimulant properties have a particular affinity for the immune system and the circulation. Myrrh is an excellent choice for skin complaints such as eczema, ringworm, athlete's foot, chapped and cracked skin, stretch marks, rashes, and wrinkles.

Cautions

The use of myrrh should be limited by pregnant women because myrrh is a *mild* uterine stimulant.

Myrtle

(Myrtus communis)

Ingredient In

LeAspire, LeBalance, LeEndo Relief, LeMeditation

Therapeutic Properties

antiseptic, antibacterial, decongestant, deodorizer, immune stimulant, digestive, antitussive, balsamic, carminative, pectoral

Affinity For

digestion
bladder and kidneys
lungs
skin
thyroid
prostate
heart chakra
heart meridian

Resonance

physical, emotional, spiritual

Plant Family

Myrtaceae

Part of Plant Used

leaves

Aromatic Considerations

The aroma of myrrh essential oil is musky and almost euphoric. It is said to soothe anger and make the spirit quieter.

Application

Myrtle should be diluted and applied to any area of the body or to the feet.

Emotional/Spiritual Aspects

Myrtle oil is strong and grounding. It seems to open all of the senses. Myrtle can help us develop the organizational skills needed for success and stress-free living. Myrtle is about learning to prioritize in our lives, taking care of the necessities first. This helps us establish a sound base for further spiritual growth. Myrtle, since it removes some of the stresses in our lives through grounding and organization, is often useful for insomnia.

Physical Aspects

Myrtle is a very anti-inflammatory and decongestant oil. These properties make it useful for diarrhea, bladder infections, sinus infections, and lung complaints such as asthma, bronchitis, chronic coughs, and tuberculosis. Myrrh regulates the functions of glands in the endocrine system. This effect is seen most clearly in the stimulation of thyroid activity and in the decongestion of the prostate. Myrtle has a stabilizing effect on hormones and supports immune function. Myrtle is a powerful deodorizer. It is a good skin care oil and aids the digestive system.

General Information

The recorded use of myrtle essential oil goes back 4,000 years.

Cautions

Myrtle has some hormonal properties. It should be used with caution if pregnant.

Neroli

(Citrus aurantium)

Ingredient In

LeAcknowledge, LeEverlasting, LeExhilaration, LeWisdom

Therapeutic Properties

antibacterial, antidepressant, anti-infectious, anti-parasitic, antispasmodic, antiviral, aphrodisiac, deodorant, sedative, tonic

Affinity For

nerves
skin/tissues
2nd, 4th and 5th meridians/elements
crown chakra

Resonance

physical, mental, emotional, spiritual

Plant Family

Rutaceae

Part of Plant Used

flowers

Aromatic Considerations

The aroma of neroli has powerful effects on our minds and emotions. It is calming, relaxing, uplifting, and encourages confidence. It promotes feelings of joy, peace, and hope.

Application

Neroli is wonderful diffused! Neroli can also be diluted and applied anywhere on the body.

Emotional/Spiritual Aspects

Neroli essential oil reawakens passion and sensitivity. It can change negative outlooks and bring us renewed hope. Neroli can help us trust our own intuition and good sense in the making of choices. Neroli is renowned around the world for relieving nervous tension, promoting restful sleep, and elevating the mood. Neroli has been used successfully to treat depression, anxiety, and shock. It is calming and relaxing because it stabilizes the emotions and encourages confidence and courage.

Neroli is particularly appropriate for any one who has become timid or withdrawn. It can help with cynicism and despair. Neroli helps to alleviate feelings of 'nothing changes, nothing ever will.' Neroli fosters independence and trust in our possibilities for a good future.

Neroli is a natural sedative. It is useful for depression and anxiety. Neroli relaxes the body, mind, and spirit. It quiets the heart and soul.

Physical Aspects

Neroli is much more than just an 'emotional' oil. Like all essential oils, it is very antiseptic. What a pleasant oil to reach for when you get a cut or wound and need a disinfectant. Neroli rebuilds tissue and heals the skin, making it excellent for scars and skin damage of any kind. Neroli is one of the most emollient of the essential oils. It is prized in skin care products. Neroli is considered a weight loss oil.

Neroli has a profound influence on the action of the heart. It diminishes the amplitude of heart muscle contractions, but only if this is what is needed. Neroli is never dangerous. It is often used for palpitations, erratic heartbeat, and other types of cardiac spasm. It is a wonderful oil for panicky, hysterical, fearful people who become agitated over trifles. Neroli is a valuable remedy for shock or any situation that is putting a strain on the heart.

General Information

For centuries, the Egyptian people have regarded neroli highly for its ability to heal the mind, body, and spirit. Neroli's deep, sensuous aroma is often the 'heart' of floral blends.

Neroli is a very heady oil. Sniffed directly from the bottle, it is almost unpleasantly over-whelming. A tiny bit, diffused into the air or placed on the skin is amazingly potent and lovely.

Cautions

There are no known cautions for the use of neroli essential oil. Even the more conservative British school of thought in aromatherapy consider neroli oil to be totally non-irritating. Neroli oil may be used on the skin even where irritation or redness are present.

Niaouli

(Melaleuca viridiflora—also know as quinquenervia)

Ingredient In

LeMela Plus

Therapeutic Properties

very strong and powerful anti-fungal, antibacterial, antiviral; digestive tonic, cytophylactic (tissue regenerating), analgesic, insecticide, decongestant

Affinity For

immune system respiratory/pulmonary skin/muscles central and governing meridians

Resonance	**Plant Family**	**Part of Plant Used**
physical, emotional, spiritual	Myrtaceae	leaves

Aromatic Considerations

Niaouli is a member of the melaleuca (tea tree) species, but has a sweeter, more delicate scent than the *alternafolia* variety that we are most familiar with. The aroma of this oil can clear the mind and help us stay alert. Niaouli is a great aid to concentration.

Application

Niaouli can be diluted and applied to any area of the body. It makes a very good disinfectant.

Emotional/Spiritual Aspects

Niaouli is said to open the inner vision of the soul and direct our thoughts toward heaven. Niaouli can help us focus on higher values and more worthy goals. Niaouli can help us see the bigger picture of our lives and find those things that we were born to do.

Physical Aspects

Niaouli has been shown in studies to be a general immune system booster and effective as a response to allergic reactions. This oil is an excellent antiseptic for treating pulmonary infections, bronchitis, coughs, sinus congestion, and sore throats. The anti-inflammatory properties of this oil make it useful for muscle aches. Naiouli, being a member of the tea tree family, is very antiseptic. It is useful for skin conditions such as cuts, boils, burns, insect bites, and acne.

General Information

Niaouli is often found in pharmaceutical preparations such as gargles, cough drops, toothpastes, and mouth sprays.

Cautions

Niaouli is photo-toxic. Avoid direct sunlight on skin to which niaouli oil has been applied in the last 24 hours.

Nutmeg

(Myristica fragrans)

Ingredient In

LeEndo Relief, LeEnergy, LeFocus

Therapeutic Properties

antiseptic, anti-parasitic, general cerebral and circulatory stimulant

Affinity For

digestion	adrenal glands	sacral chakra
joints, muscles	hormones	liver meridian
nervous system	immune system	circulation

Resonance	**Plant Family**	**Part of Plant Used**
physical, emotional	Myrtaceae	seeds

Aromatic Considerations

Nutmeg essential oil is not appropriate for use by itself in a diffuser and care should be taken when inhaling the aroma into the nostrils.

Application

Nutmeg should always be diluted well before applying to the feet or to the body.

Emotional/Spiritual Aspects

Emotional stability is one of the characteristics of nutmeg essential oil. Nutmeg rekindles the fire within our souls and helps us to regain our lost passion for life. It seems to lift the weight of the world off our shoulders, letting us rise above situations and challenges. Nutmeg oil, added to a blend, can be an essential ingredient for relieving nervous fatigue. Nutmeg oil seems to accentuate our ability to comfort, heal, and understand other people's emotional traumas and struggles.

Physical Aspects

Nutmeg supports the adrenal glands, giving one increased vitality and ability to cope with stress. Nutmeg's affinity for the digestive system makes it useful for bacterial infections, chronic diarrhea, gallstones, sluggish digestions, poor assimilation of nutrients, nausea, vomiting, loss of appetite, and bad breath. Nutmeg is also effective for gout.

Nutmeg supports and strengthens the immune function. The improvement in circulation that nutmeg can bring about is often helpful for vertigo and fainting spells. This increased circulation can improve the function of joints and muscles and improve concentration and mental alertness. Nutmeg supports the nervous system. ***Blends which contain nutmeg are excellent choices for people with chronic illnesses.***

Cautions

Nutmeg must be used with extreme caution. If over-used or diffused for too long a period of time, nutmeg has been known to cause confusion, delirium, or even convulsions. It can over-stimulate the heart and cardiovascular system if used too frequently or too long. It should be used with extreme caution, or not at all, during pregnancy and never if epileptic. **ALWAYS** dilute well! In other words, nutmeg is a really great oil when used in a blend!

Opoponax Myrrh - Sweet Myrrh

(Commiphora guidottii)

Ingredient In

[Le]Mariah

Therapeutic Properties

antiseptic, anti-parasitic, general cerebral and circulatory stimulant

Affinity For

mucous membranes
muscles

Resonance	**Plant Family**	**Part of Plant Used**
physical, mental	Bruseraceae	gum

Aromatic Considerations

Opoponax is sweet, spicy, and warming with herbaceous undertones. It has a more pleasing aroma than regular myrrh.

Application

Opoponax can be applied anywhere on the body. As with most essential oils, it is best diluted.

Emotional/Spiritual Aspects

Opoponax is an oil for precision and logic. Opoponax clears fuzzy thinking and helps daydreamers come down from the clouds. It is a good addition to blends which will be used to stimulate clarity of thought and attention to detail. Opoponax can help us make desired changes in our lives and in ourselves because it helps us see situations with more clarity. Opoponax can give us direction and purpose. Emotionally, this oils supports our ability to sort truth from error. It can help us see the way to justice and responsibility in our daily lives.

Physical Aspects

Opoponax has a drying action on mucous build-up in the lungs. It can be used for bronchitis, colds, sore throats, and coughs. Opoponax is effective as a muscle relaxant and anti-inflammatory, making it useful for arthritis. It may help purge stagnant blood from the uterus. Opoponax is an excellent insect repellent.

General Information

Opoponax is sometimes used as a base note in blends where it stabilizes and sweetens the aroma.

Cautions

Opoponax should be avoided if pregnant and this essential oil may be photo-toxic, although regular myrrh certainly is not.

Orange, Bitter

(Citrus aurantium)

Ingredient In

[Le]Bountiful, [Le]Everlasting, [Le]Holiday Spirit, [Le]Unity

Therapeutic Properties

antiseptic, anti-parasitic, general cerebral and circulatory stimulant, antidepressant, antispasmodic, tonic

Affinity For

digestion

nervous system

wood element

Resonance

physical, emotional

Plant Family

Rutaceae

Part of Plant Used

fruit

Aromatic Considerations

Orange, bitter essential oil has the sweet, citrus smell that is characteristic of orange, sweet (*Citrus sinensis)*, but orange, bitter has an underlying touch of tart bitterness which is reminiscent of grapefruit oil. It is very nice diffused, and makes a pleasant change from the heady sweetness of orange, sweet or neroli essential oils.

Application

Orange, bitter should be diluted and applied to the feet or to the body.

Emotional/Spiritual Aspects

Orange, bitter, like all citrus oils, is wonderful diffused during the winter months. Citrus oils seem to release a few rays of sunshine into the air. They are subtly energizing. They brighten the outlook and lift the spirits. Orange, bitter is an effective treatment for depression, especially when it is made worse by cloudy or winter weather and lack of sunlight. Orange, bitter, though considered a stimulant, can also help one relax at the end of a long day.

Physical Aspects

Orange, bitter is used in blends to promote weight loss, helping to curb the appetite and dissolve cellulite. The keynote features of this oil, however, are on digestion. Orange, bitter is used in the treatment of heartburn, flatulence, and diarrhea. It also seems to aid in the absorption of vitamin C.

General Information

Many parts of this plant, *Citrus aurantium,* are extracted for use as essential oils. Orange, bitter essential oil is made from the fruit, bergamot is extracted from the peel, petitgrain is extracted from the foliage and twigs, and neroli is distilled from the blossoms. Even though all of these oils are made from the same plant, they are very different in aroma and therapeutic properties.

Cautions

Orange, bitter is photo-toxic. You should avoid direct sunlight on skin to which this oil has been applied for at least 12 hours.

Orange, Sweet

(Citrus sinensis)

Ingredient In

LeAngel, LeBelieve, LeBeloved, LeBountiful, LeDiscernment, LeEternity, LeEverlasting, LeEZ-Traveler, LeHeart Song, LeHoliday Spirit, LeInsight, LeMoonlight, LeSolitude, LeSunburst, LeTranquility, LeVisibility, LeVitality, LeWake-Up, LeWisdom

Therapeutic Properties

disinfectant, diuretic, calmative, anticoagulant, sedative, stomachic, cholagogue (encourages the production of bile and the digestion of fats), diuretic, tonic, antispasmodic, antiseptic, antibiotic, depurative, anti-inflammatory

Affinity For

digestive system
respiratory system
skin
wood element
sacral chakra
spleen meridian

Resonance

physical, emotional

Plant Family

Rutaceae

Part of Plant Used

fruit

Aromatic Considerations

Orange, sweet has a delightful fragrance. It promotes feelings of well-being and happiness. By itself, or as an ingredient in a essential oil blend, orange, sweet promotes restful sleep.

Application

The aroma of orange, sweet is an excellent remedy to alleviate nausea or morning sickness. It is sometimes helpful with these conditions to apply a drop or two of the oil behind the ears. Orange, sweet oil can be diluted and applied anywhere on the body. It is also a lovely oil to diffuse in your home or workplace.

Emotional/Spiritual Aspects

The emotions of frustration and discouragement block the flow of energy to and from the liver. Any block in energy creates tension. The tension created by blocked energy in the liver results in moodiness, irritability, nausea, headaches, insomnia, and expecting more of ourselves and others than is reasonable. Orange, sweet is an excellent oil for all of these conditions and emotions.

Orange, sweet essential oil brings peace and happiness to the mind and body and joy to the heart. It provides emotional support to overcome sadness and courage to escape emotional and physical abuse. This oil re-establishes optimism and a sense of humor when they have become lost through abuse or sadness. Orange, sweet can make even the most mundane practical task flow along easily and enjoyably.

Physical Aspects

Orange, sweet can relieve cardiac spasms and false angina that are the result of stress or depression. The nicer, lighter attitude produced by orange, sweet oil improves overall immune function, aids respiration, increases lymphatic drainage, improves digestive function, and raises low blood sugar levels. Orange, sweet is particularly effective when a complaint has anxiety, depression, or nerve weakness at its core. Sweet orange is one of the essential oils used in programs to treat eating disorders. The astringent properties of orange, sweet oil improves a dull, oily complexion. It is of benefit in the treatment of wrinkles as it hydrates and strengthens the cells of the epidermis.

General Information

This is a very versatile and inexpensive essential oil. It works very well as a cleaner, removing sticky adhesive residue from most surfaces.

Cautions

This oil is very mild. Although orange, sweet is a citrus, it is ***not*** considered photo-toxic.

Oregano

(Origanum vulgare)

Ingredient In

[Le]Deliverance, [Le]Life Force, [Le]No-More

Therapeutic Properties

anti-infectious, antibiotic, antiviral, antiseptic, stimulant, anti-aphrodisiac, emmenagogue, anti-parasitic, expectorant, rebufacient, anti-fungal, immunostimulant

Affinity For

immune system
digestive system
sacral chakra
respiratory system

Resonance

physical

Plant Family

Labiatae

Part of Plant Used

leaves

Aromatic Considerations

Oregano is not pleasant diffused by itself. However, the antimicrobial properties can be pleasantly diffused into the air as part of a blended oil formula.

Application

Be sure to dilute very well before applying to the feet or to the body.

Emotional/Spiritual Aspects

Oregano essential oil promotes a feeling of strength and stability.

Physical Aspects

Oregano, in either herbal or essential oil form, has strong antiseptic and antimicrobial properties. Oregano essential oil balances metabolism, strengthens the vital centers of the body, and is an immune stimulant. In the respiratory tract, oregano is useful for treating chronic bronchitis, respiratory infections, pneumonia, pulmonary tuberculosis, colds, and flu.

General Information

Oregano is an extremely beneficial and effective oil which has received some attention from the media lately. Unfortunately, too many reporters and announcers do not know the difference between therapeutic grade essential oils and oils which have been diluted with carrier type oils. ***DO NOT follow their suggestions and use large quantities at once***. 2 or 3 drops of a pure essential oil is always sufficient.

Cautions

Oregano should be avoided or used very cautiously during pregnancy. This oil can cause extreme skin irritation if applied repeatedly without dilution. Oregano should be used with a little bit of caution when diffused. Oregano is probably too strong for use in baths. Be sure to dilute well when applying to body.

Oregano, Wild

(Origanum vulgare)

This is the same plant and species as the oregano listed above, but it is harvested in the wild rather than cultivated for use. There are those who believe that wild-crafted oils (and herbals) are stronger and more medicinal than cultivated ones. I have found that growing conditions vary from place to place in both cultivated beds and in the wild. The differences in quality may have more to do with the conditions under which the harvested plants grew rather than whether or not the plant grew wild or was cultivated.

In a Biblical sense, when man left Eden he was given dominion over the earth and expected to till, cultivate, and improve it somewhat. Good essential oil growers are careful to grow the most vital and therapeutic plants possible. Their livelihood and reputation depend on their ability to optimize the medicinal value of their products.

Often, wildcrated oils are not up to the standards of loved and cared for (cultivated) plants. Wild Oregano is often the exception. It can be better.

Palmarosa

(Cymbopogon martinii)

Ingredient In

LeAcknowledge, LeBaby Me, LeBelieve, LeEverlasting, LeInner Peace, LeTranquility, LeTrust, LeTurmoil, LeUnity, LeVitality

Therapeutic Properties

antibiotic, anti-fungal, antiviral, tonic, antiseptic, emollient, digestive and circulatory stimulant, hydrating

Affinity For

cardiovascular system	yin energy	heart chakra
thyroid gland	bladder meridian	solar plexus chakra
skin care		

Resonance	**Plant Family**	**Part of Plant Used**
physical	Graminae	leaves

Aromatic Considerations

Rose *(not palmarosa)* is a very expensive and fragrant essential oil but, in a blend of oils, the aroma of rose can be overpowered by the other ingredients. The medicinal value is still there, but much of the aroma of the rose is lost. Palmarosa, when added to a blend which has rose as one of the ingredients, emphasizes the scent of *roses.* This vastly improves the bouquet of the blend.

Palmarosa reduces stress and tension while relaxing tight muscles and lessening pain.

Application

Palmarosa, though a very mild essential oil, should still be diluted before applying to the body. A drop or two, however, may be worn, undiluted, as a perfume.

Emotional/Spiritual Aspects

Sometimes, in an attempt to cover insecurities within ourselves or to cover past hurts, we hold onto to situations or people so tightly that they feel they must struggle to be free. Palmarosa helps us to embrace change and let go. Since we live in an ever changing world, there are many times when we must let go of the 'old' way of doing and being in order to move forward and grow. If we are constantly 'letting go and letting God' direct our lives for our good, we will not just be changing, we will be growing toward the best we can be. Our success and happiness will be inevitable and assured.

Palmarosa can help us ***enjoy*** being versatile and adaptable, as we move through the changes that life always brings. This strength within oneself reduces stress and tension and eliminates the sort of nervous exhaustion that resisting life creates. If you have already exhausted yourself in the struggle against change, try palmarosa—or blends containing it—to balance and strengthen yourself. The lovely aroma of this essential oil promotes recovery and strengthens resolve.

Those who believe that a plant's shape and environment denote its medicinal value would say that the long stem of this aromatic grass waving with the breeze indicates flexibility and freedom of movement. This adaptability (going with the flow) is yin in nature. But palmarosa is firmly rooted in the earth, giving it both adaptability and a feeling of security. Palmarosa is suited for people who cannot abide change, the frequent absence of loved ones, or who frequently suffer from homesickness. This would be a good oil to try for children who get very upset when their mother must leave them for a few minutes.

Physical Aspects

Palmarosa is used in skin care regimens for all types of skin. This essential oil ***balances*** the production of sebum, making it effective for both oily and dry skin types. Palmarosa stimulates new cell growth, making it an effective oil in the treatment of scarring from acne or injury. Palmarosa seems to have a beneficial effect on thyroid hormones and acts as a uterine and vaginal tonic. This essential oil acts against fungal infections, bacterial infections, and candida.

Cautions

Palmarosa is a very mild essential oil. There are no known contra-indications for its use.

Parsley

(Petroselinum sativum)

Ingredient In

LeVallee *(this blend was created for rebuilding skin after a serious 3rd degree burn)*

Therapeutic Properties

antimicrobial, antiseptic, astringent, diuretic, emmenagogue, laxative, stomachic, uterine tonic

Affinity For

cellular structure
urinary tract

Resonance	**Plant Family**	**Part of Plant Used**
physical, emotional	Umbelliferae	seeds

Aromatic Considerations

Parsley essential oil is not recommended for diffusing as a single oil.

Application

Parsley should be diluted extra carefully before being applied to skin. It is far better used in a blend of essential oils than used by itself.

Emotional/Spiritual Aspects

Parsley essential oil helps us move from wishing things were different, to actually thriving in challenging conditions and after demanding events. It has a marked effect on people who, regardless of the circumstances of their lives, are perpetually dissatisfied with how things are. They may live out their entire lives wishing things could be different so they could, at least, be happy.

Physical Aspects

Parsley's ability to strengthen the integrity of cell membranes makes it a useful and versatile oil. It is widely used to promote hair follicle health to stimulate hair growth. Parsley, as part of a blended oil, can be a good tonic for the scalp. Parsley essential oil helps clear bruises and repair broken blood vessels and capillaries. It can be useful in repairing damaged skin and reducing cellulite. Parsley has a toning effect on the urinary tract and a diuretic effect on cells and tissues. This essential oil is often used in treatments for cystitis and urinary infections.

Cautions

Parsley is a concentrated, almost caustic, essential oil. ***It should be used with extreme caution as a single oil. Pregnant women should avoid the use of parsley oil altogether.*** Parsley is best used as part of an essential oil blend such as LeVallee.

While useful for mild urinary tract infections, *parsley is contra-indicated for more severe forms of kidney disease and degeneration.*

Some recent studies indicate the continual over-use of parsley may stress the liver.

Patchouli

(Pogostemon cablin)

Ingredient In

LeBountiful, LeExhilaration, LeFocus, LeInside-Out, LeMoonlight, LeNo-More, LeRefresh-Mint, LeTranquility, LeWoman Wise

Therapeutic Properties

anti-inflammatory, tissue regenerative, tonic, cytophylactic, antiseptic, decongestant, antibiotic, anti-fungal, antidepressant, aphrodisiac, astringent, calmative, nervine

Affinity For

reproductive system	hormones	sacral chakra	yang energy
urinary tract	liver	stomach meridian	

Resonance	**Plant Family**	**Part of Plant Used**
physical, emotional	Labiatae	leaves, flowers

Aromatic Considerations

The aroma of patchouli oil is very calming and centering. It helps bring about a cooperative effort between your heart and your head. Self-imposed barriers and limitations seem to melt away. Patchouli can relieve anxiety, fear, and indecision.

Application

Patchouli is a great skin oil. Dilute and apply it everywhere!

Emotional/Spiritual Aspects

Patchouli encourages us to dream of new horizons and work toward new goals. Patchouli is a vital ingredient in any essential oil blend that targets our perspective on money, material possessions, or lack of abundance issues of any kind. Patchouli is especially suited to people with strong constitutions who rarely pay any attention to their health as they pursue their material goals. Almost without warning, they eventually collapse, both mentally and physically. Patchouli is a valuable aid to their recovery and helps them achieve a balance in their lives that prevents a reoccurrence of this pattern.

Physical Aspects

Patchouli is an oil I have come to love for its effect on physical exhaustion and chronic fatigue. Patchouli is a tissue regenerating oil. It aids with scarring, rashes, eczema, and bacterial and fungal infections. Patchouli is especially good for vaginal infections such as candida and others. Patchouli essential oil improves hormone balance and aids the liver and kidneys by discharging toxins. Patchouli can help with constipation when the emotional roots are holding on to every material thing and element of safety that we can. This essential oil has been used in programs for substance addiction. It is a very good oil for chapped skin, athlete's feet, ringworm, and weeping wounds. Patchouli's affinity for liver function makes it a valuable oil for allergies and mild auto-immune disorders.

Cautions

There are no known cautions for therapeutic grade patchouli essential oil.

Peppermint

(Wild Mint or Field Mint)

(Mentha arvensis)

Ingredient In

LeTenda Care, LePaine, LeCrystal Clear

Aromatic Considerations

Peppermint arvensis is similar to peppermint piperita, but is more reminiscent of candy canes.

	Plant Family	**Part of Plant Used**
Therapeutic Aspects	Labiatae	stems, leaves, flower buds

The properties and actions for peppermint arvensis, are very similar to mentha piperita.

Cautions

Arvensis has a higher menthol content than piperita, making it slightly more potent therapeutically, and a little more caustic.

Peppermint

(Mentha piperita)

Ingredient In

LeAspire, LeBalance, LeBreezey, LeCrystal Clear, LeCypernium, LeDeeper, LeInside-Out, LeEZ-Traveler, LeMy-Graine, LePaine, LePatches, LeTenda Care, LeTherma Care, LeWake-Up

Therapeutic Properties

tonic, cytophylactic, anti-infectious, antiseptic, decongestant, antibiotic, anti-fungal, antidepressant, anti-toxic, aphrodisiac, astringent, calmative, nervine, anti-inflammatory to the nerves and the prostate.

Affinity For

digestive system
tissues
mind
nerves
earth element
wood element
lung meridian
small intestine meridian
yang energy
throat chakra

Resonance

physical, mental

Plant Family

Labiatae

Part of Plant Used

stems. leaves, flower buds

Aromatic Considerations

Peppermint oil stimulates the mind, increasing the ability to focus and concentrate. When inhaled, it restores the sense of taste by stimulating the trigeminal nerve. Oddly, inhaling peppermint oil can also curb the appetite.

Application

Peppermint oil should be diluted well before applying to the skin. Placing one drop of peppermint under the tongue and breathing past it (the peppermint oil) has been known to stop an asthma attack or clear the nasal passages and sinus cavities. Vocal performers often use this trick to dispel mucous from their throats and stimulate their vocal cords.

Peppermint is a good massage oil for stimulating circulation. Peppermint is too strong to be added to a bath.

Emotional/Spiritual/ Aspects

Peppermint is like a rush of fresh energy into the system. It allows us to relax instead of letting anxiety build up in our body or mind. Peppermint oil is specific for people who move between highs and lows, sadness and happiness, until the ever-widening mood swings settle into lethargy, intolerance, and frustration. Just as peppermint strengthens the digestion and aids the absorption of nutrients on a physical level, it enhances our ability to 'digest' new ideas and impressions.

Physica/Mental Aspects

Dr. Dembar of the University of Cincinnati discovered in a research study that inhaling peppermint oil increased the mental accuracy of the students tested by up to 28%. Peppermint oil can also be used for headaches and nerve regeneration.

Peppermint is renowned for action on the digestive system and for use in bowel disorders. It is one of the best essential oils for nausea, vomiting, morning sickness (small amounts only), mouth or gum infections, fainting, and motion sickness.

Peppermint oil is strongly anti-inflammatory and analgesic. Peppermint oil increases circulation. All varieties of peppermint essential oil are useful for muscle pain, inflamed joints, and arthritis. The anti-inflammatory properties make peppermint essential oil supportive of prostate function.

General Information

Peppermint, like lavender, is soothing in small amounts and strongly stimulating in larger amounts.

Cautions

Peppermint oil is stimulating to the uterus. Extreme caution, mostly as to the amount used, should be taken with peppermint oils if pregnant.

Petitgrain

(Citrus aurantium)

Ingredient In

LeEndo Relief

Therapeutic Properties

anti-inflammatory, antispasmodic, antidepressant, stimulant, tonic, calmative, anti-infectious, antiseptic, nervine, re-establishes nerve equilibrium

Affinity For

hormones
cardiovascular system
skin
throat chakra
liver meridian

Resonance	Plant Family	Part of Plant Used
physical, emotional	Rutaceae	leaves

Aromatic Considerations

Petitgrain has a fresh and revitalizing orange aroma that almost sparkles through the air. Because petitgrain is made from the bark and twigs of the tree, the aroma of petitgrain is stronger and stays in the air longer than other citrus oils.

Application

Petitgrain is an excellent choice for diffusing. It can be diluted and applied anywhere on the body.

Emotional/Spiritual Aspects

Emotionally, petitgrain presents us with new ideas and new beginnings. Petitgrain brings us to a state of mind where calm, natural growth, without feelings of being pressured, can occur. It is powerfully stabilizing to high-strung temperaments and volatile dispositions. Petitgrain seems to help lower the defenses and harsh qualities that are often seen in people who are insecure about their worth or place. Petitgrain helps overcome pessimism and insomnia due to anger from feelings of betrayal. It re-establishes equilibrium in the nerves. Petitgrain stimulates the mind, supports memory, and gladdens the heart.

Physical Aspects

Petitgrain promotes hormone balance in both men and women, especially when combined with clary sage. It is excellent for relieving rapid or erratic heart palpitations. Petitgrain is often used in substance abuse programs to aid in detoxification. Petitgrain is useful in the convalescent stage of illness. It is an excellent oil for stabilizing oil production of the skin and coping with excessive perspiration.

General Information

Petitgrain essential oil is made from the bark and twigs of *citrus aurantium*. This is the same plant that neroli and orange, bitter are made from.

Cautions

Petitgrain is listed by most authorities as photo-toxic, so care should be taken not to expose skin to sunlight after topical application.

Pine Needle

(Pinus pinaster)

Ingredient In

LeAspire, LeEnergy, LeGrateful Heart, LeSanctuary

Therapeutic Properties

anti-infectious, anti-fungal, tonic, pectoral, expectorant, diuretic, balsamic, stimulant, depurative, restorative

Affinity For

respiratory system
metabolism
circulation
skin care
brow chakra
crown chakra
governing vessel meridian
stomach meridian
lung meridian

Resonance	Plant Family	Part of Plant Used
physical, emotional	Coniferae	needles, leaves

Aromatic Considerations

The aroma of pine needle essential oil can bring us true wisdom through acceptance of what was and acknowledgement of what is and what can be.

Application

Pine needle is especially nice in a bath or sauna. Dilute to apply to the feet or the body.

Emotional/Spiritual Aspects

Pine needle essential oil is useful for moving on from regrets and self-judgement. It can bring relief from feeling the necessity to 'carry the whole world' on our own shoulders. Pine needle helps us to establish a healthy respect for our own needs, including the need to rest and rejuvenate from time to time. Pine needle is also for those who confuse the acquisition of more and more 'facts' as wisdom.

Physical Aspects

When pine needle essential oil is massaged into the skin, it promotes healthy circulation and brings comfort to sore joints and muscles. Pine is an excellent massage oil for arthritis.

Pine oil increases metabolism and nutrient absorption. Pine has a beneficial action on both the kidneys and the intestines, aiding them in their function of removing cellular waste and toxins from the body.

This essential oil is a pleasant way to disinfect the air or any surface.

General Information

Pine needles were used by the ancient Romans and Greeks and by the American Indians to treat respiratory problems, relieve muscle aches, and prevent scurvy.

Cautions

Pine needle essential oil may irritate the skin if used undiluted or for prolonged periods of time.

Ravensara

(Agathophyllum aromatica i.e. Ravensara aromatica)

Ingredient In

LeBreezey, LeLife Force, LeMariah, LeVallee

Therapeutic Properties

antiseptic, antiviral, antibiotic, anti-fungal, expectorant, febrifuge

Affinity For

immune system
endocrine system
particularly adrenal glands
respiratory system
muscles
brow chakra

Resonance

physical, emotional

Plant Family

Lauraceae

Part of Plant Used

wood, leaves

Aromatic Considerations

The aroma of ravensara can help us unlock and unblock negative emotions, and then banish their effects from our lives. It is similar to eucalyptus, but milder and more pleasant.

Application

Ravensara can be diffused as a single oil, but it is most therapeutic and delightful as part of a blend. Ravensara can be diluted and applied to the feet or the body.

Emotional/Spiritual Aspects

Emotionally, ravensara is like a spiritual disinfectant. It goes through our minds and memories and blasts away negative emotions and responses. Ravensara does this gently, letting us know every step of the way that we are doing all right and will soon be doing even better.

Physical Aspects

Ravensara is strongly antiviral. It really gets in and kills 'critters.' It then supports the kidneys and lymphatic system in getting rid of the 'dead bodies' of the invaders. Ravensara has an affinity for the lungs and is useful in chronic respiratory conditions.

Ravensara is often used to bring relief from shingles. Ravensara kills the attacking viruses and brings relief from the pain.

Ravensara is listed throughout the literature for use with chicken pox, measles, and all viral infections. Ravensara has brought relief from mononucleosis and chronic fatigue syndrome. Ravensara acts as an expectorant and helps to promote a healthy fever. A blend containing ravensara would be a good thing to dilute and rub on yourself if you are showing any signs of coming down with the flu.

Cautions

This oil is considered completely safe and non-toxic, but care should always be taken during pregnancy.

Rose, absolute

(*Rosa damascena*)

Ingredient In

[Le]Angel, [Le]Baby Me, [Le]Believe, [Le]Benediction, [Le]Discernment, [Le]Expressions, [Le]Everlasting, [Le]Faith, [Le]Heart Song, [Le]Tomorrow, [Le]Trust, [Le]Turmoil, [Le]Unity

Therapeutic Properties

anti-infectious, antiseptic, astringent, tonic, stimulant, aphrodisiac, emollient, nervine, cytophylactic

Affinity For

cardiovascular system	genito-urinary system	central vessel meridian
nervous system	yin energy	spleen meridian
digestive system	heart chakra	

Resonance	Plant Family	Part of Plant Used
physical, emotional	Rosaceae	flowers

Rose is the highest frequency essential oil. As the frequency of the body raises to meet this amazing oil, wonderful things happen in the body.

Aromatic Considerations

Rose is an almost annoyingly intoxicating fragrance, but when you need it, the aroma is absolutely divine.

Application

There is no wrong way to use rose. Simply enjoy it as often as you can.

Emotional/Spiritual Aspects

Rose is an outstanding remedy for those times when we feel trapped by our responsibilities or by the past. Sometimes we need help to let go and move forward into the future easily and with delight. The best way that I know to describe rose oil is to tell you a story that was told to me.

A very wise man was walking along the edge of the river one day. He heard faint calls for help coming from just over the edge of the rushing river. As he looked over the edge he saw a person, so very afraid, clinging to an old dead branch with all of his might.

"Help me," the poor person calls out to him. "Please, give me your hand. I can't hold on another moment." The wise man looks around him and spots a beautiful rose growing on the side of the riverbed. Picking it, he holds it out to the distraught person, saying, "Take hold of this rose. It is the most magic of flowers. You will be saved and all will be well with you."

The person immediately reaches for the magic flower, losing his grip on the old dead branch—and the rushing river instantly carries him away.

The wise man smiles and walks down the riverbank for a short way. There he finds the person, wet and shaken, but washed ashore quite safely. The wise man hands the person the flower and says gently, with compassion and understanding in his voice, "You only needed to trust and let go."

We ***choose*** our attitudes and beliefs based on our ***perceptions*** of the experiences in our past. Rose oil can help us understand that nothing from the past needs to hamper our futures.

Physical Aspects

Rose is one of the very best oils for use in any emotional crisis. It is useful in extreme debility and fatigue. Rose has a four-fold action on nerves, digestion, vascular, and urinary systems. This action is one of cleansing, rather than stimulation. Rose oil, surprisingly, is one of the most antiseptic essential oils. This antiseptic action, combined with its action on capillaries and its soothing and emollient qualities, make it a wonderful oil for nearly all types of skin.

General Information

All absolutes, because of their concentration and intensity, should be evaluated in extremely small quantities. Large amounts of these oils can overcome the receptor sites in the nose. The complexity of the fragrance, especially the rare and exotic notes, become entirely lost to our sense of smell.

Rose Geranium

(Pelargonium roseum)

Ingredient In

^{Le}Angel, ^{Le}Baby Me, ^{Le}Balance, ^{Le}Benediction, ^{Le}Everlasting, ^{Le}Heart Song, ^{Le}Unity

Therapeutic Properties

antidepressant, antiseptic, astringent, cicatrisant, cytophylactic, diuretic, deodorant, haemostatic, styptic, tonic, vermifuge, and vulnerary.

Affinity For

nervous system
adrenal cortex
hormones
lymphatic system
skin
chakras:
solar plexus, brow, heart
yin energy

Resonance

physical, emotional

Plant Family

Geraniaceae

Part of Plant Used

leaves

Aromatic Considerations

Rose geranium has quite a lovely aroma. It is sweeter and lighter than geranium. It has an herbal undertone and a rosy overtone that geranium lacks. When diffused, rose geranium can help us feel joy in our journey.

Application

Rose geranium can be worn as perfume, used in a bath, or diluted and massaged anywhere on the body.

Emotional/Spiritual Aspects

One aspect of rose geranium is for emotional work with those who feel burdened by, or resentful of, the necessity to work *so very hard*. This situation may be perception or reality. Rose geranium can benefit those who have found themselves in a real position of neverending work, with no rest, no pause, and maybe even with very little reward.

Rose geranium is a call to attention. It requires us to analyze our lives, streamline them, and then enables us to do with joy those things that are required of us. Rose geranium soothes the nervous system. It relieves depression and anxiety, making the world look like a much friendlier and supportive place.

Physical Aspects

Rose geranium stimulates the lymphatic system, relieving congestion and pain throughout the body. As the body detoxifies, symptoms of PMS such as water retention, bloating, and headache disappear. Rose geranium is useful for treating jaundice and gallstones. On the skin, rose geranium balances the secretion of sebum. It is antiseptic and healing to the skin for acne, burns, and wounds.

General Information

The uses of rose geranium are very similar to those of geranium.

Cautions

Rose geranium has mild hormonal properties; care should be used during pregnancy.

Rosemary

(Rosmarinus officinalis)

Ingredient In

LeAspire, LeCandila, LeCrystal Clear, LeDandy, LeDelicate, LeDeliverance, LeEnergy, LeLife Force, LeMela Plus, LeRevitalize, LeTurmoil, LeSimplicity, LeSpice-C, LeWake-Up, LeWith-In

Therapeutic Properties

antibacterial, anti-catarrhal, anti-infectious, antispasmodic, analgesic, balances the endocrine system, mucolytic, tonic, astringent, aphrodisiac, cicatrisive, cytophylactic, pectoral, antidepressant, sedative, calmative, emollient, antiseptic

Affinity For

brain
central nervous system
digestive system
liver
cardiovascular system
urinary tract
respiratory system
skin
yang energy
solar plexus chakra
liver meridian
small intestine meridian
heart meridian

Resonance	Plant Family	Part of Plant Used
physical, emotional	Labiatae	flowering plant

Aromatic Considerations

Rosemary, diffused, stimulates memory function and helps to organize the thought process.

Application

Rosemary can be diluted and applied anywhere on the body. It can be added to shampoo or conditioner to cover gray in darker hair colors.

Emotional/Spiritual Aspects

In emotional work using essential oils, often the influence of the oil is to create a haven of safety from which the person can relearn how to relate to their world. This is not the case with rosemary. Rosemary fosters an inquisitive spirit. Rosemary sends us out in all directions, looking for light and understanding. Understanding truth is energy in its essential form. Understanding ourselves and what is expected of us by Heaven is the most important truth. This understanding is light, and lidght is knowledge.

Rosemary balances heart function and energizes the solar plexus. Rosemary is specific for people who are usually vibrant, organized, industrious, and sensitive. They have become apathetic due to dwelling on perceived hurts or injustices. People needing rosemary rarely become imbalanced from stress or too much work; they thrive on work. Rosemary essential oil can send them on a quest to understand what happened and why. With understanding, or even just beginning to ask the questions that will lead to understanding, comes peace.

Physical Aspects

A glance at the list of physical and energy systems in the ***Affinity For*** section above gives you some idea of the wide range of action of this amazingly versatile essential oil. Every body system listed above impacts other body systems until rosemary's influence resonates throughout the entire system. We will detail just a few of rosemary's many therapeutic qualities here.

Rosemary's action on the brain and nervous system makes it useful for loss of memory, learning difficulties, indecisiveness, and mental fatigue. The antiseptic action of rosemary oil is particularly strong for intestinal infections, colitis, flatulence, liver disorders, and respiratory complaints such as sinus congestion and bronchitis.

Being antispasmodic and analgesic, rosemary is useful for arthritis, muscle pain and weakness, and headaches. In the cardiovascular area, rosemary assists with arteriosclerosis, palpitations, poor circulation, migraine headaches, and low blood pressure.

Rosemary has an affinity for skin care, hair care, and the dissolving of cellulite. Rosemary is used to minimize gray in the hair of brunettes. The astringent properties of rosemary make it effective for dandruff, hair loss, and tightening saggy areas of skin.

Rosemary is an excellent oil for exhaustion and general debility, overindulgence in food or drink, and hangovers. Rosemary is mentioned in the literature as helpful for viral hepatitis.

Cautions

Rosemary should be used cautiously or avoided if pregnant or epileptic.

Rosewood

(Aniba rosaeodora)

Ingredient In

LeAcknowledge, LeBaby Me, , LeBelieve, LeBenediction, LeDiscernment, LeEverlasting, LeExhilaration, LeFaith, LeFocus, LeGrateful Heart, LeHeart Song, LeInner Peace, LeMeditation, LeMillenia, LePatches, LeSego Lily, LeSolitude, LeTrust, LeTurmoil

Therapeutic Properties

antibacterial, anti-fungal, anti-infectious, astringent, antispasmodic, emollient, tonic, cephalic, deodorant, insecticide, mild immune stimulant

Affinity For

muscles
skin
central nervous system
central vessel meridian
bladder meridian
throat chakra

Resonance	**Plant Family**	**Part of Plant Used**
emotional, physical	Lauraceae	wood

Aromatic Considerations

The gentle aroma of rosewood creates a peaceful atmosphere when diffused.

Application

Rosewood can be worn as a perfume, diffused, or diluted and applied to the feet or anywhere on the body.

Emotional/Spiritual Aspects

Rosewood's action on the central nervous system can help us balance our emotions, maintaining evenness of mood instead of wide fluctuations from moment to moment. Rosewood is an excellent choice for grief of all kinds. It helps us notice and respond to the loving strength of those around us until we are able to respond again with love of our own. Rosewood helps us move past the grief, and sometimes the anger, of our losses and find the good memories and the love that we once felt.

Because rosewood's action lies in the realm of the throat chakra, it can have an effect on our ability to speak up and speak about things close to our hearts. Sometimes communication is about the things that we ***don't*** say. Rosewood can help us find a balance between speaking up and holding our tongue.

Physical Aspects

The actions of rosewood are predominantly on the skin and the nerves, but like all essential oils, rosewood is antiseptic. Rosewood is useful for skin rashes, irritations, dermatitis, scars, and skin that has become dry and inflamed. It brings balance to the secretions of the sebaceous glands, improves elasticity, and enhances the skin's ability to act as a barrier to infectious invasion. Rosewood, or essential oil blends containing it, are often used as massage oils for the prevention of stretch marks.

Rosewood is a very good oil for headaches that cause nausea, especially when the headaches are linked to nervousness and tension in the muscles of the neck and back.

General Information

Rosewood will probably become increasingly more difficult to find and more expensive as over-harvesting has caused changes in the laws of some countries. Howood is being tried throughout the world as a substitute for rosewood.

Cautions

I do not recommend the internal consumption of essential oils, but a special warning needs to be issued about rosewood. Even among authorities that do recommend internal consumption, rosewood is contra-indicated. In fact, it is considered extremely dangerous. **DO NOT** take rosewood essential oil internally.

There are no other known cautions for rosewood essential oil.

Sage

(Salvia officinalis)

Ingredient In

LeBalance, LeConnection, LeDandy, LeDelicate, LeDiscernment, LeEndo Relief, LeEverlasting, LeFocus, LeUnity, LeWeightless

Therapeutic Properties

antiseptic, antibacterial, antiviral, anti-cancerous, immune stimulant, antiseptic, antispasmodic, analgesic, diuretic, has estrogen-like properties

Affinity For

nervous system	mind	pelvic chakras and all organs within those areas	
lymphatic system	skin, tissues	throat chakra	stomach meridian

Resonance	**Plant Family**	**Part of Plant Used**
physical, spiritual	Labiatae	leaves, flowers

Aromatic Considerations

The aroma of sage clears and sharpens the mind.

Application

Sage essential oil should be diluted well before applying to the body or the feet.

Emotional/Spiritual Aspects

Sage is a good oil for alleviating the effects of prolonged stress on the body and the mind. Sage cleanses the energy grid and strengthens its ability to protect us from negative influences. Sage has a positive influence on intuition, bringing clarity and vision to our souls if we will take the time to ponder and listen.

Physical Aspects

The impact on physical health of a strong nervous system and an active lymph system cannot be over emphasized. Sage's ability to strengthen the pelvic chakra and the organs within it, gives vigor and strength to the vital centers of the body. With nerves, lymph, and pelvic organs being strengthened, it is easy to see why sage has long been considered the 'master healer.'

Sage is believed to contain constituents that stimulate the secretion of progesterone-testosterone and keep their activities balanced. Sage is useful for most glandular disorders, any complaint related to lymph congestion, and any disorders related to nerve deterioration or prolonged nervous stress. Sage also clears away cellular debri and strengthens cell wall integrity, making sage useful for arthritis, dandruff, hair loss, skin conditions, gingivitis, sprains, and firming tissues.

General Information

The Lakota Indians considered sage as the 'master healer', as did the Romans. It has been a popular ingredient in nerve tonics throughout the ages.

Cautions

Large doses or over-use of sage should be avoided by any one who suffers from any type of seizure disorder. Sage should be avoided during the early stages of pregnancy.

Sandalwood

(Santalum album)

Ingredient In

LeAcknowledge, LeBenediction, LeDreams, LeEverlasting, LeExhilaration, LeExpressions, LeFocus, LeInner Peace, LeIQ, LeLetting Go, LeMagi, LeMeditation, LeMoonlight, LeTomorrow, LeTrust, LeTurmoil, LeUnity

Therapeutic Properties

supports cardiovascular system, antiseptic, antidepressant, diuretic, tonic, aphrodisiac, astringent, emollient, calming, anti-infectious, decongestant

Affinity For

pineal
pituitary
skin
lymph

central vessel meridian
tripple warmer meridian
bladder meridian
gallbladder meridian

vibration between crown and base chakras
affecting all chakras in between

Resonance

physical, emotional, energetic, spiritual

Plant Family

Santalaceae

Part of Plant Used

wood

Aromatic Considerations

Among sandalwood's many actions is its ability to give us a sense of inner peace, even when we know that we are heading into difficult challenges.

Application

Sandalwood is the favorite essential oil of many people, including me. It should be worn on the body anywhere, at any time, and diffused everywhere.

Emotional/Spiritual Aspects

Sandalwood has a very high sesquiterpene percentage. As it crosses the blood/brain barrier it increases oxygen around the pineal and pituitary glands and stimulates the amygdala. This has a profound effect on attitude and emotion. Sandalwood can help us focus outward, loving and accepting others with a full heart. Sandalwood increases our desire to ponder and then act on the perceptions and impressions we have received. (Problem solving is an action of the amygdala.)

The energy of sandalwood vibrates between the crown chakra and the base chakra. This makes it both grounding and energizing to the physical body and to the mind. Sandalwood is often used in yoga disciplines and in meditation because it enhances our ability to look inside ourselves and be honest about what we see there. The aroma of sandalwood strengthens the astral body, which is the Chinese way of saying that it improves communication between the physical body and the energetic languages of the mind and spirit.

Sandalwood has the ability to go into the DNA of the cells and unlock emotional trauma. It can help us curb manipulative or controlling tendencies in our personalities. Sandalwood essential oil alleviates depression, anxiety, and nervous exhaustion.

Physical Aspects

Some of the many uses of sandalwood include bladder and throat infections, bronchitis, tuberculosis, cystitis, and fluid retention. Sandalwood is an excellent skin and tissue regenerating oil. Sandalwood should probably be part of any program for a chronic type illness.

General Information

Sandalwood is another resource which is being seriously depleted worldwide. It takes a minimum of 30 years to mature a sandalwood tree to its optimum value therapeutically and it is the heartwood of the tree that makes the very best essential oil. These conditions contribute to the fact that sandalwood is often adulterated with something else to extend the quantity. The price of the essential oil is beginning to reflect the difficulties in obtaining this most precious essential oil.

Cautions

Unadulterated sandalwood is absolutely non-toxic.

Spearmint

(Mentha spicata)

Ingredient In

LeMariah, LeSunburst, LeRefresh-Mint, LeWake-Up

Therapeutic Properties

antiseptic, antispasmodic, disinfectant, carminative, cephalic, emenagogue, insecticide, restorative, stimulant

Affinity For

respiratory system
digestive system
metabolism
teeth and gums

Resonance

physical, emotional, mental

Plant Family

Labiatae

Part of Plant Used

leaves

Aromatic Considerations

A blend of spearmint and peppermint oils is an excellent blend for driving. It allows you to feel both wide awake, alert, and calm.

Application

Spearmint can be diluted in water and used as a mouth wash. Spearmint essential oil, diluted with carrier oil, can be applied anywhere on the body.

Emotional/Spiritual Aspects

Spearmint essential oil is calming, relaxing, and uplifting. It is milder than peppermint and less likely to be over-stimulating if too much is used. Spearmint oil is a pleasant alternative to citrus oils for treating mental fatigue, depression, and eating disorders.

Physical Aspects

Spearmint has a relaxing and cooling effect on muscles and the nerves which feed them. This makes spearmint useful for spasmodic cough, abdominal cramps and spasms, muscle cramps, and nervous convulsions. Spearmint's disinfectant properties are particularly effective for internal infections. Spearmint helps to restore normal function to the organs and systems of the body by repairing damage that has been done to cells, tissues, and nerves. Spearmint is an excellent choice for treating wounds and injuries. Its mildly stimulating properties make it a great tonic oil following an illness. The stimulant properties of spearmint work on the nerves, brain, blood circulation, metabolism, and immune system. Spearmint is said to help the body burn fat. Spearmint, swished regularly in the mouth, helps repair the enamel on the teeth.

General Information

Many times spearmint is treated as nothing more than a milder form of peppermint, but these two essential oils have very different chemical components and very different therapeutic actions.

Cautions

Spearmint should be used cautiously with pregnant women and small children.

Spikenard

(Nardostachys jatamansi)

Ingredient In

LeEverlasting, LeJourney, LeMariah, LeMoonlight, LeNo-More, LeTenda Care, LeTurmoil, LeUnity, LeVallee, LeWoman Wise

Therapeutic Properties

antiseptic, antibiotic, anti-fungal, anti-inflammatory, calmative, sedative, deodorant, skin tonic, laxative

Affinity For

intestinal tract
reproductive system
nervous system
skin
crown chakra

Resonance
physical, emotional

Plant Family
Valerianaceae

Part of Plant Used
roots

Aromatic Considerations

Spikenard has a wet earth, animal-like or, perhaps, mossy aroma that I find pleasant only when I am really in need of the soothing, sedating qualities of this essential oil. Whether the aroma is pleasant in your opinion or not, the aroma of spikenard will create a soothing, back-to-nature atmosphere around you.

Application

Spikenard should be diluted and applied wherever it is needed.

Emotional/Spiritual Aspects

Spikenard can help us leave destructive emotional elements of the past behind. Spikenard is the emotional equivalent of packing up and leaving the old ways of thinking and reacting behind. Spikenard oil is not about 'repair' of attitudes or relationships; it is about doing a 'clean sweep' emotionally and beginning again.

Spikenard is a good oil for use at the time of approaching death. It can give one the courage needed to seek release from this life and move forward to the new. Spikenard is an oil of forgiveness. It can help us come to terms with the experiences of our life and to feel at peace with those who shared our journey with us. ***It was a flask of spikenard oil that Mary Magdaline used on the Savior's feet. There may have been several reasons for her choice of this precious and expensive ointment. Perhaps it was in preparation of his coming death, to aid him in forgiving all the injustices that had and would be done to him, or it could have been to help the mortal side of his nature find the courage to complete the great task assigned to him. Maybe it was just out of love and a desire to serve that she chose to anoint her Lord with oil of spikenard.***

Physical Aspects

Spikenard is a wonderful oil for ailments resulting from bacterial infections on the skin or in the body. Spikenard will protect wounds from bacterial infections while soothing and calming the victim. The essential oil of spikenard makes an excellent deodorant. Problems in the intestinal tract are at the root of many of our physical ailments. Spikenard has a gentle laxative action. Spikenard helps maintain proper hormone levels throughout the reproductive system. ***Spikenard has a much higher percentage of sesquiterpenes than frankincense.***

General Information

Spikenard is also known as 'false valerian.' There are a small number of people who react negatively and quite strongly to valerian, even in less concentrated herbal forms. Spikenard accomplishes many of the same things as valerian. Spikenard is a little less potent but it has always accomplished whatever I have needed it to. Spikenard presents less likelihood of a negative reaction.

Cautions

This is a non-irritant and non-toxic oil. The are no known precautions that should be taken with spikenard.

Spruce, Canadian

(Tsuga canadensis)

Ingredient In

LeAspire, LeAssurance, LeBenediction, LeConnection, LeDeeper, LeDiscernment, LeDreams, LeEverlasting, LeHoliday Spirit, LeInner Peace, LeMagi, LeMeditation, LeMillenia, LePatches, LeSanctuary, LeStefanie, LeTrust, LeUnity, LeVision, LeWhispering Hope, LeWisdom

Therapeutic Properties

anti-infectious, anti-inflammatory, antispasmodic, cortisone-like

Affinity For

bones, joints, muscles
endocrine system
especially the thyroid and thymus
solar plexus chakra
brow chakra
governing vessel meridian
heart meridian
liver meridian

Resonance
physical, emotional

Plant Family
Coniferae

Part of Plant Used
needles, leaves

Aromatic Considerations

The aroma of Canadian spruce is calming to the nervous system. It encourages communication, both the speaking and listening aspects.

Application

Spruce can be applied, diluted, to the feet or any other area of the body. Spruce is very pleasant in the bath or sauna. It is frequently used as an ingredient in room sprays, soaps, and detergents.

Emotional/Spiritual Aspects

Spruce (and other conifers) create the symbolic effect of an umbrella which protects the earth and brings energy in from the universe. At night the animals of the forest lie down under a conifer tree for the protection and rejuvenation that the tree will provide for them. Spruce grounds the solar plexus and stimulates the thymus, creating the emotional balance necessary to be gracious at both giving and receiving. Spruce can help us push through emotional blocks to further healing.

Physical Aspects

The analgesic and anti-inflammatory properties of spruce make it beneficial for bone pain, aching joints, arthritis, and sciatica. Spruce should be massaged wherever sore muscles need relaxing and re-energizing. Spruce is an excellent oil for the respiratory and endocrine systems. Spruce is a general gland and organ tonic, but it has an intrinsic affinity for balancing the thyroid function and stimulating the thymus gland.

General Information

The aroma of Canadian spruce is that of a forest of conifer trees, but with a strong balsamy vanilla undertone, which is very comforting to the emotions. *Tsuga canadensis* is Canadian spruce, not the species called black spruce, which is *Picea marianna*. *Tsuga canadensis* seems to be consistently sweeter, more mellow, and with more of the balsam and vanilla notes that I love than *Picea marianna.* Canadian spruce adds a rich depth to blends that is not usually accomplished with any other variety of spruce.

St. John's Wort

(Hypericum perforatum)

Ingredient In

LeWoman Wise

Therapeutic Properties

analgesic, anti-inflammatory, nervine

Affinity For

nerves
joints
muscles
bones

Resonance
physical, emotional, mental

Plant Family
Clusiaceae

Part of Plant Used
leaves, flowers

Aromatic Considerations

Diffused, St. John's Wort may relieve fatigue, anxiety, headache, low spirits, and sadness. The aroma of St. John's Wort is also stimulating to the mind and the memory.

Application

St. John's Wort should be diluted well and used in moderation. (See Caution section below)

Emotional/Spiritual Aspects

St. John's Wort is recommended for depression, especially following injuries, fright, or shock. The plants in this family are very hardy. They often live up to 50 years. I believe this resilience in the face of trials is a part of he nature of this essential oil.

Physical Aspects

St. John's Wort essential oil, well-diluted is used for sunburns, burns, bruises, varicose veins, and scars. The anti-inflammatory and nervine properties of this oil are particularly effective in nerve rich areas of the body such as the brain, back of the neck, fingers, toes, and coccyx (tailbone). St. John's Wort, diluted and applied along the spine, may be helpful for nerve damage and muscles spasms resulting from whiplash injuries and may be effective, especially as part of a blend, for muscle spasms and twitches in arms of legs when drifting off to sleep.

Cautions

Until further studies have been conducted on St. John's Wort essential oil, it is probably best to use it well-diluted, in moderation, or as a small percentage of a blend. St. John's Wort should be avoided if pregnant. Although St. John's Wort has been used for at least a couple of centuries as an herbal medicine and as a homeopathic remedy, very little information is available about the essential oil.

Sugandha Kokila

(Cinnamomum glaucescens)

Therapeutic Properties

analgesic, antimicrobial, antiseptic, anti-inflammatory, antispasmodic, decongestant, expectorant, mucolytic, astringent, relaxant, stomachic

Affinity For

cardiopulmonary system	respiratory system	urinary tract
digestive system	nervous system	

Resonance	**Plant Family**	**Part of Plant Used**
physical, emotional	Lauraceae	dried berries

Aromatic Considerations

Sugandha kokila has a mild cinnamon aroma. It is woody, resinous, and herbaceous all at once. The essential oils made from the berries of *cinnamomum* species are a little bit milder than oil made from the bark. Care should still be taken with inhalation and diffusion. Cinnamon in any form can be irritating to tender mucous membranes.

Application

Sugandha kokila should be diluted well before applying to areas of the body where increased circulation or pain relief are needed. Sugandha kokila can also be applied to the feet.

Emotional/Spiritual Aspects

Sugandha kokila essential oil is uplifting to the emotions and clearing to the mind. It brings a sense of being supported and cared for. Sugandha kokila is useful for anxiety and stress related swings in mood and energy.

Physical Aspecs

Sugandha kokila increases circulation, reduces pain and inflammation in the muscles and joints. It is excellent, either alone or as part of a blend for arthritis.

Cautions

Always dilute Sugandha kokila well and inhale with care.

Tagette

(Tagetes minuta)

Ingredient In

LeCandila, LeVallee

Therapeutic Properties

anti-microbial, fungicidal, antibiotic, antiseptic, insecticide, sedative, antispasmodic, diaphoretic, mucolytic

Affinity For

respiratory system	tissues and skin

Resonance	**Plant Family**	**Part of Plant Used**
physical	Compositae	flowers

Aromatic Considerations

The aroma of tagette essential oil is quite complex. The top note is sharp and bitter and has an almost unpleasant effect in the nose. This pungency is followed by a pleasant, herbaceous aroma (if you are still sniffing!). The end note is almost fruity with a citrus-like aroma. It is surprisingly pleasant when diffused. The fruit and citrus aromas seem to linger in the air.

Application

Tagette should always be diluted well to avoid skin irritation. It may be applied to the feet or anywhere that skin care and repair is needed.

Emotional/Spiritual Aspects

I have never known an essential oil not to operate on just the physical plane, with no emotional effects. However, there does not seem to be any literature on the emotional aspects of this oil.

Physical Aspects

Tagette is useful for infectious respiratory conditions where it encourages sufficient fever to burn away the infectious agent. Tagette aids in breaking up congestion, liquefying mucous and getting it flowing, and encouraging the drainage of lymph nodes. Tagette may be helpful to rid the body of toxins. Tagette is used to dissolve bunions, calluses, and corns. One of the most common uses of this essential oil is in the rebuilding of tissues and skin after burns or other injuries.

General Information

The aroma and therapeutic properties of tagette improves with age. At best, tagette should be aged for at least 6 months after distillation before being used in an essential oil blend.

Cautions

This is a very powerful and potent essential oil; be sure to dilute well. It is not intended for use with children. Do not use tagette if pregnant. Tagette may cause skin irritation and be photo-toxic if overused.

Tamala

(Cinnamomum tamala)

Ingredient In

LeTranquility

Therapeutic Properties

anti-fungal, antibacterial, anti-inflammatory

Affinity For

digestive system	muscles	sacral chakra
circulation	joints	nerves
immune system	skin	

Resonance	**Plant Family**	**Part of Plant Used**
physical	Lauraceae	leaves

Aromatic Considerations

Some people claim that *cinnamomum tamala* is quite similar to *Cinnamomum verun* but the aromas are quite different. To me, that means that the composition and therapeutic properties are also quite different.

Tamala is certainly milder and a bit less pungent.

Application

Like all essential oils from the *cinnamomum* family, tamala should be diluted well before applying to the skin. Care should also be taken when diffusing this essential oil.

Emotional/Spiritual Aspects

Tamala can be beneficial at lifting the spirits and brightening the day. Tamala offers to take us to a place of emotional protection. Tamala benefits the nervous system and should be used for headache and insomnia that is brought on by stress or frayed nerves.

Physical Aspects

Tamala adds important antibacterial and anti-fungal properties to a blend that is for skin irritations and infections. When blending with tamala, it is good to add an oil or two that nourishes the skin such as sandalwood or patchouli. The synergy of this combination will quell the potential skin irritating effects of the tamala.

Tamala improves circulation and is useful in the treatment of sore muscles and inflamed joints. This essential oil can bring relief from the pain of arthritis and sprains. Tamala benefits the digestive system and helps to improve appetite. One of the best actions of tamala is on the immune system. It is not an immune stimulant, but nourishes and supports the immune system for the long-term.

General Information

Tamala was used to make a fragrant ointment in ancient Greece. The leaves of this plant are mentioned in a Greek text dating back to the 1st century. Tamala is in the same family as the plant from which laurel leaf essential oil is distilled. Tamala is another plant that is mistakenly referred to and confused with both laurel leaf and bay.

Cautions

Tamala oil is best used in low doses or as part of a blend of essential oils. This essential oil is too strong for use in the tub or shower. It should be used cautiously with children and people with sensitive skin.

Tangerine

(Citrus reticulata)

Ingredient In

[Le]Everlasting, [Le]Heart Song, [Le]Holiday Spirit, [Le]Insight, [Le]Sunburst, [Le]Tranquility

Therapeutic Properties

anti-coagulant, anti-inflammatory, laxative, sedative, calmative, nervine, cytophylactic

Affinity For

respiratory system
nervous system
spleen meridian
digestive system

Resonance

physical, emotional

Plant Family

Rutaceae

Part of Plant Used

fruit

Aromatic Considerations

Like all citrus oils, tangerine promotes feelings of happiness and peace. It encourages us to reach out to others with kindness and compassion.

Application

Tangerine should be diluted before applying to the skin.

Emotional/Spiritual Aspects

Tangerine essential oil is a very pleasant sedative. It soothes all types of hyperactivity, whether in the body or the mind. Tangerine can have a substantial effect on anger, depression, and impulsive behaviors.

Physical Aspects

Tangerine has been proven effective against Staphylococcus aureus. This is the species of bacteria which is responsible when wounds become septic. A septic wound quickly spreads to other parts of the body, even if there is no wound there. Tangerine oil contains components which kill the bacteria and stop it from spreading.

Tangerine's antispasmodic actions are effective all over the body. This essential oil can be used for spasms in the respiratory and digestive systems, as well as in muscle groups. Tangerine essential oil is an effective blood purifier and it increases the oxygen carrying capacity of red blood cells. Tangerine is helpful in removing excess water from body tissues and is a mild lymphatic decongestant.

General Information

Tangerine essential oil and mandarin essential oil are distilled, in different countries, from plants that are identified by the same latin name, *citrus reticulata.* That is very strange, since the plants, themselves, are quite different, as are the fruits. The fruit, the juice, *and the essential oil* of tangerine are much more orange in color than those of mandarin. They are harvested at different times of year, and this has a subtle effect on aroma and therapeutic properties.

Cautions

Tangerine essential oil is photo-toxic. Avoid direct sunlight on skin to which this oil has been applied in the last 12 hours.

Tarragon

(Artemisia dracunculus)

Ingredient In

[Le]Everlasting, [Le]Inside Out

Therapeutic Properties

anti-arthritic, digestive, emmenagogue, menstrual regulator; stimulant, vermifuge; anti-inflammatory, antiseptic, antiviral, antispasmodic, diuretic, laxative, neuromuscular sedative

Affinity For

digestive system	nervous system	autonomic nervous system
lymphatic system	urinary tract	

Resonance	**Plant Family**	**Part of Plant Used**
physical, emotional	Compositae	leaves

Aromatic Considerations

Tarragon is especially nice when diffused with marjoram. Tarragon can soothe emotions and bring relief from grief, anger, and shock.

Application

Tarragon should be diluted well before applying to the skin of the body or the feet.

Emotional/Spiritual Aspects

Tarragon helps us to draw in the energy of life that is all around us. It fosters more than just the desire for health or the will to live; it inspires us to seek for, and find, energy enough (and some to spare) for us to accomplish all that we desire.

Physical Aspects

Tarragon aids digestion by stimulating the secretion of digestive acids and bile into the stomach. This increases the appetite and improves the absorption of nutrients into the bloodstream. Tarragon also increases the peristaltic motion of the intestines, eliminating bouts of constipation. Tarragon acts to increase circulation, liquefy and drain lymphatic mucous. Tarragon's antiseptic properties have a special affinity for urinary tract infections. Stubborn infections in weeping wounds often respond to washing with a very dilute solution of tarragon essential oil.

Tarragon stimulates and balances the autonomic nervous system which is responsible for such things as the heartbeat, the function of the kidneys, and the flow of hormones.

Cautions

Depending on conditions at the time of harvest, tarragon essential oil can have quite a high concentration of methyl chavicol, which can be toxic taken internally and irritating externally. Use of tarragon as a single oil should be avoided; at the very least, extreme care and caution should be used. Tarragon should be avoided if you are pregnant.

Tea Tree

(Melaleuca alternifolia)

Ingredient In

LeCandila, LeMela Plus, LePurify, LeSimplicity

Therapeutic Properties

antibacterial, anti-fungal, antiseptic, antiviral, immune stimulant, antibiotic, anti-parasitic, vulnerary, anti-inflammatory, expectorant, decongestant, analgesic

Affinity For

tissue and skin | brow and sacral chakras | metal and fire elements

Resonance

physical, emotional

Plant Family

Myrtaceae

Part of Plant Used

leaves

Aromatic Considerations

Tea tree is a very strong and pungent oil. It is very effective in killing air-borne bacteria.

Application

Tea tree should be diluted before applying to the skin except in the case of insect bites, where it is best applied neat.

Emotional/Spiritual Aspects

The aroma of tea tree can help us replace a victim mentality with a desire to understand why events and circumstances happen. Tea tree can be used to bring both tolerance and growth into our lives. Tea tree starts the process of spiritual and emotional cleansing. It can help us turn toward the positive and find refreshment for our spirit. The aroma of tea tree essential oil has the feel of a good friend who has come to help us 'clean house.' The cleaning up and throwing out will be good for us and will be far less painful than we have imagined it would be.

Physical Aspects

Tea tree essential oil is effective against some of the nastiest microbes on the planet. Tea tree can prevent sepsis in wounds and it (or something else effective) should be used to treat wounds, boils, sores, cuts, insect bites, and stings. The only way to kill a virus is to weaken or rupture its protective shell—called a cyst. Tea tree oil has been shown effective in this capacity, which greatly shortens the duration of viral infections. Tea tree is also a mild tissue regenerator, making it a sensible choice for rashes, nail or skin fungal infections. wounds, cold sores, acne, athlete's foot, ringworm, head lice, vaginal thrush (dilute very well here), and candida.

General Information

Tea tree has been in use as an antiseptic for centuries. It was used by soldiers and sailors in World War II in the treatment of tropical infections.

Thyme

(Thymus zygis var vulgaris)

Ingredient In

LeBountiful, LeDandy, LeDelicate, LeDeliverance, LeEnergy, LeEternity, LeInside-Out, LeLife Force, LeMariah, LeSimplicity, LeTenda Care

Therapeutic Properties

antibacterial, anti-parasitic, anti-fungal, anti-infectious, antiseptic, antiviral, antibiotic, pectoral, analgesic, expectorant, balsamic, stimulant, tonic, rubefacient, diuretic, emmenagogue, vermifuge, anti-venomous, anti-putrescent, immune stimulant

Affinity For

digestive system
immune system
circulatory system
lymphatic system
muscles
bones
base chakra
water element
metal element
heart meridian

Resonance
physical, emotional

Plant Family
Labiatae

Part of Plant Used
leaves, stems, flowers

Aromatic Considerations

Thyme should be diffused, either by itself, or as part of a synergistic blend, to purify the air of your home or office during the cold and flu season. (A blend would probably have a better aroma.)

Application

Dilute well to apply to the feet or body.

Emotional/Spiritual Aspects

Thyme is revitalizing and nourishing to the nerves and emotions. It can help us overcome mental and emotional exhaustion, inability to concentrate, apathy, and uneasy feelings that have no cause. Thyme can aid us in finding a fresh view of a situation or a new way of doing something. It is specific for physical exhaustion, especially when there seems to be a lack of direction and motivation more than overwork. Thyme can give us strength, self-confidence, and will power. It can help us think positively, allowing us to give ourselves credit for every little bit of will power we possess, instead of berating ourselves when we display less of it than we think we should have.

Physical Aspects

As a general tonic for the stomach, thyme's carminative properties alleviate gas and bloating. Gas is an indication of poorly digested food. It can interfere with sleep, raise your blood pressure, become a threat to your cardiovascular system, cause severe stomach aches, cramps, and vomiting, as well as headaches and nausea. Thyme has a beneficial effect on heart valves. It relaxes the veins and arteries, reducing blood pressure and, as a result, reducing stress on the heart. It should be mentioned that, like nearly all natural remedies, thyme balances blood pressure, bringing it back to normal whether it is high or low.

The antiseptic and antiviral properties of thyme are strong enough to handle most situations. Thyme is even recommended, applied along the spine, for such ailments as spinal meningitis. Thyme, along with killing the invading microbes, aids lymphatic drainage and urine output, and strengthens the immune system. Thyme should be tried for lingering coughs.

General Information

Be sure to use Thymus zygis or Thymus vulgaris as they are milder; stronger types should never be used on children or those with high blood pressure. Red thyme is a Thymus zygis but the method of extraction creates concentrations of thymol that are excessive for frequent use or for use with children.

Cautions

Thyme, when not part of a blend, should be used with great caution or avoided altogether.

Turmeric

(Cucuma longa)

Ingredient In

LeMariah

Therapeutic Properties

antiviral, antioxidant, anti-inflammatory, antiseptic, anti-coagulant, digestive tonic, cytophylactic, galactagogue, calmative, carminative, emollient, anti-parasitic

Affinity For

immune system
circulatory system
nervous system
joints, muscles

Resonance	Plant Family	Part of Plant Used
physical, emotional	Zingiberaceae	root

Aromatic Considerations

Turmeric has a warm, earthy, spicy aroma.

Application

Always dilute turmeric especially well. It can cause skin irritation if applied without dilution or applied too frequently.

Emotional/Spiritual Aspects

The emotional energy of turmeric involves the proper exchange of time, talents, attention, money and material goods, or love and gratitude in our lives. These imbalances can exist between us and other people, or they may exist within ourselves and be manifesting as an eating disorder or a victim/servant mentality. However or wherever it may be expressed, the core emotion is usually lack of self-confidence or feelings of unworthiness. It may also stem from a misinterpretation of childhood teachings about service and love.

Physical Aspects

Turmeric is valuable as an antiseptic for cuts and scrapes. It is also an anti-inflammatory, making it helpful with arthritis and fybromyalgia. Turmeric is a strong anti-oxidant, helping protect the body from free radical damage. Some studies suggest that turmeric helps increase the productions of natural cortisone by the adrenal glands.

Turmeric has been shown to help reduce platelets from clumping together and clogging the arteries. Turmeric also increases circulation. These actions lessen the likelihood and minimizes the effects of atherosclerosis.

Turmeric is also beneficial in fighting influenza viruses, lessening the possibilities of an acute infection developing into an auto-immune disease.

General Information

Turmeric comes from the root, or rhizome, of the plant, and is in the same family as ginger.

Cautions

Turmeric may stimulate uterine contractions, so should be avoided or used sparingly during pregnancy.

Valerian Root

(Valeriana officinalis)

Ingredient In

LeStefanie

Therapeutic Properties

analgesic, antispasmodic, nervine, sedative

Affinity For

nerves

Resonance	Plant Family	Part of Plant Used
physical, emotional	Valerianaceae	root

Aromatic Considerations

Valerian root has an earthy aroma, which is *much* more pleasant than the aroma of the fresh root would lead you to expect. I think the fresh root smells like a dead mouse in a very dirty sock!! The essential oil has none of that aroma!

Application

Valerian root is an excellent essential oil to add to the bath. It is even quite pleasant diffused.

Emotional/Spiritual Aspects

Valerian root is an oil of understanding, forgiveness, and reconciliation. It is of particular value to those who are too hard on themselves. Valerian root can help us move away from unhealthy forms of guilt, understand that we have learned the lessons of the past, accept who we were and who we are, and forgive ourselves for the foolishness (or even stupidity) that is in our past.

Physical Aspects

Valerian root essential oil contains some volatile components not found in any other essential oil currently produced for sale. These components are useful for an incredibly long list of conditions related to nerves and nervous tension. This is a versatile essential oil that can soothe your spirit, calm your nerves, and help you cope with the stresses of our modern world. It is useful for headache, irritability, pre-menstrual symptoms, any type of cramping or spasms, insomnia, heart palpitations, panic attacks, and neuralgia.

General Information

While valerian acts as a sedative and nervine on most people, there are a small percentage of people who react just the opposite. Valerian 'wires' them, making them irritable and aggressive. This effect wears off quickly, but should be accepted as a clear indication that this oil is not for you—at least, not at this time.

Cautions

Valerian, as a single, should be avoided during pregnancy and by children. There is some documentation indicating that overuse may cause lethargy but, in low doses or in blends, valerian appears to be non-toxic and non-irritating to most people (see general information above).

Vanilla

(Vanilla planifolia)

Ingredient In

LeSanctuary, LeSego Lily, LeBelieve

Therapeutic Properties

antioxidant, aphrodisiac, anti-carcinogenic, febrifuge, antidepressant, sedative, tranquilizing

Affinity For

hormone balance
immune system
nerves
governing vessel meridian
liver meridian

Resonance

physical, emotional

Plant Family

Orchidaceae

Part of Plant Used

fruit

Aromatic Considerations

The aroma of vanilla is one of the most calming and uplifting of scents. Vanilla has such a wonderful aroma that even if it had no therapeutic properties at all, I would use it every day for the scent alone.

Application

Vanilla is usually diffused or used in candles and soaps.

Emotional/Spiritual Aspects

The aroma of vanilla helps us feel confidenct that the future will be full of promise and hope. Vanilla can give us hope, perspective, and confidence in our ability to listen to inspiration and seek guidance from the Spirit. Vanilla is a very welcoming and warming oil. It can set a very romantic tone.

Physical Aspects

The removal of free radicals from the body will gradually result in a stronger immune system, better memory, improved vision and hearing, more stable emotions, improved mental acuity, and overall repair of body systems, organs, and tissues. Vanilla, used regularly, can accomplish all this and with such a pleasant aroma! Vanilla can reduce the heat and the inflammation of a fever, while calming the patient into a peaceful sleep. Vanilla is one of the best oils for hyperactivity in any body system or organ. It is a great oil for insomnia or high blood pressure. Vanilla activates certain precursors that are necessary for hormone balance.

General Information

Vanilla essential oil is heavy and dark colored. Blends to which it has been added need to be shaken well before use. Even if you faithfully shake the blend, there will always be a dark pool in the bottom of the bottle, but the energy, aroma, and therapeutic properties of the vanilla have infused into the entire blend.

Vetiver

(Vetivera zizanioides)

Ingredient In

LeVallee

Therapeutic Properties

antiseptic, calming, immune stimulant, sedative, rubefacient

Affinity For

hormones
skin, joints, muscles
red blood cells
balances yin and yang energies —male and female hormones

Resonance

physical, emotional

Plant Family

Graminae

Part of Plant Used

roots

Aromatic Considerations

The aroma of vetiver is reminiscent of patchouli and lemongrass, but is not a pleasant aroma by itself, in my opinion. Vetiver is physically, mentally, and psychologically grounding.

Application

Vetiver can be added to a bath. You can dilute vetiver and apply to the body.

Emotional/Spiritual Aspects

Vetiver is a useful oil for emotional and energy work. It helps us connect the past to the present, learning from the things we have experienced and using the present to heal the past. Vetiver builds bridges between our memories and experiences, our mental capacities, and our physical bodies. It transforms our memories and experiences into wisdom and maturity. Vetiver can be good for us when a 'dose of reality' is needed in our lives.

Physical Aspects

Vetiver is an excellent oil for skin care. It speeds up the disappearance of scars from accidents or acne by promoting the growth of new cells patterned after the original blueprint of cellular structure rather than replicating the damaged pattern. The anti-inflammatory and sedative properties of vetiver make it useful with arthritis, sprains, and muscle spasms. Vetiver is said to aid in the production of healthy red cells in the blood. Vetiver is considered a tonic oil. It is, to our bodies and minds, a bit like the complete overhaul and servicing that we routinely give our vehicles.

General Information

Vetiver is known in India as 'the oil of tranquility.'

Cautions

This essential oil is said to be completely safe. Caution is still advised in pregnancy, as it is with any essential oil.

Wintergreen

(Gaultheria procumbens)

Ingredient In

LeDeeper, LeMariah, LeRefresh-Mint, LeTenda Care LeVallee, LeWarm Down

Therapeutic Properties

analgesic, anti-inflammatory, anti-rheumatic, antiseptic, antispasmodic, disinfectant, diuretic, warming

Affinity For

nerves
bones, joints, muscles
kidneys
respiratory system

Resonance

physical, emotional

Plant Family

Ericaceae

Part of Plant Used

leaves

Aromatic Considerations

Wintergreen has a wonderful aroma. It is stimulating, but deeper and more grounding than the essential oils of the mint family. Wintergreen is cleansing and opening to the physical senses.

Application

Wintergreen can be applied to any area of the body where it is needed. Be sure to dilute well. Wintergreen essential oil is very pleasant diffused.

Emotional/Spiritual Aspects

Wintergreen essential oil is a very aggressive essence which stimulates very powerful responses in return. Wintergreen promotes change on a profound level as the mind/body complex responds. Wintergreen shakes up and wakes up the mind and every system of the body.

Physical Aspects

Wintergreen produces an analgesic, numbing effect on the nerves present in whatever tissue it is applied to. Wintergreen clears obstructions to the flow of blood in the tissues and in the veins and arteries. This increases circulation in general and brings warmth to the area. This warmth is as strong and as healing as anything you will experience with commercial athletic rub products. This warmth also relaxes the muscles in the area to which it was applied. As the circulatory system works more efficiently, many health problems are alleviated.

The stimulant properties of wintergreen apply to all systems and organs of the body. Wintergreen increases the activity of the kidneys, preventing toxins, uric acid, fats, and liquids from building up in body tissues. Wintergreen essential oil aids digestion by stimulating proper secretion of gastric juices and bile. It stimulates the activity of the lungs, intestines, and other organs, preventing the accumulation of congestion and waste materials.

Cautions

Wingergreen essential oil has a high methyl salicylate content. Nevertheless, it is safe to use. Please see Chapter 14, page 9, (the last of the section on birch) for safety information about this constituent. Birch and wintergreen often receive very bad press because of misunderstandings about the effects of this 'supposed' toxic ingredient.

Wintergreen should be used cautiously if pregnant and always diluted well.

Yarrow

(Achillea millefolium)

Ingredient In

^Le^Balance, ^Le^Cypernium, ^Le^Vallee

Therapeutic Properties

anti-inflammatory, anti-arthritic, antiseptic, antispasmodic, astringent, carminative, cicatrisant, diaphoretic, digestive, expectorant, haemostatic, hypotensive, stomachic and tonic.

Affinity For

skin, tissue, and scalp
respiratory system
digestive system
stomach meridian
bladder meridian
wood element
metal element

Resonance

physical, emotionl, spiritual

Plant Family

Compositae

Part of Plant Used

flowering tops

Application

Yarrow essential oil is applied neat (without a carrier oil) to close a wound. It should be applied diluted for other applications and circumstances.

Aromatic Considerations

The aroma of yarrow oil balances our highs and lows, externally and internally, physically and mentally.

Emotional/Spiritual Aspects

In Chinese folklore, the aroma of yarrow is said to bring about the meeting of Heaven and Earth in our lives. With our head in the clouds, we have far-reaching vision and inspiration to guide us, but we have the stability and common sense of having our feet firmly planted on the ground.

Just as yarrow oil pulls together the edges of a deep wound, yarrow pulls together and heals the damaged places in our energy and psyche. Yarrow, emotionally, is for those times when we feel that there are important parts of ourselves that have become lost or fragmented. We feel the pain of loss, like the pain of a wound. Yarrow pulls the emotional and energetic edges together and allows us to heal.

Folklore of several countries states that yarrow is associated with love and fidelity.

Physical Aspects

Yarrow is one of the truly great healing oils! Applied topically to a cut, even a very deep one, yarrow will pull the edges together and help the cut to heal almost miraculously. Yarrow's antiseptic properties are strong enough to prevent infection, no matter how dirty or contaminated conditions were at the time of the injury. Yarrow, known for centuries as an herb to stop bleeding, is even more effective in the concentrated essential oil form.

The anti-inflammatory properties of yarrow are effective whether the inflammation is in the nasal or respiratory passages, the digestive tract, along the gum line, the uterus or ovaries, or anywhere else in the body.

Like the anti-inflammatory properties of this essential oil, the astringent properties of yarrow work throughout the body. Astringents cause the tightening of tissues. This makes yarrow very helpful for such things as dandruff, hair loss, setting the teeth firmly into the gums, or firming up areas of sagging skin. Astringent oils such as yarrow are beneficial as face washes for oily skin and acne. Yarrow is an excellent oil for the female reproductive system where astringency and a mild hormonal action combine to make this oil vital in treatment programs for ovarian cysts and uterine fibroid tumors.

It has been reported recently in several publications that yarrow's use with cancer and diabetes has been known throughout the ages. I can find no scientific studies to back these claims, but anecdotal evidence is certainly abundant. Yarrow essential oil also acts on the bone marrow to stimulate the creation of red blood cells and enhance the coagulation of the blood.

Yarrow is gently diaphoretic and a febrifuge. When you are ill, the use of yarrow holds the fever from getting dangerously high and stimulates perspiration. Fever and perspiration are the body's way of killing the microbes and then carrying them out of the system.

Yarrow improves digestion by stimulating the secretion of bile and restoring the liver and other organs. I could go on for several more pages about yarrow. It has been one of my favorite herbs for many years and is one of my favorite essential oils. Enough cannot be said about the benefits of this amazingly versatile healing oil.

Cautions

Reasonable caution should be taken during pregnancy. There are no other cautions connected to this oil. It is possible to find a use for it every day of our lives.

General Information

Many essential oil companies carry more than one yarrow essential oil. A yarrow oil which has a pale green color seems to be slightly stronger in hormone balancing properties than a deeper blue one. This pale green one is the one added in LeBalance and LeCypernium.

Yellow yarrow is an ingredient in LeTherma-care and is a particularly good febrifuge (reduces fever and produces a sweat).

Deeper blue yarrow oils have an advantage as an astringent and in pulling the edges of wounds together. The blue one is the one sought after most frequently as a single oil.

Ylang Ylang - Complete

(Cananga odorata)

Ingredient In

LeAngel, LeAssurance, LeBaby Me, LeBalance, LeBelieve, LeBeloved, LeBenediction, LeCandila, LeConnection, LeEverlasting, LeEZ-Traveler, LeGood-Nite, LeGrateful Heart, LeHeart Song, LeInner Peace, LeKadence, LeLetting Go, LeMoonlight, LeRefresh-Mint, LeSanctuary, LeTomorrow, LeTranquility, LeUnity, LeVitality, LeWhispering Hope, LeWisdom

Therapeutic Properties

sedative, antiseptic, aphrodisiac, nervine, antidepressant, calmative

Affinity For

adrenals and thymus
nerves
heart chakra
yin energy

Resonance

emotional, physical

Plant Family

Anonaceae

Part of Plant Used

flowers

Application

Ylang is an excellent oil for diffusing. Diluted, it can be worn anywhere on the body.

Aromatic Considerations

The aroma of ylang ylang can bring back feelings of confidence, joy, and peace.

Emotional/Spiritual Aspects

The aromatic focus of ylang ylang is spirituality. It fosters a desire in our souls for deeper and more meaningful communication with heaven. As we develop the emotional, caring, nurturing, intuitive, spiritual side of our natures, many things shift for us. We find that we are able to block or filter the negativity and 'garbage' around us. We are better able to focus our thoughts and our drive.

One of the behaviors that signals a need for ylang ylang is throwing temper tantrums that, if we are honest with ourselves, have the underlying intent of getting us our own way. Another indication for ylang ylang is sudden loss of interest in work, personal appearance, and even in family members and friends. Ylang ylang may also be helpful for insecurity, low self-esteem, anger, rage, and dare-devil tendencies.

Physical Aspects

Ylang ylang balances the male-female energies and hormones in the body by stimulating the adrenals and thymus glands. This can balance sexual energy and bring joy, harmony, and passion to relationships. The hormonal support properties of ylang ylang make it useful for the symptoms of PMS and many other hormone related complaints. Ylang ylang is a uterine tonic. Dilute and apply to the abdomen for this function.

As ylang ylang's hormonal properties work in conjunction with its nervine properties, ylang ylang becomes exceptionally effective for depression, irritability, anxiety, rapid breathing, heart palpitations, high blood pressure, hypertension, nervous tension, physical and mental exhaustion, nervousness, and insomnia. Ylang ylang is also excellent for routine skin care, more serious skin problems, and hair loss. Ylang ylang is also used to regulate circulation, fight intestinal infections, and alleviate constipation.

General Information

The distillation of the delicate flowers of ylang ylang is a complex process. The product that is extracted two hours after the distillation process begins is referred to in the industry as the 'extra.' This distillation is extremely heady, potent, and overly-sweet, and is not used in aromatherapy applications but is used by the perfume industry because a little goes a long way and the aroma remains stable longer.

This 'extra' is combined with the first and second distillations to form Ylang Ylang Complete. The 1st and 2nd distillations are the same flowers continuing the distillation process for longer periods of time before being 'pulled.' The first and second distillations are more subtle and less sweet in aroma. They are often used in therapeutic applications, but the complete is generally preferred.

Zanthoxylum

(Zanthoxylum armatum)

Ingredient In

[Le]My-Graine, [Le]Turmoil, [Le]With-In

Therapeutic Properties

antimicrobial, antibacterial, anti-fungal, antidepressant, antispasmodic, analgesic, anti-inflammatory, sedating and stimulating, tonic, carminative, stomachic, immune support, deodorant

Affinity For

circulatory system	digestive system	sacral chakra
respiratory system	nervous system	

Resonance	**Plant Family**	**Part of Plant Used**
physical, emotional	Rutaceae	fruit

Application

Zanthoxylum should be diluted for application to the body. It can also be diffused.

Aromatic Considerations

Zanthoxylum has a refreshing, spicy aroma. It calms the nerves and assists in meditation.

Emotional/Spiritual Aspects

The aromatic influence of zanthoxylum helps us to accept that we, in ourselves, are enough and that what we can do is enough. We are not 'broken' or 'damaged' and no one needs to 'fix' or 'heal' us. This attitude is acceptance of ourselves, not apathy or lack of direction and inner drive. We will know more clearly what we need to be doing and what direction we need to be going in. This place of peace and acceptance is created by finally understanding that we are loved for who we are, not for what we know or the things we do. This acceptance puts wind beneath our wings and allows us to soar. Because this is sacral chakra energy, this acceptance also corrects structural problems in our sacrum and lower back. The world suddenly feels much less demanding and stressful. Sitting down and taking a break becomes possible for us.

Physical Aspects

The analgesic and antispasmodic properties of zanthoxylum make it useful for arthritis, inflamed joints and other joint problems. Zanthoxylum increases circulation, relieves muscle cramps, and is of benefit in the treatment of varicose veins and varicose ulcers. Zanthoxylum is sedating and calming to the nervous system, making it useful in the treatment of stress related conditions such as headache, insomnia, and nervous tension. This essential oil aids the digestive system and increases the appetite during convalescent stages of illness. Zanthoxylum is used for tooth problems and gum diseases.

One of the most exciting scientific studies that I have found showed clearly that zanthoxylum prevents free radical damage throughout the body, but particularly in the liver. This study was conducted in the Department of Pharmacy, Bharat Institue of Technology, India. The data collected was for use of zanthoylum ***in essential oil form***. The study included data for unborn babies where liver damage in the mother or complications of pregnancy necessitated the use of drug therapies that would normally have compromised the liver of the fetus. The testing clearly showed that zanthoxylum essential oil protected and supported the fetal liver. This is absolutely amazing news!! (For a little bit more information on the liver, see information under Ledum.)

Cautions

Zanthoxylum has been used for centuries in Nepal, but is new to the world essential oil market. Care should be taken with pregnancy, at least until there is more information available.

The essential oils referred to throughout this document are distributed by Butterfly Express, llc.

Synergy and Blended Oils

A blended essential oil combines two or more pure single essential oils in such a manner that the result is an oil blend that is more effective than if those oils had been used separately. When oils are mixed together in the correct order and in the correct proportions, a chemical compound is created that is very particular and very powerful. The frequencies of each single oil seem to act both separately and as part of the unique frequency of the blend. Often a drop or two of the blended oil will accomplish what a drop or two of each of the singles oils would do. It will also give you the unique healing properties of the blend itself. As a simple example: the anti-inflammatory properties of chamomile are greatly increased by adding lavender in the correct proportion. This cooperative effort by the ingredients in a blend is referred to as *synergy* or *synergism*. The interaction of particular essential oils upon each other gives a dynamism to the blend which could not be achieved by using the single oils separately.

There are several factors that contribute to the effect that oils have on one another. One factor that drastically affects the properties of an essential oil blend is what kind of 'note' the individual single oils are. The term note, at least in part, refers to the evaporation rate of a single essential oil. Top notes are those oils which evaporate (diffuse into the air) most quickly. Oils that disperse more slowly are considered middle notes and then, finally, base notes are those oils which evaporate the slowest.

In general, base notes are considered to ground our energies. These oils, especially those from the conifer family, ground us to earth while allowing us to keep our vision lofty and pointed toward Heaven. Their impact is often on the lower chakras, or on the energy that vibrates between the crown and the sacral chakra. This energy must vibrate smoothly if we are to be vibrant and healthy.

Middle notes are usually essential oils that are derived from the leaves, seeds, spices, or herbs, and are healing to the individual organs and systems of our bodies. They bring nutrition and balance to us physically. The higher notes, usually fruit or floral oils, resonate with us on emotional and spiritual levels. Individual essential oils contain constituents which cover a limited range of frequencies, and operate on all three levels. A well-done blend operates deeply at many frequency levels in the body. A comparison can be made to listening to 3 violins playing well together, or listening (and responding to) music played by a famous orchestra.

The notes of the individual components of a blend enable it to work on all aspects of a problem and a person in the most correct and effective order. A well-blended oil, comprised of several individual essential oils, works in layers when applied to the body or inhaled. The top note oils clear the spiritual aspects of the situation and then evaporate off. The middle notes, according to their various diffusion rates, clear the emotions and begin working on the digestion, respiration, and metabolism before they evaporate off. Finally, the deeper notes finish the process by stabilizing the physical body and grounding the emotions.

Blended oils have the added advantage of being less likely to cause a reaction or any kind of problem. For example, there is quite a long list of cautions associated with the use of clary sage. However, in a blend, there is rarely more than a very small percentage of this oil. All the best effects of the use of clary sage can be accomplished, along with the benefits of the other oils in the blend, with much less risk of side effects or over-dose of any one oil. This is a very great advantage when working with pregnant women, children, the elderly or those who suffer from seizure disorders or other major health concerns.

It should be noted, before a discussion of essential oil blends begins, that there really is no such thing as an essential oil that works only on the emotions or only on the physical body. Every physical ailment either has its roots in the emotions, or because of the stress and disruption to life that it has caused, has created emotional components that need to be dealt with.

There are a few blends discussed in the remainder of this chapter that have few physical aspects listed. This is not because they do not affect the physical body. Negative emotions can wreak havoc anywhere in the body. It would be almost impossible to list all of the organs and systems that may have been affected by those emotions. Always keep an eye out for an emotional description of an oil that seems to match you (or the person you are working with). Pay attention, after you have used the oil for a little while, to what has improved physically in the body.

This chapter provides in-depth descriptions and information about specific essential oil blends created by the author, LaRee Westover, and currently marketed by Butterfly Express, llc.

Using Essential Oil Blends Other Than Those From Butterfly Express, llc.

This book talks about blends that are for sale at Butterfly Express. That is because those are the oil blends with which I am most familiar. I should be. I created the majority of them, and I use and love them everyday. I know, first hand, of their quality and the love and careful handling that they receive.

There are many excellent essential oil blends on the market, and there is a lot to be learned from comparing the ingredients of one blend to the ingredients of another, similar blend. If you have a blend that you like, whose intended use is similar to a Butterfly Express blend, it will be educational to compare their ingredients. Make a note of the single oils that are found in ***both*** blends. Study what these oils do by themselves and ponder on what they are meant to accomplish in the blends. Then, make a note of the component oils that are different in each blend. Study what those oils do as singles. Here again, try to decide why each oil was added to the blend. Ask yourself what each oil brings to the blend that makes it unique and different from the other blend. By the time you have done this, you will have a good idea of the subtle differences in the therapeutic action and direction of each blend. You will also have expanded your knowledge of essential oils and how they work together. Then, take a whiff of each one and decide on your own aroma preference. You are now ready to decide which blend is best for you in different situations.

Making Your Own Blends

Perhaps, you would like to try your hand at making your own blends. In blending, there is just no substitute for experience. Learning to blend can be expensive, but it very fun and rewarding. But even your mistakes will bless you in ways you may not see at the time. Here are a few tips to help you get started (and, hopefully, save you a little bit of money):

The first thing your blend will need will be a stabilizer. Conifer oils such as spruce or cedarwood are often used here. The part of the plant used to make the essential oil will usually be the wood, the root, or the resin. If a resin or a root, the percentage will be quite small; the conifers are often quite a large percentae of a blend. Myrrh, as a stabilizer, increases the shelf life and stability of a blend. Be careful; keep the percentage low, and make sure you really want myrrh's aroma in your blend.

The next level of your blend, usually comprising more than one oil, will be essential oils made from the leaves, seeds, spices, and herbal parts of the plants. Which specific oils you chose will depend completely on what you are trying to accomplish and how 'medicinal' you can tolerate letting the blend become. Pay attention to plant families and the part of the plant the various essential oils were derived from. This, and the medicinal properties of the plant, can guide your thinking and make your blend more effective.

The top, and final, notes of a blend will be either florals or fruits. These are the most volatile oils and have the highest frequency. They go in last so their fragile molecules will not be destroyed by the heavier molecules of the stabilizer oils. Florals and fruits are the crowning achievement of the plant. These essential oils are considered to operate on the emotional and spiritual level in our bodies.

When blending essential oils together, work slowly. 'Feel' your way. When the right amount has been added for a synergistic and harmonious blend, the energy will shift; you will feel it, if you are working slowly and feeling with your heart. A deep yawn or the urge to let your mind wander and think about something else is often a sign of energy shifting.

If the proportions of each oil were right and the oils were added in a reasonably correct order, there will be harmony in the blend. The aroma and energy of each individual oil will not bombard you all at once. Such a bombardment of disassociated energies is referred to in blending as 'clattering.' and you will know when you are feeling it! The blend will feel 'unpleasant,' and won't 'open' the energy of the body like a well-done blend does. Just try again. With each experience, you will have learned something about the characteristics and personalities of essential oils.

One last thing: Everything is relative in blending. An essential oil that was a middle 'note' in one blend, may be the 'top' note of another blend, depending on what else is in the blend and what you were trying to accomplish in the first place. Study blends that you like as clues for new blends that you might make.

LeAcknowledge

Ingredients

bergamot, frankincense, geranium, melissa blend, neroli, palmarosa, rosewood, sandalwood,

Affinity for

nervous system	heart chakra	liver meridian
liver	throat chakra	
	sacral chakra	

Resonance

physical, emotional, spiritual

Application

LeAcknowledge should be applied over the liver when the liver is toxic and the mind and emotions are sluggish or slow. Other particularly effective places for application are behind the ears, on the face, neck, thymus, or wrists. I especially like applying oils to the wrists because I frequently wave my wrists in front of my face for one reason or another.

Aromatic Considerations

This blend has a pleasant enough aroma to be worn as a perfume and is especially nice used in a bath when one is feeling overwhelmed or discouraged by life. The aroma of this blend can promote feelings of calmness, courage, and increased self-confidence.

Emotional/Spiritual Aspects

LeAcknowledge nourishes and strengthens the nervous system, helping to quiet feelings of fear and discouragement. Another benefit of this blend is in enabling us to see the 'reality' of life or health situations. Accepting what will be or will not be in our lives can allow us to move forward with healing and peace instead of discouragement and despair. Recognizing what it is that we are feeling, and knowing that it is acceptable to feel that way for the moment, often allows us to move through that feeling and move on with our lives. LeAcknowledge may also give us increased confidence in social situations and enhanced creativity in our attitudes and skills. One aspect of this blend concerns a better balance in attitudes and desires in sexual matters. LeAcknowledge is also one of the great oils for depression.

Because it balances the heart and sacral chakras, LeAcknowledge can help us recognize and accept the love and sympathy that people around us are trying to express. For those of us with very independent natures, it may help us with the ability to let others be of service to us. Increased balance in the throat chakra allows us to express our own feelings and needs and to express feelings of appreciation and gratitude for the services we receive. Balance in these areas may also bring relief from feelings of frustration, self-pity, insecurity, hopelessness, inadequacy and feeling that we are being overwhelmed by the responsibilities of our lives. This allows us to feel enthusiasm for new things and to expect to find joy and abundance in our lives.

LeAcknowledge, like LeBountiful, may change the way that we feel toward material possessions, making us both more appreciative of them and less focused on their acquisition.

Physical Aspects

Because LeAcknowledge has a cleansing effect on the liver it may be useful for allergies and other mild immune system dysfunctions. Any ailment that has anger as an underlying emotional component, which many physical ailments do, would benefit from the use of LeAcknowledge. Kidney and bladder problems such as frequent infections and cystitis, with their emotional connection to fear and feelings of inadequacy, often respond favorably to this blend. The use of this essential oil blend may not only relieve the discomfort of the moment, but will also help lessen the likelihood and frequency of future attacks. LeAcknowledge is an excellent oil when applied as a deodorant and is considered a mild hormone balancer.

^{Le}Angel

Ingredients

blue tansy, copaiba balsam, cedarwood, lavender, geranium, orange sweet, rose, rose geranium, ylang ylang

Affinity for

all of the energy centers (chakras), especially if the imbalance is the result of childhood abuse—absolutely amazing in this regard!

Resonance

emotional, spiritual

Application

^{Le}Angel should be applied, diluted in a carrier oil, over the energy centers (chakras) or on the temples. It is very pleasant when diffused and can be used in a bath or worn as a perfume. ^{Le}Angel is a simple, yet beautiful fragrance.

Aromatic Considerations

Use of this blend often brings memories of a time or place when one felt safe and loved. Often the person will wish to express these feelings or talk about a loved one from their past with whom they felt particularly loved, accepted, and safe.

Emotional/Spiritual Aspects

^{Le}Angel is specific for use in releasing traumatic memories connected to negative experiences of various kinds. It is particularly effective for feelings of insecurity, helplessness, and rage resulting from childhood abuse, both sexual and otherwise. Adults who were abused as children often feel confusion, anger at themselves, and misplaced guilt because 'they let ***it*** happen.' ^{Le}Angel can bring them to a place of safety where they can acknowledge these feelings and sort through them. The releasing and processing of these memories has a cleansing effect on the stored anger that is often held in the liver meridian. ^{Le}Angel does not erase the memory of these events. It allows one to move through the anger, validate themselves, let go, and move forward rather than let past experiences dictate their actions and their decisions in the present. ^{Le}Angel is helpful in the relief of anxiety and can protect us from the negative energy and unprocessed emotions of others. ^{Le}Angel is one of the best essential oil blends for stabilizing mood swings, especially in children.

Physical Aspects

There are some behavior patterns and illnesses that are common to people who feel a lot of anger. This is true whether the roots of the anger lie in childhood abuse or in some other event or cause. Some of these physical symptoms are vascular headaches and migraines, high blood pressure, tension and stiffness in the neck and shoulders, muscle cramping, inflammation of the nerves, and distress in the gall bladder and liver. Because ^{Le}Angel helps to cleanse the liver, it can be of benefit in many of these ailments.

^{Le}Aspire

Ingredients

cypress, eucalyptus, laurel, marjoram, myrtle, peppermint, pine needle, rosemary, spruce

Affinity for

respiratory system
uptake of calcium
liver meridian

Resonance

physical

Application

LeAspire should be applied diluted with a carrier oil on the chest and neck for respiratory ailments. Using LeAspire, with or without herbs, as a compress or poultice can be particularly effective. This blend can also be applied to the energy points on the ears and to the bottoms of the feet. LeAspire can be applied alternately with LeBreezey. Although the oils in LeAspire are quite effective against infectious agents, LeDeliverance, which is strongly antiviral and antibacterial, is often applied simultaneously to aid in the fight against infection. LeAspire is used to open the airways and relieve the congestion in the lungs.

Aromatic Considerations

LeAspire is especially effective used in a humidifier to decongest and clear respiratory passages and to relieve coughs and sore throats.

Physical Aspects

LeAspire is used to bring relief from colds, bronchitis, pneumonia, sinusitis, respiratory congestion, allergy symptoms, deep pneumonia, pleurisy, asthma, and flu that have settled in the lungs. LeBreezey is considered by some to be more effective for upper respiratory conditions and LeAspire for use in deeper chest complaints affecting the bronchial passages and the lungs. Both LeBreezey and LeAspire have proven effective in eliminating snoring when diffused or applied, well diluted, to the face and chest areas. LeAspire is an excellent expectorant, aiding the body in the discharge of phlegm and mucus. This blend also has antispasmodic properties which help to quiet dry, hacking coughs.

The synergy of the single oils in LeAspire gives it the unique ability to dissolve bone spurs ***if*** applied frequently and faithfully. A bone spur creates bruising in the tissues surrounding it, especially if the person is on her feet and pressure is being applied when walking or wearing shoes. It is recommended that a carrier oil containing arnica be used when LeAspire is used for a bone spur. The arnica will reduce the bruising and the pain that the bone spur is causing while LeAspire works to remove the spur. It is recommended that treatment with LeAspire be continued for a few weeks after the pain is gone.

LeAssurance

Ingredients

frankincense, lavender, chamomile Roman, spruce, ylang ylang

Affinity for

nervous system
solar plexus chakra
emotions

Resonance

emotional, spiritual, physical

Application

LeAssurance should be applied to the nape of the neck to stimulate the mind and help one move foreward productively. Other areas of the body that are recommended are the solar plexus, sternum, navel, wrist, palms of the hands, and the feet—particularly on the top of the big toe and on the K1 acupressure points.

Aromatic Considerations

LeAssurance is wonderful worn as a perfume; effective for yourself and those around you when used in this way. This blend is also very pleasant when diffused.

Emotional/Spiritual Aspects

LeAssurance is an especially good choice when there is a need to overcome feelings of anxiety, fear, or apathy that leads to procrastination. This blend can aid us in getting back to the task at hand or back to life in general. It helps to sort out the reasons for the reluctance we are experiencing about working toward or achieving our goals. This blend was created to help us find self-confidence and self-assurance. It provides the enthusiasm to tackle the tasks necessary to achieve our goals.

LeAway

Ingredients

catnip, cedarwood, cinnamon berry, citronella java, clove bud, eucalyptus peppermint

Application

LeAway should be diluted in water or Miracle II Neutralizer and applied, either by misting or rubbing on, just as you would with any other insect repellent. You can also spray the diluted solution on clothing and on the bottoms of pant legs, sleeves, and hats, being careful to avoid contact with the eyes.

General Information

Insect bites can be dangerous as well as just annoying, but slathering yourself with chemicals may not be a good solution. LeAway is a blend of some of the single essential oils most often used to repel insects.

LeBaby Me

Ingredients

bergamot, palmarosa, chamomile Roman, rose, rose geranium, rosewood, ylang ylang

Affinity for

skin
endocrine system
heart chakra
emotions

Resonance

spiritual, physical, emotional

Application

LeBaby Me is usually applied diluted with distilled water or carrier oil, especially for frequent use or application over larger areas of the body. LeBaby Me is appropriate for all skin types. The type of carrier oil you will use will depend on the type of skin you have. This blend is very relaxing when added to a bath.

Aromatic Considerations

LeBaby Me helps to open the heart chakra, enabling us to give and receive love. This blend also brings a sense of calmness and competence.

Emotional/Spiritual Aspects

LeBaby Me is a special combination for mothers, expectant and otherwise, and for babies of all ages. The use of this oil brings feelings of connection and willingness to give and take in relationships, particularly in parent/child relationships. It is also recommended for use in bonding between a mother and a new baby. This blend also helps us to feel a connection with the Eternal Father of us all.

The frequency of this blend is extremely high, well into the spiritual range, but is so well balanced that notes from all three realms (physical, emotional and spiritual) can be felt and enjoyed. First the more volatile top notes do their work with the spirit and the emotions, and then the middle and lower notes kick in to ground and balance the more physical aspects. LeBaby Me is good for depression and the 'baby blues.'

Physical Aspects

LeBaby Me contains ingredients which increase skin elasticity, retard wrinkles, enhance skin tone and remove scaly patches. The synergistic effect of this blend increases the ability of the skin to act as a protective barrier against germs. LeBaby Me is effective applied on the inner ankles, lower back and abdomen to reduce cramping during menstruation and following childbirth. This blend is also used to reduce or prevent stretch marks during and after a pregnancy. Please refer to Chapter 13 for information on the many uses of this oil during pregnancy and childbirth. LeBaby Me makes an excellent diaper rash cream. It can be used, diluted of course, for a full body massage at any stage of life. LeBaby Me is wonderful for skin conditioning and makes an excellent aftershave for sensitive skin, especially when mixed with a little Miracle Salve. The oils in this blend were chosen for their cell regenerating properties. This blend has an affinity for the endocrine organs, particularly in stabilizing low blood sugar.

Cautions

Contains very mild oils but is still best diluted well, especially for use on babies and small children

LeBalance

Ingredients

chaste tree, clary sage, cypress, chamomile Egyptian, lavender, marjoram, myrtle, peppermint, rose geranium, sage, yarrow, ylang ylang

Affinity for

nervous system
endocrine system
emotions

Resonance

spiritual, emotional, physical

Application

LeBalance should be applied around the ankles on both men and women. It can also be diffused and is soothing when a drop or two is placed in the tub. If using in the shower, plug the drain and allow a couple of inches of water to accumulate in the bottom of the tub. Add your oils and continue your shower.

Aromatic Considerations

LeBalance is beneficial in the control of mood swings brought about by hormone and endocrine system imbalances in both men and women. (Yes, men have hormones that can and do get out of balance, too!)

Physical Aspects

LeBalance is a great oil for supporting the endocrine system and balancing the hormones in both men and women.

For men, LeBalance helps balance male energy, regulate prostate function, and reduce congestion and enlargement of the prostate which often re-establishes proper urinary function.

For women, LeBalance has been used successfully many times to reduce or eliminate hot flashes and headaches in women who are approaching or going through menopause.

LeBalance has antispasmodic properties. It is helpful as a digestive aid and as a diuretic, especially when the problems in these areas are linked to hormone imbalances.

General Information

LeBalance often brings quick relief from the symptoms of menopause and should be used by women age 45 and older. LeWoman Wise is a better choice for younger women of menstruating age to balance hormones and relieve the symptoms of PMS. For best results, LeWoman Wise and LeBalance should be used in conjunction with LeEndo Relief, which has a strengthening effect on the entire endocrine system.

Cautions

LeBalance, being an oil which has an effect on hormones, should definitely not be used during pregnancy!!

LeBelieve

Ingredients

copaiba balsam, frankincense, palmarosa, rose, rosewood, vanilla, ylang ylang

Affinity for

nervous system
emotions
all of the chakras
cellular memory
most of the meridians

Resonance

physical, emotional

Application

LeBelieve is beautiful diffused, is nice worn as a perfume, and exceptional when used in the bath.

Aromatic Considerations

LeBelieve should be considered whenever there is a need to forgive and release emotions from the past that are holding one back in life. This oil aids in learning to love oneself and achieve a sense of inner peace.

Emotional/Spiritual aspects

LeBelieve was created to release negative emotions and perceptions at the cellular level. This helps us to replace negativity with love, forgiveness, peace, and understanding. Working at the cellular level helps to make these changes permanent. Such changes brings us more confidence in ourselves. LeBelieve can help us see that we have the abilities we need and that we will be led to where we need to be at appropriate times in our lives. LeBelieve is a great oil to aid us in being more optimistic, more motivated, and more tenacious.

This blend can help us balance the need we feel to protect ourselves and be ready for anything that may come along, while providing us with a healthy trust in the future. We can feel confidence in our ability to thrive as we cope with the circumstances and situations of our lives. LeBelieve helps us to forgive ourselves for mistakes made in the past and returns our heart to a state of joyous anticipation for whatever experiences life may have in store for us next.

This blend seems to have the ability to help the dying accept death as the next phase of life, moving peacefully and calmly toward death when the time has come. LeBelieve can also be of benefit to those left behind in finding solace and relief from loneliness.

As LeBelieve helps us move into a more self-forgiving and self-confident state, we should feel more generous, cooperative, and compassionate towards others. We will also find contentment and inner strength. LeBelieve seems to have a beneficial effect on our intuition and out ability to act upon it.

Physical Aspects

LeBelieve can reach into the core of a cell and release traumas and negative emotions on a cellular level. This blend is also useful in energy corrections that reset cellular memory. When the cell reproduces itself through mitosis, it will begin to reproduce the original undamaged and untraumatized version of the cell instead of the cell in its traumatized state. This is very valuable in healing following accidents, burns, and other physical traumas.

LeBeloved

Ingredients

bergamot, geranium, lemon, mandarin, orange sweet, ylang ylang

Affinity for

spiritual side of our natures
emotions
heart chakra

Resonance

spiritual, emotional, physical

Application

LeBeloved should be applied over the heart chakra using the palms of the hands. It can also be diffused.

Aromatic Considerations

The aroma of LeBeloved is like a breath of fresh air for our hearts and souls. When we feel out of sync with our loved ones or overwhelmed by our responsibilities to them, this oil helps bring us back to what is most important in our lives.

Emotional/Spiritual Aspects

LeBeloved profoundly affects the heart chakra and is a beautiful oil for relationships—both romantic and with family and friends. It opens our hearts and our spirits to recognize that we are loved more than we can possibly comprehend. Understanding the great love that God has for us can help us to heal our own emotional wounds. From our wholeness of heart, we can then see clearly and respond generously in just the right way.

LeBeloved is helpful in developing inner strength and fortitude. The oils is this blend are of benefit when we are feeling overwhelmed or must accept changes in the circumstances of our lives. LeBeloved has been of value with mood swings and panic attacks.

Physical Aspects

The negative emotions found in dysfunctional and destructive relationships can manifest in a variety of ways, making this blend effective for a broad spectrum of physical complaints. This list may include bed-wetting, a tendency for cystits and urinary tract infections, headaches, heart palpitations, menstrual cramps and just about anything else. The important thing to pay attention to is the emotional drivers of physical pain.

LeBenediction

Ingredients

angelica, bay, geranium, hyssop, lemon, melissa blend, myrrh, rose, rose geranium, rosewood, sandalwood, spruce, ylang ylang

Affinity for

energy system
establishing emotional balance
bilary ducts
liver
respiratory system
endocrine system
pineal gland
pituitary gland
central vessel meridian
bladder meridian
throat chakra
crown chakra

Resonance

spiritual, physical

Application

LeBenediction should be placed on shoulders, wrists, and thymus area and is also of great benefit when diffused into a room that is highly charged with energy.

Aromatic Considerations

The aroma of LeBenediction can increase the integrity of the auric field, strengthening our personal energy barriers. This blend is particularly useful for meditation and gospel study.

Emotional/Spiritual Aspects

LeBenediction is a favorite among massage and energy therapists. It strengthens one's own energy boundaries and protects against 'energy drains' that sometimes occur when working with other people's energy fields. This blend should be used at times when you are feeling particularly vulnerable and 'energy sensitive' and easily drained by people and situations.

LeBenediction can help us speak up and express our needs clearly without blaming or whining, especially if we are sensitive to or over-awed by the person we are addressing. This blend can also temper our tendency to judge unkindly when we feel that a person has created the mess they are in and we are justified in leaving them alone to fix it.

LeBenediction also aids us in learning to acknowledge the role that blessings from above have played in our own successes and achievements. Gratitude to heaven is a very healing emotion; probably the best thing you can do to balance your own chakra centers. Try this blend any time you are feeling angry, stressed, or depressed.

LeBenediction is also very effective after an illness for returning energy levels to normal and getting us back on our feet both physically and emotionally.

Physical Aspects

LeBenediction is often useful for tension headaches, heart palpitations, and high blood pressure where picking up on the energies of others is a contributing factor. LeBenediction makes an effective deodorant.

Unique Characteristics

Frequently utilized to create an energy 'bubble barrier' which allows us to interact with others without compromising our 'self.' This is true whether we are being drained by others or are at a low point ourselves and having a draining effect on those around us.

Cautions: Avoid exposing areas of skin where LeBenediction was applied to direct sunlight for 3 to 6 hours.

LeBountiful

Ingredients

orange bitter, cassia, cinnamon, clove, frankincense, myrrh, patchouli, orange sweet, thyme

Affinity for

immune system
respiratory system
body's external magnetic field
emotional balance
stomach meridian
pericardium meridian

Resonance

physical, mental—the frequency of this blend is similar to that of a healthy brain

Application

LeBountiful can be diluted and worn on the wrist, behind the ears, or as a perfume or cologne. It is sometimes helpful to place a drop or two on the checkbook, on the car dashboard, on a phone or a wallet. The results are often quite profound.

Aromatic Considerations

The intent of this blend is to create feelings of security, generosity, and thankfulness. These feelings then bring the 'blessings of heaven' down on our heads.

Emotional/Spiritual Aspects

LeBountiful is specifically designed to affect the energy fields around us and to help us achieve a frequency that attracts goodness into our lives. It is an aid to our thinking clearly about money issues and lessens the stress in these areas. One of the most outstanding effects of this blend is the feeling of abundance that it creates in our minds and spirits. It simply moderates, or evaporates altogether, any feeling that there is never going to be enough and that there is certainly not enough for everybody to have what they think they need. The absence of these fearful feelings helps us eliminate even the slightest tendencies to greed and selfishness in our natures. Benevolence is the best word I can find to describe the feeling this blend creates. We find ourselves able to let go of our fear of trusting others, being dependent on them, or needing to ask for help. LeBountiful has a profound effect on the things we worry about and how we choose to respond to these situations.

Physical Aspects

LeBountiful is also beneficial to the brain in other ways. It seems to clear the mind and rejuvenate sluggish thought processes. This blend can be stimulating and energizing if we are feeling tired and worn down. LeBountiful is also an immune support and stimulant. LeBountiful can be used as a decongestant for the lungs during bronchitis or pneumonia. Use of LeBountiful at these times provides a needed boost in energy and mood.

General Information

This is an oil of 'attraction.' As we develop an attitude of abundance we find that we receive what we need to make us balanced, whether it is physical, emotional, or spiritual. In other words, the more you give, the more you receive.

LeBreezey

Ingredients

birch, eucalyptus, lemon, peppermint, ravensara

Affinity for

respiratory system
immune system
skin
muscles

Resonance

physical

Application

LeBreezey should be diluted and rubbed on the chest or back. It can also be diffused or placed on your pillow at night.

Aromatic Considerations

LeBreezey opens bronchial and sinus passages very effectively and has been successful in alleviating snoring.

Emotional/Spiritual Aspects

While generally thought of as an oil for physical illness, the aroma of LeBreezey lifts the spirits and brings a sense of confidence and self-worth.

Physical Aspects

LeBreezey, besides being very effective in times of illness, is an excellent respiratory tonic and immune stimulant. The inclusion of ravensara oil creates viral fighting and tissue rebuilding properties, especially for the lung and bronchial tissues. This blend should also be tried for conditions such as colds, asthma, allergies, sinus congestion, and flu. LeBreezey is an immune stimulant. LeBreezey makes an excellent muscle relaxant and pain reliever when you do not have LeWarm Down or LeDeeper handy and you have strained a muscle.

General Information

LeBreezey is often used alternately with LeAspire.

LeCandila

Ingredients

cypress, lavender, manuka, tagette, tea tree, rosemary, ylang ylang

Affinity for

immune system
reproductive system
digestive system
skin

Resonance

physical

Application

LeCandila should be diluted well and applied to affected areas. If you use this blend as a douche for vaginal candida, be sure to dilute very well!

Physical Aspects

LeCandila was created for use against thrush, candida, and vaginal yeast type infections. LeCandila is not a 'magic bullet'—there is no such thing, really. To eradicate a candida overgrowth you ***must*** make dietary changes. The use of a good quality acidophilus or pro-biotic is also recommended. A Vitamin E supplement in your diet may also be of benefit.

General Information

Most of us will have some sort of systemic yeast overgrowth at one time or another during our lives. This will probably be due to a diet which is too acidic or taking antibiotics. Even a brief period of an acidic diet, such as during the holiday season, can produce an acidic enough environment to cause an outbreak of candida. A round of anti-biotics, if we find it necessary to subject ourselves to such a regimen, can also create the optimal environment for a candida overgrowth. Candila, and a product carried by Butterfly Express, llc, called Candidase, can be very beneficial in keeping yeast from multiplying out of control.

LeConnection

Ingredients

angelica, cedarwood, fir, sage, spruce, ylang ylang

Affinity for

root/base chakra
solar plexus chakra
emotional balance

Resonance

spiritual and emotional

Application

LeConnection is very nice applied to the back of the neck, on the temples, or just about any where that you can imagine.

Aromatic Considerations

LeConnection has a delightful aroma which is centering, grounding, and emotionally balancing.

Emotional/Spiritual Aspects

LeConnection is designed for people who are characteristically over-enthusiastic and have unrealistic expectations of themselves, of others, or of life in general. This blend is helpful in moderating a tendency to make hasty decisions and choices. It is also of benefit to those who escape too often into their own fantasy world.

The spruce in this blend has an affinity for the solar plexus chakra. The solar plexus chakra connects us to divine energy and gives us balance and joy in our service to others. LeConnection is an excellent oil to use as part of a journal or prayer session. LeConnection can help us see where our perceptions have parted company with reality and truth. If we have been basing our decisions and behaviors on our mis-perceptions, this oil can help us make more appropriate decisions and behave in more appropriate ways.

Physical Aspects

The sage in this blend has an affinity for the pelvic area chakras and the organs contained in the pelvic region. This is an important thing to remember when trouble in these areas is connected to emotions and mis-perceptions.

LeCrystal Clear

Ingredients

basil, peppermint arvensis, peppermint piperata, rosemary

Affinity for

brain
nervous system
brow chakra
solar plexus chakra
emotional balancing

Resonance
emotional, mental
Application
LeCrystal Clear can be applied on the brow, along the back of the neck, on the wrists, and on the temples. It is also useful diffused or placed, 1 or 2 drops only, in a bath. A few drops on a cotton ball placed next to you will help keep you alert and awake for a project that needs finishing.
Aromatic Considerations
LeCrystal Clear diffused or inhaled clears and energizes the mind and increases mental alertness.
Emotional/Mental Aspects
This blend is very effective when studying or needing to remember difficult or complicated data. It helps to organize the thought processes, allowing more accurate recall later.
Physical Aspects
LeCrystal Clear is nourishing to the nerves, the adrenal cortex, and the cardiovascular system. This is one of the best essential oil blends for the treatment of impending shock. LeCrystal Clear can help to balance hormones and bring relief from headaches that are associated with hormone imbalances.
General Information
There are three blends by Butterfly Express, llc, which help with mental alertness. These are LeCrystal Clear, LeFocus, LeIQ.

LeCypernium

Ingredients
cypress, geranium, peppermint
Affinity for
circulatory system
vascular system
vein and capillary health
Resonance
physical
Application
LeCypernium is diluted (4 - 5 drops to 1 Tablespoon of carrier oil, almond oil, or KY jelly) and applied specifically to areas of trouble such as varicose veins, spider veins, and hemorrhoids.
Physical Aspects
LeCypernium was created for the relief of hemorrhoids but has proven useful for varicose veins and overall vein health. LeCypernium increases the circulation and vascular strength in any area to which it is applied. LeCypernium makes an excellent anti-inflammatory.

LeDandy

Ingredients
basil, cypress, lavender, rosemary, sage, thyme
Affinity for
hair, scalp, skin
Resonance
physical
Application
LeDandy is applied by adding 2-3 drops to your shampoo each time you wash your hair. It is often beneficial to follow this treatment with LeDelicate and LeEternity. LeDelicate and LeEternity both seem to help with the absorption of the nutrients necessary for scalp and hair health.

Physical Aspects

This is a formula for general scalp and hair health and works well for eliminating dandruff. Regular use adds attractive natural highlights to the hair and costs much less than regular appointments at the salon.

Cautions

Avoid contact with the eyes.

LeDeeper

Ingredients

birch, eucalyptus, helichrysum, fir, lemongrass, myrrh, peppermint, spruce, wintergreen

Affinity for

muscles
bones
nerves

Resonance

physical

Application

LeDeeper should be diluted whenever it is applied to the skin. This is an excellent oil for use in the bath.

Physical Aspects

LeDeeper contains deep penetrating, anti-inflammatory oils which are effective in relieving pain that is deep in the tissues and nerves. It is useful for sciatica, arthritis, osteoarthritis, the pain of osteoporosis, sprains, and injuries where there is bruising and/or nerve damage. LeDeeper increases blood and lymph circulation to the extremities, making it an effective choice for conditions such as neuropathy and fibromyalgia. This blend often brings instant relief when applied to the abdomen and back for pre-menstrual cramps. Other important uses for LeDeeper include pain relief with shingles and bursitis.

Cautions

Always remember to dilute essential oils when applying them to the skin.

LeDelicate

Ingredients

cypress, lavender, rosemary, sage, thyme

Affinity for

hair
scalp

Resonance

physical

Application

LeDelicate can be applied by adding 3-4 drops to the shampoo when washing your hair. For hair loss, try placing 3-4 drops of LeDelicate in your conditioner. Leave the conditioner/ LeDelicate blend in your hair and wrap entire head in a warm towel for 10-15 minutes. Afterwards rinse hair gently. This process should be repeated several times a week until the problem has disappeared.

Aromatic Considerations

The aroma of this blend is pleasant and has an uplifting effect on the mind and the spirit.

Physical Aspects

LeDelicate is a wonderful blend for overall hair health. It seems to help the scalp absorb nutrients so that the hair becomes more healthy and vibrant with each use. LeDelicate adds attractive natural highlights to the hair. For babies with cradle cap, LeDelicate, diluted with almond oil, should be massaged gently into the scalp. Use a very soft brush to dislodge the scaly patches and then rinse or wipe away gently.

LeDeliverance

Ingredients

clove, eucalyptus, cinnamon, lemon, rosemary, thyme, oregano, wild oregano

Affinity for

immune system
lymphatic system
the skin

Resonance

physical, spiritual

Application

LeDeliverance can be used in so many ways, I am sure that I will not manage to list them all here. Some common methods of use are soak the family toothbrushes in LeDeliverance mixed with water, place a drop on your toothbrush at least one time per day, and place on a cotton ball or in an inhaler and carry with you, inhaling frequently, during the cold and flu season. A particularly effective way to fight a very virulent illness is to apply LeDeliverance alternately with LeLife Force. In the evening put one of these essential oils on the K1's (accupressure points on the feet) and the other on the thymus. First thing in the morning, put the oils on again, then put them in opposite positions. If LeDeliverance was on the thymus area the night before, it should go on the feet in the morning. This method is ***very effective against really nasty stuff***.

Aromatic Considerations

An excellent use for this blend is to diffuse it every day during the cold and flu season to eliminate air-borne bacteria and viruses.

Physical Aspects

LeDeliverance is one of the most potent antiviral, antibacterial, anti-fungal combinations available. Its many uses include respiratory infections, sore throats, strep throats, dental diseases and infections, cold sores, canker sores, cuts, any type of infections, athlete's foot fungus, ***toe nail fungus***, and infection from slivers. Apply faithfully undiluted to get rid of a wart (this takes a little time so be patient). Frequent and consistent use also strengthens the immune system. LeDeliverance is an expectorant and helps the lymph system to drain. ***This is a very effective oil. Everyone should have it on hand.***

General Information

LeDeliverance can be used, diluted, or diffused, in the home as a cleaner and air purifier to fight viruses, and air borne bacteria.

Cautions

Care should also be taken to dilute well, especially if frequent use is anticipated. The clove, cinnamon, thyme and oregano in this blend make it a possible skin irritant.

LeDiscernment

Ingredients

geranium, hinoki, lavender, rose, rosewood, sage, spruce, orange sweet

Affinity for

emotional balance
brow chakra
crown chakra
heart chakra

Resonance

physical and emotional

Application

LeDiscernment can be diffused, applied to wrists or temples, added to a bath, or used with almond oil for massage.

Aromatic Considerations

Because this blend dissipates negative emotions, it helps us move forward with renewed vigor and enthusiasm to achieve our dreams.

Emotional/Spiritual Aspects

LeDiscernment promotes feelings of faith in the future and renewed enthusiasm for the pursuit of our goals and dreams. This blend can help us discern the path best suited for us and most likely to bring happiness and contentment to our lives. LeDiscernment is also helpful in bolstering decision making abilities.

LeDiscernment can help us achieve a healthy balance between the analytical left brain and the intuitive right brain. Its special function seems to be helping us maintain a balance between preparations for the future and living with joy and peace today.

LeDiscernment has a special place for those who struggle with pride or arrogance, or who fail to credit heaven and other people with any part in their successes. This blend can be particularly useful for those in leadership positions. It can aid them to see past the physical appearances and circumstances of others, while giving them the ability to discern the strengths and intrinsic worth of those they serve. The skill of seeing the worth of another soul is also a valuable asset among family members, members of a community, or work group.

Physical Aspects

All essential oils are antibacterial, antiseptic, and antiviral. LeDiscernment is no exception and it has a pleasant aroma. It can be used to disinfect almost anything. LeDiscernment is effective against canker sores.

Cautions

This blend contains a small amount of sage, which is strongly contra-indicated for use during pregnancy; it may be wise to exercise a bit of caution with this blend when pregnant, epileptic, or suffering from high blood pressure.

LeDreams

Ingredients

benzoin, bergamot, blue tansy, chamomile German, juniper, sandalwood, spruce, orange sweet dark

Affinity for

emotional balance	brow chakra and 3rd eye	pericardium meridian
	throat chakra	
	crown chakra	

Resonance

spiritual, physical, emotional

Application

LeDreams can be applied to the forehead, eyebrows, temples, behind the ears, on the base of the neck, and worn as perfume or cologne. For restful sleep, diffuse in the bedroom or apply 1 or 2 drops to your pillow. This essential oil blend makes a relaxing evening bath.

Aromatic Considerations

LeDreams has a beautiful aroma. It can be diffused during the day for pleasure or meditation, and at night to promote restful and dreamless sleep.

Emotional/Spiritual Aspects

This blend was formulated for helping us keep our dreams in sight and realize our potential without becoming self-centered or selfish. LeDreams is one of the best oils for insomnia due to negative emotions or nightmares. It is a favorite of children who are nervous in the dark or when left alone. If nightmares persist while using LeDreams, continue to use it in conjunction with energy work modalities. Finding the disturbing emotion, processing it, and letting it go is the only way to achieve lasting healing. LeDreams can help you do that. This blend has been beneficial for bedwetting if the root cause is fear or anxiousness.

LeEndo Relief

Ingredients

cumin, cypress, coriander, dill, geranium, myrtle, nutmeg, oregano, petitgrain, sage

Affinity for

endocrine system
lymph system
emotional boundaries
pineal gland
pituitary gland

Resonance

physical, emotional, spiritual

Application

LeEndo Relief should be applied to the lymph glands of the neck, chest, and armpits whenever a cold, sore throat, or flu is suspected. Using LeEndo Relief early, before the illness is fully developed will lessen its severity.

Aromatic Considerations

This blend is best applied to the body.

Emotional/Spiritual Aspects

LeEndo Relief aids our emotional health because it strengthens and balances the wide range of organs and glands that make up the endocrine system. As our bodies and minds begin to function better, we feel more secure in ourselves. We are able to establish (or re-establish) boundaries between ourselves and others. This does not mean that we become prickly or rude; it enables us to be tactful and firm while still being kind and concerned.

Physical Aspects

With improved endocrine function comes improved vitality and metabolism. Our weight naturally balances and we have enough energy to last through the day (and into the night, if we need to). As an endocrine system balancer, LeEndo Relief can have a beneficial effect on any ailment that is related to endocrine organs such as the thyroid, pancreas, pineal and pituitary glands, parathyroid, thymus and adrenal glands. This makes LeEndo Relief useful for such things as diabetes, hypoglycemia, bladder and kidney infections, candida, and so much more. Support of the thyroid and parathyroids aid the proper absorption of calcium. Calcium absorption affects such things as the prevention of gallstones, kidney stones, arthritis, and osteoporosis. LeEndo Relief regulates hot flashes and moderates the other symptoms of menopause because the hormones balance as the endocrine system function improves.

LeEnergy

Ingredients

black pepper, cinnamon, clove, juniper berry, lemongrass, nutmeg, pine, rosemary, thyme

Affinity for

endocrine system
hormone balancing
heart chakra
solar plexus chakra

Resonance

physical, emotional, spiritual

Application

LeEnergy ***must*** be diluted well before applying to the skin. It should be applied over the thyroid, kidneys, liver, pancreas, or any gland that is struggling. LeEnergy may also be applied, diluted, to the feet and is an energizing massage oil. For massage, be sure to dilute very well.

Aromatic Considerations

Blends with a cinnamon should be diffused and inhaled with caution; cinnamon can burn the sensitive tissues of the nostrils if care is not taken.

Emotional/Spiritual Aspects

LeEnergy can aid us in making decisions and taking responsibility for our own lives and actions. It moderates our need for the attention and approval of others. Sometimes, in our zeal to keep those around us safe and happy, we have a tendency to become overly controlling. LeEnergy can help us temper these tendencies with a dose of reality. Energy in the solar plexus chakra manifests as vitality and radiance. When we are balanced and energized here, we have such a giving spirit that we are almost magnetically attractive to other people. We will be very much liked and loved by all, and we will be more effective in our parental and leadership roles.

Physical Aspects

LeEnergy increases circulation, strengthens the adrenal glands, improves energy levels and mental alertness naturally without the side effects of drugs. This blend also balances the mechanical and electrical functions of the heart.

LeEternity

Ingredients

ajowan, allspice, clove, frankincense, orange sweet, thyme

Affinity for

cardiovascular health
metabolism of vitamins and minerals

Resonance

emotional, physical

Application

LeEternity should be applied, diluted, on the chest along the sternum. It can also be diffused.

Aromatic Considerations

The aroma of LeEternity balances energy and improves both mood and mental outlook.

Physical Aspects

LeEternity has powerful anti-oxidant properties. It enhances vitamin and mineral absorption for the overall improvement of health and vitality. LeEternity, because it helps the body absorb calcium, can help prevent such things as osteoporosis. The oils in this blend have been used traditionally for various problems related to the cardiovascular system.

LeEverlasting

Ingredients

A very unusual oil—it is a blend of 5 other blends: LeDreams, LeHeart Song, LeTrust, LeUnity, LeWisdom

Affinity for

emotional and spiritual health

Resonance

emotional, spiritual, physical

Application

LeEverlasting can be applied, diluted, to the chest, over the heart, on the forehead, and down the sternum (for allergy relief). This blend is very nice worn as a perfume or diluted as a massage oil. LeEverlasting is relaxing in a tub, especially when life is being a little stressful.

Aromatic Considerations

The aroma of LeEverlasting balances energy and improves both mood and mental outlook. Diffuse LeEverlasting while sleeping for a restful night's sleep and to wake up refreshed and invigorated. LeEverlasting helps one to see and seek their highest potential and best good for themselves and others.

Emotional/Spiritual Aspects

Each of the five blends contained in LeEverlasting is in the mid to very high frequency range. Each one targets a specific range of emotions. Blending these five blends together into another essential oil blend is an amazing example of synergy. LeEverlasting is a lower frequency (physical range) blend which displays the ability to act on the emotions. A person using LeEverlasting receives the emotional impact of each separate high frequency blend. At the same time, the lower frequency of the whole carries the healing more deeply into the physical body. The negative emotions are released clear down to the cellular level. This amazing mixture relieves feelings of hopelessness and self-pity.

Physical Aspects

LeEverlasting promotes a most wonderful relaxation that is followed by high levels of optimism, vigor, and energy.

LeExhilaration

Ingredients

cedarwood, clary sage, ginger, helichrysum, jasmine, melissa blend, neroli, patchouli, rosewood, sandalwood, orange sweet

Affinity for

nervous system | emotional balance | stimulation of the amygdala

Resonance

spiritual, physical

Application

LeExhilaration is beneficial applied on the wrists, temples, heart chakra area, and forehead. It can also be added to the bath. The aroma is very pleasant as a perfume or cologne.

Aromatic Considerations

The aroma of this essential oil blend can aid us in maintaining confidence and courage while it helps us improve our overall attitude. It is almost like being given a fresh new outlook and start in life.

Emotional/Spiritual Aspects

LeExhilaration is especially beneficial in those situations which appear hopeless and discouraging. With the use of this blend we find our emotions strengthening and stabilizing until we are able to see new and different solutions to old problems. It is as if there are now several paths available to us, but we previously could only see one way out of the woods. Suddenly we are able to see our surroundings in a more comprehensive way. LeExhilaration is also used to release emotional blocks and help us let go of negative feelings and perceptions.

Recent studies have shown that it is in the amygdala (located in the temporal lobes of the brain) where solutions to problems are developed. When we look at a situation, wanting to know what we should do, the amygdala 'lights up' and begins to present our minds with possible solutions. Activity in the amygdala increases with the use of LeExhilaration. This increased brain activity gives us more ability to see various new solutions to old problems.

Physical Aspects

Several of the oils in this blend are oils that profoundly affect physical body systems. Some are anti-inflammatories and others target specific organs or functions. If your physical body has been strained or weakened by situations that are testing your courage and confidence, LeExhilaration can be of benefit to you. It may have an impact on physical things that you did not realize were connected to the emotions you were feeling.

LeExpressions

Ingredients

frankincense, jasmine, rose, sandalwood, ylang ylang

Affinity for

heart chakra
throat chakra

Resonance

spiritual, physical, emotional

Application

LeExpressions is very nice diffused, wonderful for a relaxing bath and can be diluted with a carrier oil and used for a truly wonderful massage.

Aromatic Considerations

The aroma of this blend is amazing—sensuous and heady, almost euphoric and very healing to the heart.

Emotional/Spiritual Aspects

LeExpressions contains many of the highest frequency spiritual and emotionally healing essential oils. It is very nice for pampering yourself a little. LeExpressions is healing to the heart. This oil is used to enhance communication and connection in romantic relationships and is most definitely an aphrodisiac.

LeEZ-Traveler

Ingredients

birch, chamomile Roman, frankincense, lavender, myrrh, orange sweet, peppermint, ylang ylang

Affinity for

digestive system
nervous system

Resonance

physical, emotional

Application

LeEZ-Traveler should be carried with you whenever you are traveling if you are inclined to motion sickness. An inhaler is a convenient way to carry LeEZ-Traveler or you can place a few drops on a cotton ball and carry it in a small plastic bag. You can also apply this oil diluted to the soft areas of the skin such as the wrists, inner thighs, or behind the ears. It can also be diffused or added to the tub.

Aromatic Considerations

The aroma alone is often enough to stop the symptoms of motion sickness. This oil is calming and restful, providing a hint of humor and a sense of gladness to be alive.

Emotional/Spiritual Aspects

Besides alleviating the physical symptoms of motion sickness, LeEZ-Traveler promotes feelings of calmness, emotional strength, and the ability to cope with the day's events and responsibilities. It has been used to treat anorexia.

Physical Aspects

LeEZ-Traveler was originally created to assist with motion sickness during airplane travel. It has proven effective against other forms of motion sickness and unrelated incidences of nausea, dizziness, and vertigo. LeEZ-Traveler can be used as a preventative or to calm the symptoms once they have begun. It often brings relief from the symptoms of morning sickness that some women experience during pregnancy. This is a good oil to use in the days ***before*** traveling to ***avoid*** sickness while traveling.

LeFaith

Ingredients

bergamot, cabreuva, frankincense carterii, frankincense serrata, melissa blend, rose, rosewood

Affinity for

heart chakra | throat chakra | kidney meridian

Resonance

spiritual, physical, emotional

Application

LeFaith is very nice diffused, relaxing in a bath, can be diluted with a carrier oil and used for massage.

Aromatic Considerations

The aroma of this blend promotes feelings of self-worth and a desire to heal. It makes one want to be truly well, happy, and content. LeFaith turns our thoughts to gratitude for the blessings we have received.

Emotional/Spiritual Aspects

LeFaith is very much a blend specific for emotional healing. It seems to bring self-awareness without burying us in negativity or guilt concerning past mistakes. LeFaith promotes a healthy acceptance of the past and a desire to move forward into the future. This blend is specific for dealing with fears concerning being abandoned or left to cope with situations totally on one's own. If you are prone to useless worrying, you may find this blend helpful. As its name implies, it generates feeling of faith and self-confidence within us. Humility and teachableness are also gifts of this blend.

Physical Aspects

Although this blend is very much in the emotional realm, it has proven helpful for menstrual cramps and for lowering high blood pressure. In situations for which this blend proves useful, you will see the underlying emotional patterns described above.

LeFocus

Ingredients

cinnamon, cinnamon berry, ginger, nutmeg, patchouli, rosewood, sage, sandalwood

Affinity for

nervous system | emotional balance | governing vessel meridian

Resonance

physical, emotional

Application

This blend can be applied to the acupressure points on the feet that relate to the neck, head, and brain. These are found on the big toe, both top and bottom. LeFocus can also be applied to the wrists and temples.

Aromatic Considerations

I like to inhale LeFocus at times when I am studying and need to be extra alert. I also find it useful in the afternoons at the computer if my mind is slow or I am having difficulty concentrating. This blend can be diffused, but it is best to do so for short periods of time only; cinnamon, cinnamon berry, and ginger are very strong oils for diffusing. They may cause headache or a burning sensation in the nostrils.

Emotional/Spiritual Aspects

LeFocus is useful in overcoming negative thought patterns and self-defeating behaviors. Sometimes we choose to see ourselves as victims where life and everyone we know is 'out to get us.' This pattern of behavior gets in the way of our ability to take responsibility for ourselves. It can also keep us from accomplishing our goals. When LeFocus has helped us become aware of our self-defeating patterns, we can choose to change them.

Physical Aspects

This blend increases mental alertness, clears that 'foggy' feeling, and helps to alleviate mental confusion. It is a great aid to students and others when they face the need to commit something to memory quickly and be able to recall it with ease later.

General Information

LeFocus has much the same uses as LeCrystal Clear and LeIQ, but the aromas of these three blends are very dissimilar. These blends are classic examples of the wide range of plants that can accomplish similar healing tasks in the human body. Each person is unique with their own way of reacting to things. One of these three blends may work better for you and another one may work better for someone else. You may find all of them helpful, giving you the opportunity to choose one according to your preferred aroma or according to the price.

Cautions

This blend contains nutmeg, cinnamon, and sage. It should be used with care if you are susceptible to seizures or if you are pregnant. Repeated use on the skin could result in skin irritation, even when diluted.

LeGood-Nite

Ingredients

cedarwood, orange sweet, ylang ylang

Affinity for

throat chakra
immune system (use faithfully during the cough and cold season)

Resonance

physical, emotional

Application

This blend can be diffused, placed on the pillow at night, or applied, diluted, to sinus areas any time.

Aromatic Considerations

LeGood-Nite can be diffused in the home during the evening to promote restful sleep.

Emotional/Spiritual Aspects

Part of the reason that LeGood-Nite promotes restful sleep is because it encourages feelings of peace. We feel assurance that all will be well in our world even though we are sleeping and not actively watching over it. LeGood-Nite seems to help us process, painlessly, deep emotions during our sleep. In the morning we will be able to express our deep feelings about these emotions clearly and without the usual stress.

Physical Aspects

LeGood-Nite is effective for insomnia and snoring and soothes inflamed or swollen nasal and sinus passages while promoting deep and restful sleep.

LeGrateful Heart

Ingredients

coriander, frankincense, geranium, howood, melissa blend, myrrh, pine needle, rosewood, ylang ylang

Affinity for

nervous system
immune system
muscles
bones
emotional balance

Resonance

physical, emotional, spiritual

Application

LeGrateful Heart should be applied over the heart, on the forehead, or the temples. It is very pleasant diffused and smells nice enough to wear as perfume or cologne.

Aromatic Considerations

LeGrateful Heart is relaxing and creates tender feelings of empathy, gratitude, tolerance, and compassion.

Emotional/Spiritual Aspects

This blend promotes feelings of gratitude for all that we have and all that others do for us. It has a marked effect on the dark clouds of depression. It can be used to help us achieve relaxation of mind and body.

Physical Aspects

Dissatisfaction and discontentment are destructive to the nervous and immune systems. LeGrateful Heart addresses these imbalances and can provide support and healing for these feelings. LeGrateful Heart is used to stabilize the blood sugar lows of hypoglycemia. It has been used effectively in the treatment of some auto-immune disorders.

LeHeart Song

Ingredients

bergamot, geranium, grapefruit, lemon, mandarin, rose, rose geranium, rosewood, orange sweet, ylang ylang

Affinity for

emotional balance
adrenal gland
electrical system
heart chakra
throat chakra
brow chakra
crown chakra

Resonance

LeHeart Song allows the heart to find its joy and learn to sing again. It is a very high frequency spiritual and emotional blend. LeHeart Song is the #1 blend for the treatment of depression.

Application

If you have the time, LeHeart Song is very effective applied in a clockwise motion over each chakra. It is usually best to begin at the base chakra and work up the body to the crown chakra. This may be done on either the front or the back of the body. (I prefer the back, but that requires the help of a friend.) LeHeart Song can also be applied over the heart, on the ears, and to any area of poor circulation. This is a beautiful oil to diffuse, and may be worn as a perfume or as cologne.

Aromatic Considerations

The aroma of LeHeart Song can be offensive if there are emotional blockages to loving and being loved. If this occurs, apply the blend LeUnity to the palms of the hands and place the hands over the navel and thymus. Hold for 20 seconds and then reverse the hand positions and hold for another 20 seconds or more. The combination of these two oils will balance all the chakras and meridians, bringing a great feeling of peace.

Emotional/Spiritual Aspects

This high frequency blend reminds us that we are loved and cherished by many people, and certainly by Heaven. It has a multitude of uses. LeHeart Song has been of great benefit in treating depression. It is also useful in overcoming grief and trauma. Because it is a remedy for deep sorrow and grief, it makes a wonderful gift for anyone who has recently lost a loved one.

LeTranquility is the first line of defense against anxiety and panic attacks, but if it fails to work or needs a follow up, LeHeart Song is the blend to use. LeHeart Song is also helpful in stabilizing mood swings, relieving stress and tension, and helping one to relax.

You do not need to be suffering from depression or a recent loss to enjoy LeHeart Song. This blend is wonderful for getting through a tough time or just making it to the end of a difficult day. It is also quite effective as a protection against negative energy.

Because of its effect on both the heart and the throat chakras, LeHeart Song is of benefit to those who have difficulty expressing deep emotions or tend to laugh inappropriately when trying to express themselves about these things.

Physical Aspects

LeHeart Song is balancing to the electrical fields of the body and stabilizing to energy levels. Oddly enough, it brings relief from the pain and congestion of pleurisy and makes an excellent deodorant.

LeHoliday Spirit

Ingredients

benzoin, cinnamon, fir siberica, orange sweet, spruce

Affinity for

respiratory system | emotions

Resonance

emotional, spiritual, physical

Application

LeHoliday Spirit is especially appropriate applied to the crown of the head. It can also be placed on pine boughs and cones, cedar chips, logs to burn in the fireplace, and used to scent potpourri.

Aromatic Considerations

When diffused, LeHoliday Spirit creates a delightful holiday atmosphere. It reminds us of fond family events and emotions. LeHoliday Spirit is a great blend when diffused for purifying the air at any time of the year.

Emotional/Spiritual Aspects

The aroma of LeHoliday Spirit is reminiscent of Christmas. For most people this blend brings feelings of happiness and security. LeHoliday Spirit brings a desire to hold on to and build relationships with family and friends. The holiday season seems less stressful and more enjoyable when this blend is kept diffused in the house. LeHoliday Spirit can help us deal with the stress of Christmases past if our memories are of things that were not just as we wished them to be. This blend really increases the Christmas Spirit in your home—or in your favorite Christmas Scrooge!

Physical Aspects

Besides all of its wonderful emotional aspects, LeHoliday Spirit has shown itself to be beneficial at purifying the air, killing airborne 'bugs', and soothing respiratory ailments. It has also been used successfully in the treatment of anorexia.

Cautions

LeHoliday Spirit contains cinnamon and can irritate the skin if used topically undiluted.

LeInner Peace

Ingredients

angelica, cinnamon, copaiba balsam, frankincense, lavender, palmarosa, rosewood, sandalwood, spruce, ylang ylang

Affinity for

emotional balance | heart chakra | small intestine meridian
pineal gland
pituitary gland

Resonance

emotional, spiritual, physical

Application

One specific and effective way to apply LeInner Peace is across the forehead, moving from the right temple to the left temple. It can also be placed on the chest to cover the heart and the thymus. This blend is very good in the tub or as a perfume, if your mood is right. (See *unique information* section below.)

Aromatic Considerations

LeInner Peace helps to collect our thoughts and connect our heart and mind. This connection to ourselves creates a solid and balanced center from which we can connect to others.

Emotional/Spiritual Aspects

LeInner Peace can aid us in staying focused and clear, particularly about the direction of our lives. It promotes harmony between ourselves and others, and between ourselves and God. This blend helps us feel genuine compassion for others, and aids us in forming rewarding relationships.

Much like LeBenediction, LeInner Peace protects the energies of our bodies and minds from attack and depletion by the energies of others. Though protected energetically, LeInner Peace leaves us open, compassionate, and willing to be of service if we desire. It can also be helpful if we fear or hate being alone.

LeInner Peace can help us with acceptance of ourselves and others and with the calm acceptance of the changes that life brings to us all. For emotional work, use with LeSanctuary and LeMagi.

Physical Aspects

LeInner Peace affects the pineal and pituitary glands. The pineal gland regulates blood pressure, body temperature, motor function, sleep patterns, and any cyclical activity in the body. The pineal gland directly affects every other gland and organ in the body. It also regulates the cardiovascular system. The pituitary gland is considered a 'master' gland by the body. It instructs the other glands how much of their particular hormone or enzyme to produce. A blend like LeInner Peace, which has an affinity for these two glands, can balance and heal the physical body on a multitude of levels.

Unique Information

LeInner Peace can enhance whatever state you are in. If you want to feel more gratitude or contentment, you must already be feeling some of those emotions—or, at the very least, desiring with all your heart to feel them. ***You must use this blend with caution when angry or when caught up in negative emotions as this essential oil blend acts as an amplifier.*** It may amplify negative emotions as well as positive ones. It is sometimes necessary to diffuse LeSanctuary or another of your favorite uplifting emotional blends for a little while before using LeInner Peace. This is one of my favorite blends for really deep emotional or spiritual work!

LeInside-Out

Ingredients

aniseseed, cardamom, fennel, juniper, lemon, lemongrass, patchouli, peppermint piperita, tarragon, thyme, cilantro

Affinity for

digestive system | stomach meridian

Resonance

physical, emotional

Application

Apply one drop behind the ears for nausea, motion sickness, or morning sickness. LeInside-Out can also be applied over the abdomen either by diluting with a carrier oil or as a compress.

Emotional/Spiritual Aspects

LeInside-Out is primarily considered an oil which works on the physical body. Whenever you use an essential oil, you will be working on underlying emotional roots as well as physical complaints. LeInside-Out can be helpful in discovering and sorting through the emotions underlying the digestive problems. LeInside-Out can help calm the obsessive worry that sometimes contributes to digestive difficulties.

Physical Aspects

LeInside-Out improves the function of the digestive system. It helps with upset stomach, belching, bloating, stomach cramps, heartburn, constipation, and diarrhea. LeInside-Out's ability to be effective for both constipation and diarrhea may seem odd; it is not. Natural remedies work with the body to return systems to balanced and healthy states. They are not the administration of an 'opposing' remedy or force. This is true in every aspect of the body and mind when working with natural healers.

LeInside-Out should be used for any bout of intestinal flu or food poisoning. It is useful for most types of nausea, either by inhaling the aroma or putting a drop behind each ear. This blend should be applied over the abdomen for colon problems and for candida overgrowth. LeInside-Out has been useful in the treatment of parasites in animals and humans. For humans, place LeInside-Out on the feet and massage across abdomen. For animals, dilute a few drops in water and massage into soft tissues.

Cautions

LeInside-Out contains a small amount of fennel which is, when used by itself, contra-indicated for use during pregnancy. This is an example of blended oils being safer to use than single essential oils. This essential oil blend is safe to use for morning sickness in the manner described, but proper care, prudence, and judgement should be exercised.

LeInsight

Ingredients

clementine, jasmine, orange sweet, sandalwood, tangerine, vanilla

Affinity for

emotional balance

cellular memory

Resonance

physical, emotional

Application

This blend can be diffused, diluted to create a massage oil, applied to the navel, chest, or temples.

Aromatic Considerations

The aroma of LeInsight calms the nerves and grounds the emotions.

Emotional/Spiritual Aspects

LeInsight is powerful in working with personalities that have been fragmented by the terror and confusion felt as the result of abuse. A child should be able to put their trust in the adults in their lives. When this trust is betrayed, there is often deep rifts in the psyche. LeInsight is often used in Inner Child work to reconnect fragmented parts of a personality or soul. This blend is useful to release negative emotions from the past, whether the memories are conscious or not. The essential oils in this blend combine to clear patterns held in the memory of each cell. When these emotions clear, there is often an increase in intuition, organizational skills, mental faculties, and flexibility of thoughts and reactions.

Physical Aspects

Whenever layers of pain are scarred over in the mind and emotions, physical symptoms will manifest themselves in the body. They are a natural result of anger, fear, and confusion. A blend such as LeInsight can have a healing and renewing effect anywhere in the body.

It is rarely necessary for a person to relive, or even remember, terrible things that were done to them in the past in order for healing to occur. It is only when our actions have harmed another that we need to face them, figure out where our thinking went wrong, and take steps to change. Unfortunately, this is sometimes true of the actions and reactions we took as a result of abuse or mistreatment. In that situation, our own behavior needs remembrance and understanding in order for us to repent, but we do not need to 'repent' of the things that were wrongly done to us. Someone else is willingly carrying that burden for us already.

LeIQ

Ingredients

cabreuva, cedarwood, copaiba balsam, coriander, cypress, frankincense, helichrysum, laurel, lavender, lemon, melissa blend, sandalwood

Affinity for

emotional balance
nervous system

Resonance

physical, emotional

Application

This blend can be diffused, applied to the neck and throat or under the nose. It has a deep and pleasant aroma, making it appropriate as a perfume or cologne.

Aromatic Considerations

LeIQ has the most pleasing aroma and the highest frequency of all the blends for mental alertness; it is my personal favorite.

Emotional/Spiritual Aspects

LeIQ alleviates mental fatigue and increases mental alertness. It aids in concentration and memory. LeIQ is powerfully stimulating and helpful when feeling faint, going into shock, and for recovery from jet lag. It is particularly useful when one is over-tired but must continue on until a project is completed.

Physical Aspects

LeIQ contains frankincense, sandalwood, and helichrysum. These oils are high in sesquiterpenes and cross the blood/brain barrier to cleanse, nourish, and carry oxygen to the brain. This blend seems to dissolve some types of chemicals and clear them from the receptor sites feeding the pituitary, pineal, and hypothalamus glands.

LeJourney

Ingredients

basil, calamus, cassia, cinnamon bark, frankincense, hyssop, myrrh, spikenard

Affinity for

immune system

Resonance

this is a high frequency spiritual oil which acts dramatically in the physical plane.

Application

Careful dilution is recommended because this blend contains cinnamon and cassia. It should be applied to the feet or the chest.

Aromatic Considerations

Because of the cinnamon, cassia, and calamus contained in this blend, LeJourney is recommended for only short periods of diffusing at any given time. Care should be taken not to 'burn' the nostrils when inhaling or diffusing this blend of oils.

Emotional/Spiritual aspects

LeJourney gives us a sense of harmony with ourselves and an increased ability to learn from the experiences of our lives.

Physical Aspects

LeJourney is comprised of essential oils mentioned in the Bible (see Exodus, chapter 30). It is strongly antiviral and is used to expel disease and dead tissue from the body. LeJourney is an immune stimulant and is effective against colds and flu.

LeKadence

Ingredients

allspice, cedarwood, orange sweet, ylang ylang

Affinity for

nerves
cardiovascular system
heart chakra
throat chakra
brow chakra
all aspects of the 5th meridian
gallbladder meridian
liver meridian

Resonance

physical, emotional, spiritual

Application

LeKadence is delightful as a perfume or cologne. It can be added to a bath or diffused. It is appropriate to dilute and apply anywhere on the body.

Aromatic Considerations

The components of LeKadence are similar to LeGood-Nite, but with a delightful spicy twist that completely changes its aroma, use, and frequency.

Emotional/Spiritual Aspects

The focus of LeKadence is the exhaustion, both mental and physical, that is associated with too much work and worry.

Physical Aspects

LeKadence improves the uptake of nutrients to the brain and nervous system. It can help alleviate exhaustion in whatever form it has taken in the body and mind. LeKadence is especially useful for recovering from deep seated or extended illnesses. Sometimes sleep patterns are interrupted by nervous exhaustion, physical weakness, and worry. The body needs sleep ***so*** badly, but just cannot seem to rest. LeKadence, with the same oils that make LeGood-Nite effective, can be helpful here. The addition of allspice aids the rejuvenation of the cells as the body rests.

LeKadence brings vitality to the heart chakra and the heart muscle. It reduces inflammation in and around the heart and pericardial sac. LeKadence is often effective for quieting heart palpitations, especially those brought on by worrying. This blend is useful for dizziness and vertigo. LeKadence can be helpful if one is having difficulty concentrating or keeping the mind focused on a thought or project.

LeLetting Go

Ingredients

blue tansy, hinoki, lavender, lemon, geranium, sandalwood, ylang ylang

Affinity for

emotions
digestive system
urinary tract

Resonance

physical, emotional

Application

LeLetting Go should be applied directly over the liver, on the bottom of the feet, or behind the ears. This blend is very nice in a bath or diffused.

Aromatic Considerations

LeLetting Go is a favorite blend of many people. By letting go of negative emotions, we can create feelings of tolerance and compassion towards the faults & foibles of the human race, including ourselves. Regular use of this essential oil blend can help us develop feelings of trust, safety, and security.

Emotional/Spiritual Aspects

LeLetting Go is literally for what the name implies. It is for 'letting go' of negative emotions that we are holding onto in the physical tissues of our bodies. You can use LeLetting Go to aid in the release of anger, frustration, resentment, despair, grief, insecurity, or any other emotion that is not serving you well. This blend is appropriate when your forward progress in emotional or physical healing seems to be halted. This oil is beneficial when used for the rebellious spirit sometimes seen in teens and others of us from time to time.

Physical Aspects

LeLetting Go of the emotional baggage that we don't need can have an energizing effect on the colon, kidneys, liver and gall-bladder in particular.

LeLife Force

Ingredients

blue tansy, caraway, clove bud, dill, frankincense, galbanum, geranium, hyssop, lemon, oregano, ravensara, rosemary, thyme

Affinity for

nervous system
immune system

Resonance

physical, emotional

Application

One of the best places to apply this blend is along the spine. Other good places are all over the feet and on the thymus area of the chest.

Aromatic Considerations

LeLife Force should be diffused to strengthen the immune system and increase energy levels. It will also disinfect and purify the air, eliminating germs and bacteria.

Emotional/Spiritual Aspects

LeLife Force immediately raises the over-all frequency of the body, improving outlook and response to stress and trauma.

Physical Aspects

LeLife Force should be used following any illness or traumatic experience that has left one feeling weak, shaky, or on edge. This blend can make a big difference in the recovery period of accidents and illnesses. LeLife Force builds, strengthens, and protects the body because it is an immune and adrenal gland stimulant and toner. Use it with LeEndo Relief during the cold and flu season. You may avoid getting sick altogether, and, if you do catch something, the illness will have a shorter duration and recovery period.

For fever, dilute and apply along the spine. For bronchitis, use LeLife Force with LeAspire or LeBreezey applied to the chest. For an earache, put 1 drop of LeLife Force in carrier oil and put into the ear. In addition I like to put 2 or 3 drops of BBL tincture in the ear. BBL will numb the pain and cause any inflammation to dissipate through a multitude of small holes which heal quickly (instead of in one large rupture which is the way ears usually deal with inflammation).

Soaking your feet in very hot water to which 2 or 3 drops of LeLife Force has been added, can assist the body to detoxify, especially from environmental poisons and medications. The combination of immune stimulant properties and detoxifying capabilities make LeLife Force effective against allergies and other mild auto-immune dysfunctions.

LeMagi

Ingredients

angelica, birch, frankincense, juniper berry, myrrh, sandalwood, spruce

Affinity for

emotions solar plexus chakra crown chakra

Resonance

This is a low frequency, physical range essential oil blend, but has profound effects on the emotional and spiritual planes. Like all oils with an affinity for the solar plexus chakra, changes are made deep in the cellular memory.

Application

For work with the crown chakra, apply on the top of the head, preferably in a clockwise motion. LeMagi can also be applied just above the eyebrows, on the solar plexus, and thymus, also in a clockwise direction. LeMagi would make a unique statement as a perfume or cologne, but not an offensive one.

Aromatic Considerations

LeMagi should be diffused after a spiritual or energy work session to complete the changes, carry them deeply, and make them permanent. When diffused, LeMagi creates feelings of reverence and heightened spirituality. It can help one overcome doubt and negative feelings about one's abilities.

Emotional/Spiritual Aspects

LeMagi is a favorite of many people because it seems to clarify intuition and heighten the ability to hear the whisperings of divine inspiration. Among the many emotional blends, LeMagi stands out for those with low self-esteem who are unable to feel really confident about themselves and their contribution, even after a job well done. This blend is comforting in times of despair. LeMagi is helpful in coping with the fear of being left alone or with feelings of loneliness and isolation.

General information

LeMagi derives its name from the frankincense and myrrh it contains and the Wise Men (also known as the Magi) who brought them as gifts to the Christ Child. I believe this blend increases our own wisdom and ability to look at our world with clarity. That is a true gift.

LeMariah

Ingredients

bay, helichrysum, Idaho tansy, spearmint, opopanax, ravensara, spikenard, spearmint, thyme, turmeric, wintergreen

Affinity for

respiratory system immune system

Resonance

physical

Application

LeMariah should be applied, diluted, to the chest and back at frequent intervals.

Aromatic Considerations

LeMariah should be diffused near the patient to aid in clearing the lungs.

Physical Aspects

This blend was specifically designed for use against the new flu strains that are giving people such a scare today. It seems to be the nature of these new strains to manifest very differently from one person to another. One person may sustain more damage to the circulatory system while another person may be hit hardest in the lung and respiratory areas. The strength of this blend lies in its antiviral/antibacterial properties and in its ability to clear and support the lungs. LeMariah should be used in conjunction with LeRevitalize for endocrine support to increase energy and stamina. Use LeMariah in conjunction with LeVitality to strengthen the heart.

LeMeditation

Ingredients

frankincense, myrrh, myrtle, rosewood, sandalwood, spruce

Affinity for

emotional and spiritual balance
root chakra
throat chakra
brow chakra
crown chakra

Resonance

high spiritual range

Application

LeMeditation should be applied to the slight bumps on both the right and left sides of the forehead, on the crown of the head, on the shoulders, and on the back of the neck.

Aromatic Considerations

LeMeditation creates a spiritual environment conducive to prayer and meditation; diffuse when seeking inspiration, reading scriptures, and seeking the answers from above.

Emotional/Spiritual Aspects

LeMeditation can help bring us to a state where we are more receptive of divine inspiration. This blend can aid us when meditating, pondering, or studying spiritual things. LeMeditation can help us discover and walk away from negative thought patterns. It will aid us in decision making by bringing us to a place where we can discern heavenly input.

LeMeditation is useful for calming ourselves, finding compassion for others, and lifting ourselves out of depression. This blend can help us find the motivation to make any changes in our lives that we know need to be made.

LeMela Plus

Ingredients

cajeput, clove, niaouli, rosemary, tea tree

Affinity for

skin
respiratory system

Resonance

physical—very low frequency

Application

LeMela Plus should be applied topically on insect bites and stings. LeMela Plus can also be diluted and massaged over the liver. Add a few drops of LeMela Plus to Miracle Salve, sold at Butterfly Express, LLC, to make an antibacterial ointment for cuts and abrasions.

Aromatic Considerations

LeMela Plus can be diffused to dispel odors.

Physical Aspects

LeMela Plus is strongly antiseptic. It prevents the growth of bacteria, fungus, and other infectious agents. LeMela plus can be used for athlete's foot and toe nail fungal infections. It can also be used for disinfecting cuts, scrapes, and wounds. A drop applied to insect bites will keep them from infecting. Rosemary and tea tree, major ingredients in LeMela Plus, are said to be effective in treating infections.

LeMillenia

Ingredients

blue tansy, elemi, fir, frankincense, geranium, chamomile German, lavender, rosewood, spruce

Affinity for

body structure and alignment
muscles
skin
energy/electrical system
nervous system
every meridian
every chakra
emotions

Resonance

LeMillenia is a very low frequency oil. This makes it very effective for working on issues of physical structure and alignment. However, LeMillenia is also an outstanding emotional blend.

Application

LeMillenia is very good applied to the bottoms of the feet or along the inside of the foot (the spine in reflexology and foot zone therapy). You can balance the energy between the left and right lobes of the brain by putting a drop of LeMillenia on your index fingers and placing your fingers on your temples. The left hand should be on the right temple, and the right hand on the left temple.

Aromatic Considerations

When diffused, LeMillenia builds courage, confidence, and self-esteem while being calming and relaxing at the same time.

Emotional/Spiritual Aspects

LeMillenia helps one find the courage to move forward with confidence and faith. It brings clarity about what is really necessary for happiness and contentment. It can help us find an equilibrium between being organized, neat, orderly, meticulous, logical, and analytical (all good traits) and being obsessively focused on perfection. LeMillenia is used to aid us with self-expression, fear of conflict and disagreement, and the ability to make decisions. This blend can foster tenacity and independence of spirit.

Physical Aspects

"Chiropractor in a bottle" is a good description of this blend except that LeMillenia aligns so much more than just physical structures. LeMillenia aligns the electrical energies of the body, balances every meridian, and energizes every chakra. In addition, LeMillenia maintains the integrity of the connective tissues that wrap, connect, and protect every organ and balances the emotions connected to each organ. LeMillenia balances the moisture and fluid levels in the body.

One of my favorite uses for LeMillenia is in working with ADHD and hyperactivity. Applying LeMillenia to the feet at least once a day can make a profound difference in a child's ability to sit still and concentrate. I use the feet because it is an excellent place to draw essential oils into the body. I also like the feet because the person (it is often a little boy) can put his shoes back on, go to school, and no one teases him because he 'smells like flowers.' Also consider using LeTranquility along with the LeMillenia.

As an agent of structural alignment, LeMillenia can be used as a diuretic, an antispasmodic, an expectorant, and a nervine, LeMillenia is helpful for some types of arthritis, for sciatica, and to improve capillary circulation. LeMillenia should be tried at the very first moment a hernia is suspected. Using LeMillenia to brush your teeth may keep your teeth aligned and prevent cavities. A drop should be diluted in almond oil and put in the ear for earache. This will realign physical structures and take the pressure off of the ear canal or ear drum. Because LeMillenia realigns physical and electrical structures, it is beneficial for some types of headaches. It is antispasmodic, analgesic and excellent where bruising has occurred.

There is not enough understanding of anorexia, but it is known that something in the way LeMillenia realigns the body systems changes the thinking and brings relief from this condition.

LeMoonlight

Ingredients

angelica, cedarwood, cinnamon, clary sage, geranium, jasmine, mandarin, neroli, patchouli, sandalwood, spikenard, orange sweet, ylang ylang

Affinity for

emotions base chakra sacral chakra heart chakra

Resonance

physical with deep emotional impact

Application

LeMoonlight can be diffused any time you like or worn as a perfume.

Aromatic Considerations

The aroma of this blend is earthy with a strong sensuous floral tone.

Emotional/Physical Aspects

LeMoonlight is a potent aphrodisiac. It sets a mood of connection to and appreciation for your romantic partner. LeMoonlight adds to the delight you feel in the sensual and passionate side of your lives together and creates emotional depth and bonding.

LeMy-graine

Ingredients

copaiba balsam, chamomile German, Grapefruit, helichrysum, lavender, marjorm, peppermint, zanthoxylum

Affinity for

nerves muscles bones

Resonance

physical

Application

LeMy-graine can be put on the temples, forehead, and back of the neck. Often the aroma will be all that is needed to back off a migraine. For really tough headaches, put 3 drops in your bath and 8-10 drops on a cold washcloth placed at the back of the neck at the same time. Try to relax as much as possible while the essential oil takes effect.

Aromatic Considerations

Usually very effective for headaches when inhaled or diffused.

Emotional/Physical Aspects

LeMy-graine is used for migraine and stress related headaches with or without accompanying nausea. This blend is also useful following neck injuries and to open the blood supplies to and from the head. LeMy-graine does its best work with headaches related to stress and circulation problems. Mild hormone oils make it effective for some women for the headache which comes at the beginning or end of their period. LeMy-graine may be useful for some types of depression. Use with LeWoman Wise or LeBalance if hormone imbalances are suspected.

LeNo-More

Ingredients

calamus, elemi, oregano, patchouli, spikenard

Affinity for

immune system
lymphatic system
skin

Resonance

physical

Application

LeNo-More is used mainly to disinfect and prevent mold growth. It can be applied diluted to the body if any type of infection has occurred. If the infection is caused by a fungus (rather than a bacteria) it is probably best to dilute with water rather than with a vegetable protein based carrier oil. A fungus can feed on vegetable protein carrier oils such as almond, olive, or grapeseed. This blend is effective against such nasties as athlete's foot and toe nail fungus.

Aromatic Considerations

Very effectively kills air-borne germs

Physical Aspects

Because of the oxygen-carrying capabilities of essential oils, they are all antibacterial, anti-fungal, antiseptic, etc. to some extent. This blend contains many of the most powerful antiseptic oils available. Having been blended synergistically, they are even more effective than any of the singles would be if used
alone. Each single oil is less likely to create any reactions or problems when it is a percentage of a blend.

LePaine

Ingredients

birch, clove bud, copaiba balsam, eucalyptus, helichrysum, peppermint

Affinity for

nervous system
muscle tissue
bones

Resonance

physical, emotional

Application

LePaine should be diluted and applied to the area where the pain is located. It can also be used very effectively as a compress. LePaine is often used in layers with LeWarm Down, LeTenda Care, LeDeeper, and LeMillenia. It should be layered with LePatches if you suspect tendon or ligament damage.

Physical Aspects

LePaine is much more than a pain reliever, although it is strongly analgesic. LePaine promotes quicker healing by bringing oxygen to the injured area and increasing circulation. LePaine is anti-inflammatory, antispasmodic, and calming to nerves. This essential oil blend can be used for sciatica, bone pain, arthritis, sports injuries, muscle spasms, torn ligaments, headaches, osteoporosis, bone spurs, bursitis, back pain, and bruising.

Cautions

If you use LePaine in the tub or shower for pain relief or muscle relaxation, use no more that 2 or 3 drops.

LePatches

Ingredients

frankincense, gingergrass, rosewood, peppermint, spruce

Affinity for

nerves
muscles, tendons, ligaments
bones, joints
all 5 subtle bodies
all of the meridians
all of the chakras

Resonance

physical
emotional

Application

LePatches should be diluted and applied on location at the site of the pain or injury. LePatches is excellent as a compress and as a general massage oil.

Physical Aspects

LePatches was designed for the repair and healing of damaged tissues, tendons, and ligaments. LePatches is strongly anti-inflammatory, making it effective in restoring motion to inflamed and swollen joints. LePatches promotes quicker and more complete healing by inducing oxygen and blood flow to the injured tissue. LePatches should be used for sports and other injuries, muscle spasms, torn ligaments and tendons, bruises, and bursitis. This blend, applied to the neck and shoulders, is useful for headaches that are produced by tension, stress, and the tightening of the muscles in the neck or upper back. LePatches is an excellent oil for improving and restoring circulation.

Emotional Aspects

LePatches heals the damaged and broken energy places in the chakras and meridians. It helps the various layers of our bodies (physical, emotional, spiritual, and mental) work together and communicate freely with each other. 'Patching' us up (actually healing us is a better description) on every level is what this essential oil blend is good for.

LePurify

Ingredients

citronella, grapefruit, lavender, lemongrass, tea tree, manuka

Affinity for

digestive system
skin
emotional stability

Resonance

physical, emotional

Application

Diffuse to purify the air, kill germs, and remove odors.

Aromatic Considerations

LePurify purifies the air, neutralizes mildew, removes the smell of cigarette smoke and many other noxious odors when diffused in a room.

Emotional/Spiritual Aspects

Some citrus oils and lavender, all of which are in this essential oil blend, are useful for anorexia and eating disorders because they moderate feelings of insecurity, self-doubt, and self-loathing.

Physical Aspects

LePurify kills odors, bacteria, molds, and fungus. It is effective when applied to spider bites and insect stings and can be used for repelling bugs, insects, and mice. LePurify sometimes brings relief from toothaches and dental abscesses; at the very least, it may relieve the problem somewhat until a dentist can be reached.

LeReconciliation

Ingredients

anthopogon, rose, ylang ylang, vanilla

Affinity for

immune system
digestive system
ligaments, bones
liver
hair
skin
all four fire meridians
wood element (1st meridian)
heart and crown chakras

Resonance

emotional, physical

Application

LeReconciliation makes a very nice perfume. It is excellent diffused, as a massage oil, or added to a bath.

Aromatic Considerations

The strength of LeReconciliation lies in helping us find perspective and peace by bringing us understanding and compassion. This empathy is like a warm blanket, covering ourselves and others.

Emotional/Spiritual Aspects

LeReconciliation can fill the deep well of loneliness we sometimes feel when our lives are being lived at a distance, physically or emotionally, from the home and heritage of our formative years. Sometimes we feel that who we have become is so different from who we were that our loved ones no longer have any idea who we are. We feel misunderstood, unappreciated, and isolated from those with whom we would like to share the depths of ourselves. The aroma of LeReconciliation helps us find peace with the past, joy in our relationships as they are today, and hope for the future of our connections to loved ones near to us or far away.

LeReconciliation is a marvelous oil for grief and loss, especially if there were hard feelings or trauma in the relationship at the time of the parting.

Physical Aspects

LeReconciliation is a good oil for skin care and massage. If there are any physical ailments with roots reaching into relationships, this blend should bring relief—both to the emotions and the physical imbalances.

Cautions

This is a very mild and pleasant oil. It has no contraindications.

LeRefresh-Mint

Ingredients

cedarwood, clove bud, cypress, eucalyptus, frankincense, juniper berry, lemongrass, myrrh, patchouli, chamomile Roman, spearmint, wintergreen, ylang ylang

Application

Place 2 to 5 drops of LeRefresh-Mint in the bottom of a small bathroom paper cup; add enough water for a mouthful or two. Stir the oil vigorously into the water. Swish in the mouth and gargle for at least 60 seconds two or more times a day to promote healthy gums.

Physical Aspects

LeRefresh-Mint contains essential oils blended synergistically to promote gum health, kill a wide variety of bacteria, and leave behind a refreshing, clean taste and sensation.

LeRevitalize

Ingredients

bergamot, blue tansy, cabreuva, chamomile Roman, carrot seed, davana, fennel, geranium, helichrysum, lemon, rosemary

Affinity for

digestive system
brain function
emotional stability

Resonance

physical, emotional

Aromatic Considerations

LeRevitalize, diffused, can give everyone in the room a boost of energy and alertness.

Application

Dilute well when applying LeRevitalize to the body. This essential oil blend is best applied over the liver or on the bottoms of the feet.

Emotional/Spiritual Aspects

LeRevitalize increases mental alertness and alleviates mental fatigue. It is a great blend for replenishing inner stores of strength and increasing stamina. LeRevitalize is especially effective for those who are worn out from chronic illness or who make a habit out of running faster than they have strength most of the time. This blend has proven useful in programs for anger management and in overcoming addictions.

Physical Aspects

LeRevitalize cleanses the liver, but does so gently and steadily. It stabilizes energy levels and improves vitality. LeRevitalize is a good digestive aid, particularly in eliminating bloating, belching, and heartburn. LeRevitalize should be applied over the abdomen, either massaged on or applied in a compress, for parasites. A compress or direct application over the gallbladder or kidneys can relieve distress and pain in these areas. This is an excellent oil for lymphatic congestion and immune stimulation.

LeSanctuary

Ingredients

cedarwood, fir, pine, spruce, vanilla, ylang ylang

Affinity for

respiratory system
nervous system
central vessel meridian
bladder meridian
all chakras
emotional balance

Resonance

LeSanctuary is a very high frequency. It can often be used in place of the very expensive single oils like rose, jasmine, or neroli with equally effective results.

Aromatic Considerations

LeSanctuary has a pleasant aroma that just wraps around you and transports you to a place of peace and calm where you may rest and gather strength for the day.

Application

This blend is meant to be diffused! It surrounds us with the feelings of contentment and faith. Alternatively, it can be worn as perfume, cologne ,or applied to the solar plexus, brain stem, crown of the head, back of the neck, behind the ears, over the thymus, or on the wrists. I like to carry this one in an inhaler so that I can let it take me to a quiet place whenever I need to.

Emotional/Spiritual Aspects

LeSanctuary promotes feelings of protection and safety. From this safe place we can examine ourselves comfortably, listening closely to the whisperings of the spirit and our own intuitive knowledge of our strengths and weaknesses. This process helps us develop wisdom and good judgement and lets us build trust in ourselves and our decisions. LeSanctuary has a special affinity for the central vessel and bladder meridians. In doing so, it can help us replace fear in our lives with faith in healthy ways. LeSanctuary brings all of the chakras into harmony with each other, balancing the energy cohesively between them.

LeSego Lily

Ingredients

copaiba balsam, grapefruit, rosewood, vanilla

Affinity for

skin
heart chakra
emotional health

Resonance

physical, emotional

Application

Diffuse or wear as a perfume. Diluted, LeSego Lily makes an excellent massage oil and is excellent in the bath.

Aromatic Considerations

LeSego Lily is light and airy with a beautiful, uplifting, and calming aroma.

Emotional/Spiritual Aspects

The aromatic influence of LeSego Lily is, in part, to bring a feeling of calmness during a crisis or when feeling anxious and out of sorts. LeSego Lily also promotes a feeling of being loved and appreciated. Its aroma often inspires us to show love and appreciation to others.

Physical Aspects

Physically, LeSego Lily is a blend for skin care and health. It promotes skin elasticity and may seem to slow the process of aging as it nourishes the skin and smooths out wrinkles. LeSego Lily is used to bring relief from the itching of hives and allergic rashes. When used for this purpose, a more emollient carrier oil containing jojoba, apricot, or rosehip oils would be beneficial.

LeSimplicity

Ingredients

lavender, lemon, manuka, melissa, oregano-wild, rosemary, tea tree, thyme

Affinity for

skin   nerves   immune system

Resonance

physical, emotional

Application

LeSimplicity should be applied to the blistered areas of a cold sore and the skin around them, usually diluted in distilled or spring water. It makes an excellent mouthwash, diluted well.

Aromatic Considerations

LeSimplicity is best used topically.

Physical Aspects

LeSimplicity is a blend of potent antiviral oils which target the HSV-1 and 2 (Herpes Simplex 1 and 2) viruses. HSV infection causes fluid-filled blisters which form in clusters and then continue to spread. Fatigue, irritability, low-grade fever, slow healing of cuts, infections around the fingernails, and whitlows are other signs of infection.

These viruses are carried from person to person in body fluids such as saliva. The initial infection often occurs during childhood when well-meaning relatives subject children to on-the-mouth kisses. Once the virus has entered the body, it 'creeps' along neural pathways and establishes a 'home-base.' HSV-1's site of latency preference is the trigeminal ganglion, a collection of nerve cells near the ear. From this spot, outbreaks tend to occur on the lower lip or face when the body is under stress or the immune system has been compromised in some way. HSV-2 seems to prefer to lodge in the nerves at the base of the spine or sacral area. This blend is designed to kill the viruses at the areas of outbreak, then follow the same neural pathways that the virus traveled until it reaches the colonies in the nerve bundles to kill it at the source.

LeSolitude

Ingredients

cabreuva, chamomile German, lavender, marjoram, rosewood, orange sweet

Affinity for

skin   heart chakra   kidney meridian
cardiovascular system
emotional health

Resonance

physical, emotional

Application

Dilute and apply to the chest and anywhere you have unsightly or uncomfortable veins. LeSolitude is excellent in the bath or diluted for a massage oil.

Aromatic Considerations

LeSolitude is calming and can help one to 'de-stress' following a stress filled day. Diffusing LeSolitude at night helps me relax into a peaceful sleep.

Emotional/Spiritual Aspects

The aroma of LeSolitude can be useful in creating an atmosphere of peace and quiet in which to regenerate and rebuild emotional reserves. This oil brings peace and happiness to mind and body. It has been useful to some in overcoming depression and coping with anxiey.

Physical Aspects

LeSolitude's affinity is for anything to do with heart or vein health. It is truly a cardiovascular oil. It should be used for varicose veins, spider veins, and to promote capillary health. LeSolitude can be used as a muscle relaxant and to relieve tension headaches. The chamomile and rosewood, in a synergistic arrangement with the stronger antiseptic oils in this blend, combine to make an oil that moisturizes dry skin and is a good treatment for eczema.

LeSpice C

Ingredients

cinnamon, clove, eucalyptus radiata, lemon, opoponax, rosemary

Affinity for

immune system
lymphatic system
respiratory system

Resonance

physical, emotional

Application

LeSpice C can be added to water to soak toothbrushes or used as a gargle for sore throats. This blend needs to be diluted well to be applied to the skin.

Aromatic Considerations

LeSpice C should be diffused periodically during the cold and flu season.

Physical Aspects

LeSpice C is similar to LeDeliverance, but has a stronger cinnamon aroma and no oregano or thyme. This blend is antiviral, antibacterial, anti-fungal, etc. LeSpice C strengthens the immune system. It (or LeDeliverance) should be used for respiratory illnesses, colds, sore throats, bronchitis, flu, and nervous exhaustion.

LeStefanie

Ingredients

cinnamon berry, cumin, helichrysum, manuka, melissa, oregano, spruce, valerian, yarrow blue,

Affinity for

immune system
respiratory system
nervous system

Resonance

physical, emotional, spiritual

Application

LeStefanie should be applied on the chest, back, and on the feet. It can also be diffused or inhaled.

Aromatic Considerations

LeStefanie is balancing and uplifting to the emotions. The melissa in this blend adds a light, lemony scent.

Emotional/Spiritual Aspects

The high percentage of melissa in this blend makes it uniquely effective for instilling a positive mental outlook on life and for improving one's ability to enjoy life to the fullest.

Physical Aspects

LeStefanie was developed to help fight antibiotic resistant pseudomonas bacteria, especially in the lungs. This blend has a great affinity for the entire respiratory system. LeStefanie should be considered for any respiratory problem, such as asthma, bronchitis, chest colds, or flu. Melissa oil is one of the strongest antiviral, antibacterial essential oils. This blend is anti-infectious, anti-inflammatory, antispasmodic, antibacterial, anti-microbial, antiviral, sedative, antidepressant, and mucolytic.

LeSunburst

Ingredients

citronella, grapefruit, lemon, lemongrass, spearmint, orange sweet, tangerine

Affinity for

skin　　muscles　　bones

Resonance

physical, emotional

Application

LeSunburst can be used as a perfume or cologne and added to bath water. It is excellent added to the dish water, dishwasher, or laundry. LeSunburst makes an excellent oil for cleaning surfaces throughout the house.

Aromatic Considerations

LeSunburst can be diffused to purify the air, remove odors, or just to enjoy a nice citrus aroma.

Emotional/Spiritual Aspects

LeSunburst is a favorite among the citrus blends because it is relaxing and calming, especially for children. This blend promotes a sense of well-being and is an excellent remedy for insomnia. LeSunburst is not a sedative. It promotes restful sleep from which you wake in the morning feeling energetic and refreshed. Some citrus oils have proven effective against eating disorders. Because of the variety of citrus oil contained in LeSunburst, it has been used in treatments for anorexia and bulimia.

Physical Aspects

LeSunburst is useful for circulatory problems, varicose veins and lymphatic congestion. It is a powerful immune stimulant. When used as a cleaner, it retards the growth of mold and mildew.

LeTenda Care

Ingredients

eucalyptus, gingergrass, juniper, lemongrass, marjoram, peppermint, spikenard, tea tree, thyme, wintergreen

Affinity for

skin　　muscles　　bones

Resonance

physical

Application

Use LeTenda Care by placing a small amount of carrier oil in the palm of your hand. Add a few drops of LeTenda Care. Use this as a massage oil for tired, overworked muscles, or to help you relax at the end of a long day. LeTenda Care can be added to a bath as an excellent muscle relaxant and over-all tonic.

Aromatic Considerations

LeTenda Care has an aroma that is pleasant and light for lifting the mood and clearing the mind.

Physical Aspects

LeTenda Care is intended to be used when muscles are tight, strained, or injured. This blend is analgesic, anti-inflammatory, antispasmodic, and has some excellent nervine properties. Besides sports injuries and muscle relaxation, LeTenda Care can be used for back pain, sciatica, bruising, and charley horses.

Comments:

Essential oils added to a carrier immediately begin to 'break down' and become less effective therapeutically. Following the method described above will insure that the essential oils are potent and effective each time you use them.

LeTherma-Care

Ingredients

coriander, litsea cubeba, peppermint, yellow yarrow

Affinity for

nervous system

fevers

Resonance

physical, emotional

Application

LeTherma-care should be diluted well and applied to the back of the neck and down the spine. It is also effective to apply LeTherma-care to the bottoms of the feet.

Aromatic Considerations

It is better to apply this essential oil blend to the body. Diffusing might be pleasant but may not give you the results in fever reduction that you need.

Physical Aspects

LeTherma-care was specifically designed to aid in gently reducing the very high fevers we have been seeing with these high-powered and quick-onset flu 'bugs.' The use of this essential oil to reduce the fever is especially nice with children. In addition to the fever reducing properties of the yarrow and the peppermint, the coriander is well renowned for giving strength both during an illness and during the convalescent stages.

LeTomorrow

Ingredients

clary sage, cypress, frankincense, geranium, lemongrass, lime, rose, sandalwood, orange sweet, ylang ylang

Affinity for

emotional balance

Resonance

physical, emotional, spiritual

Application

LeTomorrow can be applied over the heart chakra, on the wrists, behind the ears, or on the neck. This blend, mixed with a carrier oil makes an excellent massage oil. It can be diffused or worn as a perfume.

Aromatic Considerations

LeTomorrow should be diffused for the calm atmosphere that it creates. This blend creates feelings of joy, peace, and forgiveness.

Emotional/Spiritual Aspects

LeTomorrow is used in emotional work to bring the focus from the past to a happy anticipation of the potential of the future. LeTomorrow helps one to find calmness and joy in the challenges of every day living. It is useful during the changing seasons of our lives to help us maintain emotional stability. One of the most pleasing aspects of this essential oil blend is the desire that it creates within us to forgive and love others more unconditionally. I find that this blend helps people leave the past behind while attaining wisdom and acceptance.

LeTranquility

Ingredients

blue tansy, geranium, chamomile German, lavender, palmarosa, patchouli, orange sweet, tangerine, ylang ylang

Affinity for

nervous system
circulatory problems
emotional stability

Resonance

physical, emotional, spiritual

Application

LeTranquility can be used as a perfume or cologne. It is an excellent essential oil for a relaxing bath. This blend can be placed anywhere on the body.

Aromatic Considerations

Diffuse or wear LeTranquility as a perfume. Everyone around you will get to enjoy it and reap the benefits. The aroma of LeTranquility has been known to reduce or eliminate panic attacks and other anxiety based disorders.

Emotional/Spiritual Aspects

One of the best loved of the Butterfly Express, LLC blends, LeTranquility can help us develop inner strength, patience, understanding, and confidence. LeTranquility promotes relaxation, relieves anxiety, stress, tension, and depression. LeTranquility is useful as a sleep aid, especially when the problem is 'mind chatter' that just won't quit. Instead of sleeping, even though we need sleep badly, we lay there reviewing the past day in our minds or making plans for tomorrow.

LeTranquility helps us take a step back from a situation so that we may come to a fuller understanding of all aspects of the situation. From this perspective we are usually able to see solutions to our dilemmas more easily.

Physical Aspects

Physically, LeTranquility can be useful for circulatory problems to the extremities. Stress takes a high toll on the vitamin and mineral levels of the body, especially calcium. The use of LeTranquility, which promotes calmness and quells anxiety, has been helpful in cases of osteoporosis. This is one of the best blends to relieve migraine and tension headaches.

LeTranquility has been used in programs to help children and adults get off Ritalin and Prozac. Of course, it is recommended that you work closely with your doctor.

General information

This essential oil blend is the first thing you should reach for whenever someone is having a panic attack. More times than not, LeTranquility will stop the attack completely. This is a great blend for any type of anxiety disorder.

LeTrust

Ingredients

angelica, frankincense, helichrysum, lavender, lemon, melissa blend, palmarosa, rose, rosewood, sandalwood, spruce

Affinity for

emotional balance and stability
lung meridian

Resonance

LeTrust is a very high frequency essential oil blend

Application

LeTrust should be massaged over the heart or around the navel. It is also good when applied behind the ears or on the wrists

Aromatic Considerations

This blend makes a very nice perfume or cologne. LeTrust, diffused in the home, can make changes for the better in family communication, especially at meal times.

Emotional/Spiritual Aspects

LeTrust helps us be more accepting, tolerant, compassionate, and forgiving of ourselves and others. This blend can be useful in leaving behind old hurts, guilts, and frustrations. The emotions supported by LeTrust can help us evaluate our relationships and leave behind attitudes of co-dependency.

Physical Aspects

Although LeTrust is a high frequency blend and definitely a spiritual/emotional oil, it has proven useful for the relief of pain with pleurisy and gallstones. Some people report that used as a mouth rinse, this blend is good for gum disease.

LeTurmoil

Ingredients

davana, frankincense, helichrysum, lavender, lemon, lime, palmarosa, rose, rosemary, rosewood, sandalwood, spikenard, zanthoxylum

Affinity for

immune system
emotional stability

Resonance

physical, emotional

Application

'Rain drop' this blend down the spine or along the inside of the foot (the spine in foot zone therapy); then massage it in.

Aromatic Considerations

If someone is recovering from an accident or surgery, diffuse LeTurmoil near them or have them inhale it frequently.

Emotional/Spiritual Aspects

LeTurmoil helps us to view trials from a more positive perspective. This blend is useful in rebuilding the physical/emotional connection after trauma or loss. LeTurmoil should be considered for the anger stage of grief and later, if the grief seems to be settling into depression. LeTurmoil calms hyperactivity and nervousness. This remedy can calm a person who is jumping from project to project, thought to thought, and help them settle down, organize themselves, and accomplish something.

Physical Aspects

LeTurmoil is a remedy for shock and trauma, especially those that are affecting physical well-being and weakening the immune system. It stabilizes a person who is feeling faint or going into shock.

LeUnity

Ingredients

angelica, orange bitter, frankincense, geranium, hyssop, lavender, mandarin, neroli, palmarosa, rose, rose geranium, sage, sandalwood, spikenard, spruce, ylang ylang

Affinity for

emotional balance
spiritual growth
every chakra
liver meridian
small intestine meridian

Resonance

physical, emotional, spiritual

Application

LeUnity can be applied over each chakra, beginning at the base and working up to the crown. It can be applied on the feet, over the heart, and on areas of poor circulation.

Aromatic Considerations

LeUnity should be diffused in groups where incompatibility or quarrelsomeness is a problem. Use it in the home to increase peace and cooperation.

Emotional/Spiritual Aspects

LeUnity promotes harmony within ourselves, with others around us, and with our Creator. It helps us work with others in a relationship of cooperation, patience, and tolerance. This is the greatest essential oil product I know of for fostering a sense of physical and mental well-being. It can rid us of stubbornness, anger, judgement, and jealousy. Frequent use can promote unity among family members. This essential oil blend has to be experienced to be believed.

If LeBenediction is not providing enough protection from other people's energies for you, try adding LeUnity, too. This blend, like LeBountiful, fosters a sense of abundance and appreciation in our hearts.

Physical Aspects

One of the great strengths of LeUnity is its ability to balance every chakra to the extent of greatly minimizing or eliminating altogether any reaction from overuse of essential oils. This is very useful for children who get into essential oils that have been left laying around the house. Many times the balancing of all of the chakras eliminates or minimizes any allergic reaction. LeUnity makes a good deodorant.

Important information

LeUnity can be used to eliminate or minimize reactions to oils that are caused by suppressed emotions or a toxic physical body. Apply the oil to the palms of the hands and place one hand over the navel and the other hand over the thymus. Hold for 20 seconds and then reverse the position of the hands and hold for another 20 seconds or more. ***This really works!*** This procedure is also effective for grounding and balancing in a multitude of situations.

LeVallee

Ingredients

carrot seed, helichrysum, parsley, ravensara, spikenard, tagette, vetiver, wintergreen, yarrow blue

Affinity for

skin
muscle tissue
nerves

Resonance

physical

Application

LeVallee should be diluted well and applied to the area of concern.

Physical Aspects

This blend was created specifically for rebuilding skin and muscle tissue following a severe burn. It is proving useful in other conditions involving deteriorated muscle and skin tissues. LeVallee is an emollient and is soothing to damaged skin and should be used to combat dryness and skin irritation. LeVallee contains oils renowned for the rebuilding of nerve cells and networks.

LeVisibility

Ingredients

cypress, geranium, hyssop, orange sweet

Affinity for

veins, capillaries

Resonance

physical

Application

[Le]Visibility should be diluted and applied wherever there are broken capillaries or damaged veins. Be sure to dilute very well if applying to hemorrhoids.

Physical Aspects

Capillaries are the finest branches of the blood vessel system. They are fragile and can be easily damaged. [Le]Visibility promotes capillary health and reduces both the visibility and the pain of broken or weak capillaries. These broken capillaries sometimes appear on the face or as 'spider veins' on the legs. They can be quite painful because they impede proper circulation. Restless Leg Syndrome (where the legs feel tingly, 'asleep', and painful, especially when you are at rest) is caused by broken capillaries. These capillaries may be seen or unseen. [Le]Visibility, applied to the legs at bedtime, often brings relief. [Le]Visibility is also good for varicose veins. Always massage upward from the feet when working on vein health.

[Le]Vision

Ingredients

angelica, chamomile German, chamomile Roman, hyssop, lavender, lemon, spruce

Affinity for

nervous system
emotional stability and balance
stomach meridian

Resonance

physical, emotional

Application

[Le]Vision can be diffused. It is very nice in the bath, especially at the end of the day.

Aromatic Considerations

[Le]Vision, when the aroma is inhaled, can promote self-awareness, intuitiveness, and self-confidence.

Emotional/Spiritual Aspects

[Le]Vision is especially suited to dominant personality types who have become unfocused or overbearing in their personal lives. It is designed to help us see ourselves more clearly, discover our misperceptions, and grow from our mistakes. [Le]Vision may even be helpful in overcoming apathy and finding the will power to change. If we have begun to rely too much on other people's opinions and advice, [Le]Vision can help us see our own path and our own worth more clearly. This blend clears the mind, reduces anxiety and stress levels, restores inner strength, and improves decisiveness—without our needing to be overbearing or impatient. If you tend to be irritable, this may be a good blend for you.

Physical Aspects

[Le]Vision is often helpful with insomnia and, applied to the abdomen, is useful in the early treatment of gallstones.

[Le]Vitality

Ingredients

allspice, copaiba balsam, cypress, geranium, helichrysum, mandarin, marjoram, palmarosa, ylang ylang

Affinity for

cardiovascular system
pulmonary system
vein health
lymphatic system
respiratory system
urinary tract
root and crown chakras—
our connection to both Heaven and Earth
governing vessel meridian

Resonance

physical, emotional

Application

LeVitality should be diluted and applied on the chest over the heart area several times a day. LeVitality can also be applied to the acupressure heart area on the left foot, or alternatively, to the heart points found under the left ring finger and corresponding toe on the left foot. Additional points that may be of benefit are found on the arms just above the elbow. It may also be of benefit to apply LeVitality on the arteries of the neck, and to massage it along the spine between the 1st and 4th vertebrae.

Aromatic Considerations

The aroma of LeVitality is useful for shock. It also increases vitality, energy, and stamina.

Emotional/Spiritual Aspects

This blend provided me with a hopeful feeling about the state of my health. When I applied this essential oil blend, and smelled the aroma, I felt more confidence in my body's ability to heal and be strong again. LeVitality gives one more enthusiasm for life. As stamina and strength improve, there is more energy and you feel good enough to enjoy life more fully.

Physical Aspects

LeVitality is very specific for the cardiovascular, circulatory, pulmonary, and lymphatic systems. It should be tried for all heart related and circulatory conditions, but LeVitality has amazing uses in so many other areas. It is often useful for lowering high blood pressure and reducing stress levels. This blend can increase stamina among the sick or the elderly.

LeVitality is a remedy for the treatment of shock and has been used to stop or slow the progress of an oncoming stroke. For an impending stroke, LeVitality should be quickly applied to the neck and forehead. Encourage the person to breathe as deeply and calmly as possible.

Among its other uses, LeVitality is an adrenal stimulant, aids the function of the kidneys, and clears lymphatic congestion. The anti-inflammatory properties of LeVitality make it useful for arthritis, pleurisy, and sciatica. LeVitality can help balance hormones and is useful in treating toxemia during pregnancy if it is related to heart or circulation problems. LeVitality reduces the size and painfulness of hemorrhoids; be sure to dilute well here.

LeWake Up

Ingredients

grapefruit, lemongrass, orange sweet, peppermint, rosemary, spearmint

Affinity for

nervous system
emotional balance
heart chakra
spiritual side of our natures

Resonance

physical, emotional, spiritual

Application

LeWake Up is wonderful diffused. It can be diluted and applied to the bottoms of the feet, with a special emphasis on the big toe.

Aromatic Considerations

LeWake Up does exactly what the name implies. It makes us feel more energetic and wide awake to our world.

Emotional/Spiritual Aspects

LeWake Up helps us feel more energetic, enthusiastic, and even passionate about our life, the tasks we have before us, and the people around us. Somehow, it makes us want to encourage everyone around us to find the same joy that we are experiencing. This blend is a joyous vacation for our minds and spirits.

Physical Aspects

LeWake Up is helpful, both by aroma and application, for blood sugar lows (hypoglycemia) that occur just before or during the onset of the menstrual period.

LeWarm Down

Ingredients

basil, cypress, fir, lavender, marjoram, wintergreen

Affinity for

muscles bones respiratory system

Resonance

physical

Application

LeWarm Down should be applied, diluted, to any area of the body where there are sore or strained muscles. This blend makes an excellent massage oil. It is often used in conjunction with LePaine, and if there is structural misalignment, LeMillenia is added to the regimen.

Aromatic Considerations

LeWarm Down has an underlying aroma of 'black licorice.' It is the aroma of basil and is wonderful if you happen to like black licorice. If you find this aroma offensive, try LeTenda Care instead.

Physical Aspects

LeWarm Down is antispasmodic and anti-inflammatory. This makes it an excellent remedy for tight, tired, sore, and aching muscles of any description. This blend is often reached for with sports injuries, muscle strains and sprains, and for torn ligaments.

LeWarm Down seems to aid calcium absorption and distribution throughout the body. This makes it useful for charley horses and the leg cramps during pregnancy. The regular use of LeWarm Down can slow the progress of osteoporosis by improving calcium absorption.

LeWarm Down makes an excellent massage oil for back and joint pain. It often relieves stress headaches, where tight muscles in the neck and shoulders are contributing factors. LeWarm Down increases capillary circulation and protects the skin by helping it to retain moisture.

LeWeightless

Ingredients

basil, grapefruit, green pepper, lemon, lime, sage

Affinity for

digestive system emotional balance

Resonance

physical, emotional

Application

LeWeightless is pleasant diffused, where it will eliminate odors and kill bacteria while being enjoyed for its emotional properties. LeWeightless can be used in the bath; be careful to use only 2 or 3 drops. This is an excellent essential oil blend for a full body massage. Be sure to dilute well for use in a massage.

Aromatic Considerations

The aroma of LeWeightless is uplifting. It stimulates positive and creative thinking.

Emotional/Physical Aspects

This delightful blend is designed to function on both the physical and emotional planes, even more than usual for essential oils which all seem to do this to some extent. LeWeightless increases metabolism, especially fat burning, and helps to dissolve cellulite. Emotionally it lightens the weight of our own negativity which is so often the trigger for 'binge' eating or junk food consumption. LeWeightless is used in programs for eating disorders such as anorexia.

LeWeightless relieves stress, but it takes a minute. If you can remember to reach for the LeWeightless when you are craving that chocolate bar, then exercise a little self-control for a moment or two, you may find that you move on to something else in your life and the chocolate loses its allure!! This blend also has an effect on the mind, helping it to function more clearly and quickly.

LeWhispering Hope

Ingredients

chamomile Roman, juniper, lemon, melissa blend, myrrh, spruce, ylang ylang

Affinity for

emotions
gall bladder meridian

Resonance

physical, emotional

Application

LeWhispering Hope should be diluted and applied on the outer edges of the ears, on the chest, heart, temples, solar plexus, back of the neck, and wrists. It is also good in the bath, diluted and massaged over the feet or as a massage oil for the whole body. It would be a unique scent to wear as a perfume.

Aromatic Considerations

The aroma of this blend promotes feelings of peace, security, confidence, and optimism.

Emotional/Spiritual Aspects

LeWhispering Hope should be used to stimulate feelings of hope and a sense of potential and achievement if one has become discouraged. This essential oil blend can help us turn around feelings of hopelessness and helplessness. ***This is the most effective oil for suicidal thoughts.*** It is particularly helpful for feelings of frustration we may have at other peoples' choices and the impossibility of 'stepping in and doing it right for them.' LeWhispering Hope can help you find peace in just standing by their heart and praying for them.

There are many uses for this oil during a woman's childbearing years. LeWhispering Hope can help when a young mother (or any one else, really) is feeling stressed and overwhelmed. It helps to create a more positive attitude and a sense of optimism. This blend can help a young woman understand and move past feelings of ambivalence or non-acceptance of a pregnancy. LeWhispering Hope is useful during certain stages of labor and delivery. (See chapter on childbirth.)

LeWisdom

Ingredients

hinoki, lemon, neroli, orange sweet, spruce, ylang ylang

Affinity for

emotional balance and stability
throat chakra
sacral chakra
crown chakra
triple warmer meridian
kidney meridian
gall bladder meridian

Resonance

physical, emotional

Application

LeWisdom should be diluted and applied in a counter clockwise direction over the center of the chest (thymus). To go counter clockwise you start over your heart (like pledging allegiance), moving upward toward the left shoulder, across to the right shoulder, and then back down and around again. It is as though the clock is sitting on you own chest, facing out for others to see.

Aromatic Considerations

The aroma of LeWisdom is uplifting, centering, and calming to the emotions.

Emotional/Spiritual Aspects

As we experience adversity and joy in this life, our fears, frustrations, annoyances, and irritabilities should mellow into wisdom. This blend can help us do that by moving away from the negative patterns of our lives. It is of particular use for those who become distraught or discouraged because they continually pressure themselves to do more, be absolutely perfect, or to be ready for any future crisis situation that may happen. This blend is often used in Inner Child work to establish a firm presence in the present time and situation. LeWisdom can help us express and deal with repressed emotions. LeWisdom is a wonderful oil for any grieving stages of our lives. It is one of the best blends for jet lag and fatigue.

LeWith-In

Ingredients

coriander, ginger, lavender, rosemary, yarrow

Affinity for

muscles

Resonance

physical

Application

LeWith-In should be diluted with a carrier oil and applied several times a day to the area of the hernia. It can also be used effectively as a compress.

Physical Aspects

It is meant for use on inguinal and hiatal hernias. It is not applicable for surgical hernias. LeMillenia should be layered with LeWith-In for maximum structural realignment. The addition of cypress and hyssop should be considered for severe inguinal hernias. It is ***absolutely necessary*** *to* avoid strenuous exercise or anything that puts strain on the muscles involved until healing is ***complete.*** A good diet, which includes all of the nutritional needs of muscles during a repair stage, is also advised.

LeWoman Wise

Ingredients

clary sage, fennel, jasmine, lavender, marjoram, patchouli, spikenard

Affinity for

emotional balance
hormones

Resonance

physical, emotional

Application

LeWoman Wise should be diluted in a carrier oil and massaged on the lower back and abdomen. It is helpful to layer with LeDeeper if severe cramping or abdominal pain is involved during the menstrual period. LeWoman Wise can also be applied to the feet and ankles, used in the bath, and diluted for a body massage oil.

Aromatic Considerations

LeWoman Wise, even just diffused rather than applied, can help to balance hormones, stabilize mood swings, and calm irritability.

Emotional/Spiritual Aspects

There are many emotions that go completely out of whack when our hormones are out of balance. This blend can be very helpful for any of those. Sometimes trying an essential oil and seeing what changes take place can help us recognize which behaviors are hormone driven and which ones are just bad habits.

Physical Aspects

LeWoman Wise was created to help balance the hormones of younger women. It also brings a lot of relief from pre-menstrual and menstrual cramps and headaches. It may also be effective for prostate problems in men, although LeBalance is usually a better choice for men and women approaching, or in, their menopausal years. This blend should be used all month long, not just when the PMS symptoms are at their worst. Doing this will keep the symptoms from occuring.

Cautions

This blend is not for use during pregnancy!!!

The following names, in Italics, are registered trademarks of Aromatic Research Technology D.B.A. Young Living. Butterfly Express is not affiliated in any way with Young Living, nor are the compared blends replicas of each other. The comparisons are for ease of use only.

Abundance	LeBountiful
Acceptance	LeAcknowledge
Aroma Life	LeVitality
Aroma Siez	LeWarm Down
Awaken	LeEverlasting
Brain Power	LeIQ
Christmas Spirit	LeHoliday Spirit
Citrus Fresh	LeSunburst
Clarity	LeCrystal Clear
Di-Tone	LeInside-Out
Dragon Time	LeWoman Wise
Dream Catcher	LeDreams
En-r-gee	LeEnergy
Endo Flex	LeEndo Relief
Envision	LeDiscernment
Exodus	LeJourney
Forgiveness	LeTrust
Gathering	LeInner Peace
Gentle Baby	LeBaby Me
Gratitude	LeGrateful Heart
Grounding	LeConnection
Harmony	LeUnity
Hope	LeWhispering Hope
Humility	LeFaith
Immune Power	LeLife Force
Inner Child	LeInsight
Inspiration	LeMeditation
Into the Future	LeTomorrow
Joy	LeHeart Song
Juva Flex	LeRevitalize
Live with Passion	LeExhilaration
Longevity	LeEternity
Magnify/Purpose	LeFocus
Melrose	LeMela Plus
Mister	LeBalance
Motivation	LeAssurance
M-Grain	LeMy-graine
Ortho Ease	LeTenda Care
Pain Away	LePaine
Peace & Calming	LeTranquility
Present Time	LeWisdom
Purification	LePurify
R.C.	LeAspire
Raven	LeBreezey
Release	LeLetting Go
Relieve It	LeDeeper
Sacred Mountain	LeSanctuary
Sara	LeAngel
Serenity	LeSolituide
Surrender	LeVision
Thieves	LeDeliverance/LeSpice C
Three Wise Men	LeMagi
Trauma	LeTurmoil
Valor	LeMillenia
White Angelica	LeBenediction

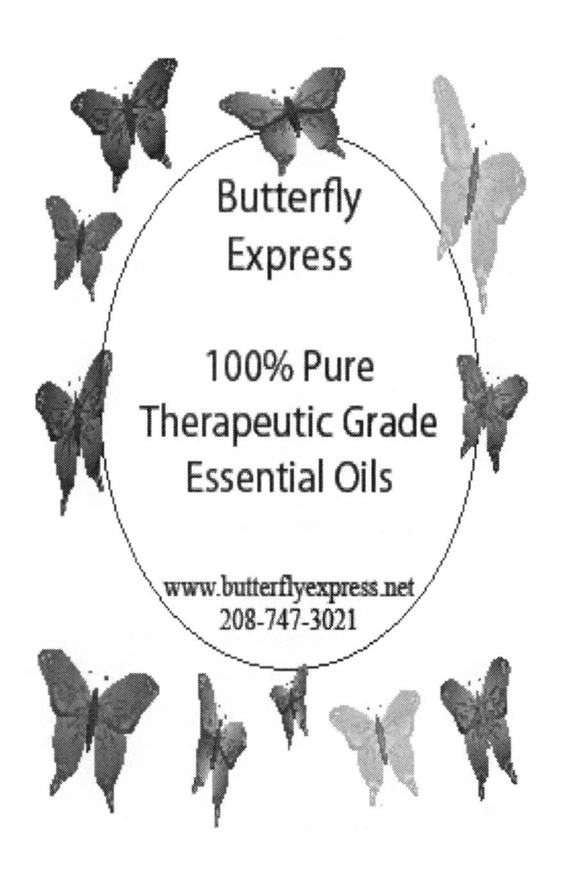

LeAway
LeBelieve
LeBeloved
LeCandila
LeCypernium
LeDandy
LeDelicate
LeExpressions
LeEZ-Traveler
LeGood-Nite
LeKadence
LeMariah
LeMoonlight
LeNo-More
LePatches
LeReconciliation
LeRefresh-Mint
LeSego Lily
LeSimplicity
LeStefanie
LeTherma Care
LeVallee
LeVisibilty
LeWake Up
LeWeightless
LeWith-In

Butterfly Miracles with Essential Oils

Ingredients of Blends

LeAcknowledge: bergamot, frankincense, geranium, melissa blend, neroli, rosewood, sandalwood, palmarosa,

LeAngel: blue tansy, cistus, copaiba balsam, cedarwood, geranium, lavender, rose, rose geranium, orange sweet, ylang ylang

LeAspire: cypress, eucalyptus, laurel, marjoram, myrtle, peppermint, pine, rosemary, spruce

LeAssurance: chamomile-Roman, frankincense, lavender, spruce, ylang ylang

LeAway: bergamot, catnip, cedarwood, cinnamon berry, citronella Java, clove bud, eucalyptus peppermint

LeBaby Me:, chamomile-Roman, palmarosa, rose, rose geranium, rosewood

LeBalance: chamomile-Egyptian, chaste tree, clary sage, cypress, lavender, marjoram, myrtle, peppermint, rose geranium, sage, yarrow green, ylang ylang,

LeBelieve: copaiba balsam, frankincense, palmarosa, rose, vanilla, vanilla, ylang ylang

LeBeloved: bergamot, lemon, mandarin, geranium, orange sweet, ylang ylang

LeBenediction: angelica, bay, geranium, hyssop, lemon, melissa blend, myrrh, rose, rosewood, rose geranium, sandalwood, spruce, ylang ylang

LeBountiful: cassia, cinnamon, clove, frankincense, myrrh, orange sweet, orange bitter, patchouli, thyme,

LeBreezey: birch, eucalyptus, lemon, ravensara, peppermint

LeCandila: cypress, tea tree, lavender, manuka, rosemary, tagette, ylang ylang,

LeConnection: angelica, cedarwood, fir, sage, spruce, ylang ylang

LeCrystal Clear: basil, peppermint piperata, peppermint arvensis, rosemary

LeCypernium: cypress, geranium, peppermint

LeDandy: basil, cypress, lavender, rosemary, sage, thyme,

LeDeeper: birch, eucalyptus, fir balsamea, helichrysum, lemongrass, myrrh, peppermint, spruce, wintergreen,

LeDelicate: cypress, lavender, rosemary, sage, thyme

LeDeliverance: clove, cinnamon, eucalyptus, lemon, oregano, oregano wild, rosemary, thyme

LeDiscernment: cistus, geranium, hinoki, lavender, orange sweet, rose, rosewood, sage, spruce

LeDreams: bergamot, blue tansy, benzoin, chamomile-German, juniper, sandalwood, spruce, sweet orange dark

LeEndo Relief: coriander, cumin, cypress, dill, geranium, myrtle, nutmeg, oregano wild, petitgrain, sage

LeEnergy: black pepper, cinnamon, clove, juniper, lemongrass, nutmeg, pine needle, rosemary, thyme

LeEternity: ajowan, allspice, clove, frankincense, orange sweet, thyme

LeEverlasting: Blended with LeDreams, LeHeart Song, LeTrust, LeUnity, LeWisdom

LeExhilaration: clary sage, cedarwood, ginger, helichrysum, jasmine, melissa blend, neroli, patchouli, rosewood, sandalwood, sweet orange

LeExpressions: frankincence, jasmine, rose, sandalwood, ylang ylang

LeEZ-Traveler: birch, chamomile-Roman, frankincense, lavender, myrrh, orange sweet, peppermint, ylang ylang

LeFaith: bergamot, cabreuva, frankincense carterii, frankincense serrata, melissa blend, rose, rosewood

LeFocus: cinnamon, cinnamon berry, ginger, nutmeg, patchouli, rosewood, sage, sandalwood

LeGood Nite: cedarwood, orange sweet, ylang ylang

LeGrateful Heart: coriander, frankincense, geranium, howood, melissa blend, myrrh, pine needle, rosewood, ylang ylang

LeHeart Song: bergamot, geranium, grapefruit, lemon, mandarin, orange sweet, rose, rose geranium, rosewood, ylang ylang,

LeHoliday Spirit: benzoin, cinnamon, fir siberica, spruce, sweet orange,

LeInner Peace: angelica, cinnamon, copaiba balsam frankincense, lavender, palmarosa, rosewood, sandalwood, spruce, ylang ylang,

LeInside-Out: aniseseed, cardamom, fennel, juniper, lemon, lemongrass, patchouli, peppermint, tarragon, thyme

LeInsight: clementine, jasmine, orange sweet, sandalwood, tangerine

LeIQ: cabreuva, copaiba balsam, cedarwood, coriander, cypress, frankincense, helichrysum, lavender, laurel, lemon, melissa blend, sandalwood

LeJourney: basil, calamus, cassia, cinnamon, frankincense, hyssop, myrrh, spikenard

LeKadence: allspice, cedarwood, orange sweet, ylang ylang

LeLetting Go: blue tansy, geranium, hinoki, lavender, lemon, sandalwood, ylang ylang
LeLife Force: blue tansy, caraway, clove bud, dill, frankincense, galbanum, geranium, hyssop, lemon, oregano, ravensara, rosemary, thyme
LeMagi: angelica, birch, frankincense, juniper, myrrh, sandalwood, spruce
LeMariah: bay, helichrysum, Idaho tansy, opopanax, ravensara, spearmint, spikenard, thyme, turmeric, wintergreen
LeMeditation: frankincense, myrrh, myrtle, rosewood, sandalwood, spruce
LeMela Plus: cajeput, clove, niaouli, rosemary, tea tree
LeMillenia: blue tansy, chamomile-German, elemi, fir balsamea, frankincense, geranium, lavender, rosewood, spruce
LeMoonlight: angelica, cedarwood, cinnamon, clary sage, geranium, jasmine, mandarin, neroli, orange sweet, orange sweet dark, patchouli, sandalwood, spikenard, ylang ylang
LeMy-graine: chamomile-German, copaiba balsam, grapefruit, helichrysum, lavender, marjoram, peppermint,
LeNo-More: calamus, elemi, oregano, patchouli, spikenard
LePaine: birch, clove, copaiba balsam, eucalyptus, helichrysum, peppermint arvensis, peppermint piperata
LePatches: frankincense, gingergrass, peppermint, rosewood, spruce
LePurify: citronella, grapefruit, lavender, lemongrass, manuka, tea tree
LeReconciliation: anthopogon, rose, ylang ylang, vanilla
LeRefresh-Mint: cedarwood, chamomile-Roman, clove bud, cypress, eucalyptus, frankincense, juniper, lemongrass, myrrh, patchouli, spearmint, wintergreen, ylang ylang,
LeRevitalize: bergamot, blue tansy, cabreuva, carrot seed, chamomile Roman, davana, fennel, geranium, helichrysum, lemon, rosemary
LeSanctuary: cedarwood, fir balsamea, pine needle, spruce, vanilla, ylang ylang
LeSego Lily: copaiba balsam, grapefruit, rosewood, vanilla
LeSimplicity: lavender, lemon, manuka, melissa, oregano wild, rosemary, tea tree, thyme
LeSolitude: cabreuva, chamomile-German, lavender, marjoram, orange sweet, rosewood
LeSpice C: cinnamon, clove, eucalyptus radiata, lemon, rosemary
LeStefanie: blue yarrow, cinnamon berry, cumin, helichrysum, manuka, melissa, oregano wild, spruce, valerian
LeSunburst: citronella, grapefruit, lemon, lemongrass, orange sweet, spearmint, tangerine
LeTenda Care: eucalyptus, gingergrass, juniper, lemongrass, marjoram, peppermint arvensis, peppermint piperita, spikenard, thyme, wintergreen,
LeTherma-care: coriander, litsea cubeba, peppermint, yarrow
LeTomorrow: clary sage, cypress, frankincense, geranium, lemongrass, lime, orange sweet, rose, sandalwood, ylang ylang
LeTranquility: blue tansy, chamomile-German, geranium, lavender, orange sweet, palmarosa, patchouli, tangerine, ylang ylang, tamala
LeTrust : angelica, frankincense, helichrysum, lavender, lemon, melissa blend, palmarosa, rose, rosewood, sandalwood, spruce
LeTurmoil: ajowan, davana, frankincense, helichrysum, lavender, lemon, lime, palmarosa, rose, rosemary, rosewood, sandalwood, spikenard
LeUnity: angelica, frankincense, geranium, hyssop, lavender, mandarin, neroli, orange bitter, palmarosa, rose, rose geranium, sage, sandalwood, spikenard, spruce, ylang ylang
LeVallee: carrot seed, helichrysum, parsley, ravensara, spikenard, tagette, vetiver, wintergreen, yarrow-blue
LeVisibility: cypress, geranium, hyssop, orange sweet
LeVision: angelica, chamomile-German, chamomile-Roman, hyssop, lavender, lemon, spruce
LeVitality: allspice, copaiba balsam, cypress, geranium, helichrysum, mandarin, marjoram, palmarosa, ylang ylang
LeWake-Up: grapefruit, lemongrass, orange sweet, peppermint, rosemary, spearmint
LeWarm Down: basil, cypress, fir balsamea, lavender, marjoram, wintergreen
LeWeightless: basil, grapefruit, green pepper, lemon, lime, sage
LeWhispering Hope: chamomile-Roman, juniper, lemon, melissa blend, myrrh, spruce, St. John's, ylang ylang
LeWisdom: hinoki, lemon, neroli, orange sweet, spruce, ylang ylang
LeWith-In: coriander, ginger, lavender, rosemary, yarrow-blue
LeWoman Wise: clary sage, jasmine, lavender, marjoram, patchouli, rue, spikenard, St. John's

Essential Oil Singles

Essential Oil	Latin Name	Plant Family	Part of Plant Used
Ajowan	Tracyspermum copticum	Umbelliferae	seeds
Allspice	Pimenta dioica	Myrtaceae	leaves, fruit
Angelica	Angelica archangelica	Umbelliferae	roots
Aniseseed	Pimpinella anisum	Umbelliferae	seeds (fruit)
Anthopogon	Rhododendron anthopogon	Ericaceae	flowers, leaves
Basil	Ocimum basilicum	Labiatae	stems, leaves, flowers
Bay	Pimenta racemosa	Myrtaceae	leaves
Benzoin	Styrax tonkinesis	Ericaceae	resin
Bergamot	Citrus bergamia	Rutaceae	fruits
Birch	Betula lenta	Betulaceae	leaves
Black Pepper	Piper nibrum	Piperaceae	fruits
Blue Tansy	Tanacetum annuum	Compositae	leaves, flowers
Cabreuva	Myocarpus fastigiatuf	Fabaceae	wood
Cajeput	Melaleuca cajuputi	Myrtaceae	leaves
Calamus	Acorus calamus	Acoraceae	roots
Caraway	Carum carvi	Umbelliferae	seeds
Cardamom	Elettaria cardamomum	Zingiberaceae	seeds
Carrot Seed	Daucus carota	Umbelliferae	seeds
Cassia	Cinnamonum cassia	Lauraceae	leaves, bark
Catnip	Nepeta cataria	Labiatae	flowers
Cedarwood	Cedrus deodora	Coniferae	bark
Celery Seed	Apium graveolens	Umbelliferae	seeds
Chamomile, Egyptian	Matricaria recutita/	Compositae	flowers
Chamomile, German absolute	Matricaria recutita/ Chamomila matricaria	Compositae	flowers
Chamomile, Roman	Chamaemelum nobile	Compositae	flowers
Chaste Tree	Vitex agnus castus	Verbenaceae	fruit
Cinnamon Bark	Cinnamomum verum/zeylanicum	Lauraceae	bark
Cinnamom Berry	Cinnamomum polyandrum	Lauraceae	fruit
Cistus - Rockrose	Cistus landaniferus	Cistaceae	leaves, twigs
Citronella Ceylon	Cymbopogon nardus	Graminae	leaf (grass)
Citronella Java	Cymbopogon winterianus	Graminae	leaf (grass)
Clary Sage	Salvia sclarea	Labiatae	plant when in flower
Clementine	Citrus nobilis	Rutaceae	fruit
Clove	Syzgium aromaticum	Myrtaceae	fruit
Copaiba Balsam	Copaifera langsdorfii	Fabaceae	resin
Coriander	Coriandrum sativum	Umbelliferae	seeds
Cumin	Cuminum cyminum	Umbelliferae	seeds
Cypress	Cupressus sempervirens	Coniferae /Cupressacea	wood, leaves
Davana	Artemisia pallens	Compositae	stems, leaves

Essential Oil	Latin Name	Plant Family	Part of Plant Used
Dill	Anethum graveolens	Umbelliferae	seeds
Elemi	Canarium luzonicum	Burseraceae	resin
Eucalyptus	Eucalyptus globulus	Myrtaceae	leaves
Eucalyptus, blue mallee	Eucalyptus polybractea	Myrtaceae	leaves
Eucalyptus, peppermint	Eucalyptus dives	Myrtaceae	leaves
Eucalyptus, radiata	Eucalyptus radiata	Myrtaceae	leaves
Fennel	Foeniculum vulgare	Umbelliferae	seeds
Fenugreek	Trigonella foenum	Fabaceae	seeds
Fir, balsam	Abies balsamea	Coniferae	needles (leaves)
Fir, sibirica	Abies siberica	Coniferae	needles (leaves)
Frankincense	Boswellia carterii	Burseraceae	resin
Frankincense, frereana	Boswellia frereana	Burseraceae	resin
Frankincense, Indian	Boswellia serrata	Burseraceae	resin
Galbanum	Ferula galbaniflua/fummosa	Umbelliferae	wood, leaves
Garlic	Allium sativum	Lilliceae	bulbs
Geranium	Pelargonium graveolens	Geraniaceae	leaves
Ginger	Zingiber officinale	Zingiberaceae	roots
Gingergrass	Cympopogan martini/sofia	Gramineae	leaves, grass
Grapefruit	Citrus paradisi	Rutaceae	fruit
Green Pepper	Piper nigrum	Piperaceae	fruit
Helichrysum	Helichrysum italicum and agustifolia	Compositae	flowers
Hinoki Wood	Chamaecyparis obtusa /Cupressacea	Coniferae	needles, twigs, leaves
Howood	Cinnamomum camphora	Lauraceae	twigs, bark
Hyssop	Hyssopus officinalis	Labiatae	stems, leaves
Idaho Tansy	Tanacetum vulgare	Compositae	leaves, flowers
Jasmine grandiflorum	Jasminum grandiflorum	Oleaceae	flowers (early morning)
Jasmine sambac	Jasminum sambac	Oleaceae	flowers (late evening)
Juniper Berry	Juniperus communis	Coniferae	fruit
Laurel	Laurus nobilis	Lauraceae	leaves
Lavender	Lavandula officinalis	Labiatae	flowering tops
Ledum	Ledum groenlandicum	Ericaceae	leaves
Lemon	Citrus limonum	Rutaceae	fruit
Lemongrass	Cymbopogon flexuosus	Graminae	leaves
Lime	Citrus aurantifolia	Rutaceae	fruit
Litsea Cubeba	Litsea cubeba (May chang)	Graminae	fruit
Mandarin	Citrus reticulata	Rutaceae	fruit
Manuka	Leptospermum scoparium	Myrtaceae	leaves, seeds
Marjoram	Origanum marjorana/hortensis	Labiatae	leaves
Melissa	Melissa officinalis	Labiatae	leaves flowers
Myrrh	Commiphora myrrha	Burseraceae	resin

Essential Oil	Latin Name	Plant Family	Part of Plant Used
Myrtle	Myrtus communis	Myrtaceae	leaves
Neroli	Citrus aurantium	Rutaceae	flowers
Niaouli	Melaleuca viridiflora/quinquenervia	Myrtaceae	leaves
Nutmeg	Myristica fragrans	Myrtaceae	seeds
Opoponax Myrrh	Commiphora guidottii	Bruseraceae	gum
Orange, bitter	Citrus aurantium	Rutaceae	fruit
Orange, sweet	Citrus sinensis	Rutaceae	fruit
Oregano	Origanum vulgare	Labiatae	leaves
Oregano, wild	Origanum vulgare	Labiatae	leaves
Palmarosa	Cymbopogon martinii	Graminae	leaves
Parsley	Petroselinum sativum	Umbelliferae	seeds
Patchouli	Pogostemon cablin	Labiatae	leaves, flowers
Peppermint	Peppermint arvensis	Labiatae	stems, leaves, flowers
Peppermint	Peppermint piperita	Labiatae	stems, leaves, flowers
Petitgrain	Citrus aurantium	Rutaceae	leaves
Pine Needle	Pinus pinaster	Coniferae	needles, leaves
Ravensara	Agathophyllum aromatica/ Ravensara aromatica	Lauraceae	wood, leaves
Rose, absolute	Rosa damascena	Rosaceae	flowers
Rose Geranium	Pelargonium roseum	Geraniaceae	leaves
Rosemary	Rosmarinus officinalis	Labiatae	flowering plant
Rosewood	Aniba rosaeodora	Lauraceae	wood
Sage	Salvia officinalis	Labiatae	leaves, flowers
Sandalwood	Santalum album	Santalaceae	wood
Spearmint	Mentha spicata	Labiatae	leaves
Spikenard	Nardostachys jatamansi	Valerianaceae	roots
Spruce, canadian	Tsuga canadensis	Coniferae	needles, leaves
Sugandha Kokila	Cinnamomum glaucescens	Lauraceae	dried berries
Tagette	Tagetes minuta	Compositae	flowers
Tamala	Cinnamomum tamala	Lauraceae	leaves
Tangerine	Citrus reticulata	Rutaceae	fruit
Tarragon	Artenisia dracunculus	Compositae	leaves
Tea Tree	Melaleuca alternifolia	Myrtaceae	leaves
Thyme	Thymus zygis/vulgaris	Labiatae	leaves, stems, flowers
Turmeric	Cucuma longa	Zingiberaceae	roots
Valerian Root	Valeriana officinalis	Valerianaceae	roots
Vanilla	Vanilla planifolia	Orchidaceae	fruit
Vetiver	Vetivera zizanioides	Graminae	roots
Wintergreen	Gaultheria procumbens	Ericaceae	leaves
Yarrow	Achillea millefolium	Compositae	flowering tops
Ylang Ylang—complete	Cananga odorata	Anonaceae	flowers
Zanthoxylum	Zanthoxylum armatum	Rutaceae	fruit

LaVergne, TN USA
28 September 2010
198859LV00002BB/2/P

9 780981 839639